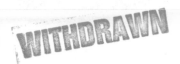

Nutrition Care
of the Older Adult

A Handbook for Dietetics
Professionals Working Throughout
the Continuum of Care

Second Edition

Consultant Dietitians in Health Care Facilities
Kathleen C. Niedert, MBA, RD, FADA,
and Becky Dorner, RD, editors

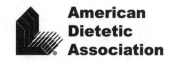
**American
Dietetic
Association**

Diana Faulhaber, Publisher
Laura Brown and Kristen Short, Development Editors
Elizabeth Nishiura, Production Editor

The views expressed in this publication are those of the authors and do not necessarily reflect policies and/or official positions of the American Dietetic Association. Mention of product names in this publication does not constitute endorsement by the authors or the American Dietetic Association. The American Dietetic Association disclaims responsibility for the application of the information contained herein.

Chapters 18 and 19 are reprinted by permission of Roche Dietitians, LLC. Copyright © Roche Dietitians.

10 9 8 7 6 5 4 3 2 1

Library of Congress Cataloging-in-Publication Data
Nutrition care of the older adult: a handbook for dietetics professionals working throughout the continuum of care / Kathleen C. Niedert and Becky Dorner, editors.—2nd ed.
     p. ; cm.
   Includes bibliographical references and index.
   ISBN 0-88091-332-0
  1. Nursing homes—Food service—Handbooks, manuals, etc. 2. Diet therapy for older people—Handbooks, manuals, etc. 3. Aged—Nutrition—Handbooks, manuals, etc.
   [DNLM: 1. Nutrition—Aged—Handbooks. 2. Dietary Services—Aged—Handbooks. 3. Eating Disorders—rehabilitation—Aged—Handbooks. 4. Long-Term Care—Aged—Handbooks. 5. Nutrition Assessment—Aged—Handbooks. 6. Risk Factors—Handbooks. WT 39 N976 2004]
I. Niedert, Kathleen C. II. Dorner, Becky.

RA999.F65N88 2004
362.17'6'0846—dc22

       2004010293

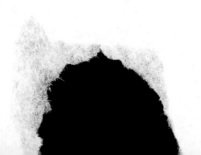

CONTENTS

Contributors   v
Foreword   vii
Preface   viii

PART I.
Introduction to Nutrition in Older Adults

1. Nutrition in Older Adults: An Overview   1
2. Risk Factors Associated With Poor Nutritional Status   8
3. Housing Options   22
4. Community-Based Nutrition Services   26

PART I.
Nutrition and Disease in Older Adults

5. Cardiovascular Disease   34
6. Diabetes   42
7. Hepatic/Liver Disease   52
8. Renal Disease   57
9. Gastrointestinal Problems   63
10. Nutritional Anemias   74
11. Neurological Diseases   80
12. Dementia   85
13. Taste and Smell   89
14. Oral Health   94
15. Cancer 100

PART III.
Nutrition Assessment

16. Nutrition Assessment   104
17. Laboratory Assessment   134
18. Drug-Nutrient Interactions   154
19. Complementary and Alternative Medicine   165
20. Skin Integrity   185
21. Hydration   196
22. Involuntary Weight Loss   202

PART IV.
Dining Challenges

23. Rehabilitating the Eating-Disabled Client   210
24. Enteral and Parenteral Nutrition Support   219
25. Nutrition Care for Palliative Care Clients   245

PART V.
Regulatory Compliance

26. Litigation and Liability Issues   261
27. Quality Management   265
28. Federal Regulations   280

Appendixes

A. Subjective Global Assessment Summary   296
B. Mini Nutritional Assessment   298
C. Nutrition Risk Assessment   300

Index   311

CONTRIBUTORS

Susan Albrecht, MS, RD
Rockland, MD

Peter L. Beyer, MS, RD
Kansas City, KS

Carolyn Breeding, MS, RD, FADA, CFSP
Richmond, KY

Sheila M. Campbell, PhD, RD
Worthington, OH

Mary Casper, MA
Toledo, OH

Jo Ann S. Carson
Dallas, TX

Ronni Chernoff, PhD, RD, FADA
Little Rock, AR

Nancy Collins, PhD, RD
Pembroke Pines, FL

Robert S. DeChicco, MS, RD, CNSD
Cleveland, OH

Sara Dicecco, MS, RD
Rochester, MN

Sylvia Escott-Stump, MA, RD
Winterville, NC

Marion J. Franz, MS, RD, CDE
Minneapolis, MN

Michelle A. Fratianne, RD, CN
Cincinnati, OH

Charlette R. Gallagher-Allred, PhD, RD
Columbus, OH

Lynda Gluch, RD
Grosse Ile, MI

Cynthia Hamilton, MS, RD, CNSD
Cleveland, OH

Pamela S. Kent, MS, RD, CSR
Cleveland, OH

Bernadette Latson
Dallas, TX

Elizabeth Lennon, MS, RD, CNSD
Cleveland, OH

Mary D. Litchford, PhD, RD
Greensboro, NC

Sandra Luthringer, RD
Erie, PA

Janet S. McKee, MS, RD
Orlando, FL

Mary Ellen Posthauer, RD, CD
Evansville, IN

Ellen Pritchett, RD, CPHQ
Naples, FL

Margaret Roche Dudek, MS, RD, FADA
Riverside, IL

Carlene Russell, MS, RD, FADA
Pleasant Hill, IA

Susan S. Schiffman, PhD
Durham, NC

Laure Stasik, MS, RN, RD, CDE
Scranton, PA

M. David Stockton, MD, MPH
Knoxville, TN

Riva Touger-Decker, PhD, RD, FADA
Newark, NJ

Jane V. White, PhD, RD, FADA
Knoxville, TN

Nickie Francisco Ziller, RD
Byron, MN

Editors
Kathleen C. Niedert, MBA, RD, FADA
Hudson, IA

Becky Dorner, RD
Akron, OH

Copy Editor
Marla Carlson
Waterloo, IA

Reviewers
Pam Brummit, MA, RD
Enid, OK

Cheryl Carson, MS, RD
Kansas City, MO

Marilyn Ferguson-Wolf, MA, RD, CD
Seattle, WA

Marolyn Steffen, RD, CD
Valparaiso, IN

George Taler, MD
Washington, DC

Georgianna Walker, MS
New Rockford, ND

FOREWORD

As the baby-boomer generation ages, the focus of American society is changing. Prognosticators predict that within the next 10 to 20 years the US population will be dominated by older adults. For this reason, the term "geriocracy" has been coined to describe the forthcoming composition of the US population.

As dietetics professionals, we must stay on the cutting edge of information to address the aging of America. In *Nutrition Care of the Older Adult,* 2nd edition, American Dietetic Association (ADA) members who are experts in their respective clinical fields share their knowledge of the nutritional implications of chronic diseases in the aging process. In this new edition, the nutrition assessment section has been updated to include the new Nutrition Care Process Model adopted by ADA in Spring 2003. And, because the aging population is looking more often to nontraditional methods for preventing and treating disease, this edition also includes a section on complementary and alternative medicine.

The aging of America also brings to the forefront the question of whether current health care models will meet the medical and social needs of older adults. *Nutrition Care of the Older Adult,* 2nd edition, provides practitioners with insight on community alternatives to the traditional long-term care facility and evaluates how each of these alternatives will address the significant issue of malnutrition in aging.

I congratulate the editors, Kathleen C. Niedert, MBA, RD, FADA and Becky Dorner, RD, for developing a manual that encompasses the total perspective of nutrition care in older adults, from nutrition and disease states to regulatory compliance in health care settings. My thanks to all the authors who graciously contributed their expertise in making this a sound, science-based, and practical guide for dietetics professionals. *Nutrition Care of the Older Adult,* 2nd edition, is an outstanding example of a product developed by ADA members to improve the nutritional well-being of American society, while also enhancing the skills of our profession.

Marianne Smith Edge, MS, RD, FADA
President
American Dietetic Association, 2003/2004

It is commonplace to think of nursing facilities and older adults together—to consider nursing facilities as the primary option for older adults who need care while regarding older adults as the population most likely to use nursing facilities. But there are good reasons to reconsider such assumptions. On the one hand, changes in health care delivery have led to the development of home health agencies and assisted living; on the other hand, there is a continued need for facilities that can handle individuals of all ages with cognitive dysfunction, spinal cord injury, or other illnesses and injuries requiring subacute or rehabilitative services. As a result, a wide range of clients with varying needs and living environments presents new challenges and opportunities for dietetics professionals.

When the American Dietetic Association (ADA) asked the Consultant Dietitians in Health Care Facilities to revise the first edition of *Nutrition Care of the Older Adult,* we jumped at the chance and enthusiastically agreed to be the editors. When we reviewed the previous edition and the two earlier editions of *Nutrition Care in Nursing Facilities,* we marveled at how the practice of medical nutrition therapy had changed since 1987, when Ann Katherine Jernigan, MS, RD, had the vision to write a handbook for the practitioner in long-term care facilities. Much progress has been made in the years between that first publication and the creation of this new edition.

The second edition of *Nutrition Care of the Older Adult* presents expanded coverage of nutrition and disease, including examinations of nutrition in dementia and in neurological disorders. The regulations chapter has been expanded, and we have included a section on litigation, an all-too-familiar issue for the dietetics profession. This new edition also emphasizes the Nutrition Care Process and Model recently developed by ADA as a road map to quality care and outcomes management.

Dietetics professionals must provide a high level of medical nutrition therapy for the individuals they assist: assessing nutrition needs, developing goals for clients, directing the implementation of nutrition plans to meet those goals, documenting relevant data, and evaluating results with outcomes research in mind. This book offers dietetics professionals up-to-date, useful material for assessing clients in this new health care environment. Although it is not intended to be all-inclusive, *Nutrition Care of the Older Adult* provides important guidance to dietetics professionals. As always, information set forth in this book should be reviewed in light of new research findings as they become available.

For this revision, we sought out professionals within our field as well as experts outside the dietetics profession to provide the information needed to take this edition into the 21st century. We are grateful to the contributors for sharing their expertise. We are also indebted to the reviewers who took the time to thoughtfully critique the content. We also want to thank Marla Carlson, a great friend, counselor, journalist, and mediator, who helped keep us both sane. She completed word processing, made hundreds of calls, conducted Internet searches, and did countless other "little" things that contributed to the final product. Finally, a special thanks to our families, who put up with midnight phone calls, weekends of microwaved meals, and numerous other inconveniences so we could meet our deadlines.

Proper nutrition care is crucial for all our clients. We urge our readers to accept the challenge to meet the nutritional needs of clients and provide excellent, quality care for all those served.

Kathleen C. Niedert, MBA, RD, FADA
Becky Dorner, RD

CHAPTER 1

Nutrition in Older Adults: An Overview

Improvements in nutrition, general health, and life expectancy are changing global demographics and the cultural, social, and economic foundations of Western society. By the year 2030, it is estimated that 1 in 5 Americans will be aged 65 years or older (1). The implications for the health care system of a demographic shift of this magnitude are just beginning to be realized.

Many diseases or conditions that would be considered abnormal or even alarming in younger adult populations are viewed as a part of the "normal aging process" in individuals aged 65 years or older. The nature of this perception will be adjusted as the number of studies that investigate the effects of aging on various body systems and processes increases and the impact of confounding factors, such as nutritional status and physical activity, is recognized.

This discussion will summarize what are currently believed to be clinically important age-related changes in physiology and their impact on the nutritional needs of older adults. Generally speaking, aging is associated with a decline in the function of most organs and tissues. However, the extent to which physiologic decline occurs varies greatly from organ system to organ system and from individual to individual.

APPETITE, FOOD INTAKE, AND THE GASTROINTESTINAL TRACT

Food intake declines as age advances. This decline is greater in men than in women. Cohort and cross-sectional US data suggest that energy intakes decline by approximately 1,000 to 1,200 kcal/day in men and by 600 to 800 kcal/day in women, resulting in declines in intakes of most nutrients (2). The US Healthy Eating Index (HEI), a summary of overall diet quality, shows that energy intakes decline by as

much as 500 kcal/day between the ages of 65 and 85 years (3). Fruit and milk consumption were low for all age groups, and declines in grain, vegetable, and meat intake were observed as age increased (3). Lower-income older adults consume significantly less energy, fewer servings from major food groups, and fewer nutrients than their higher-income counterparts (4). Minority populations consume fewer servings of most food groups, with older African-American men consuming the fewest servings of fruits and vegetables of all age groups (5). Consumption of fats, oils, and sweets was greatest in individuals 85 years and older and among denture users (5). Paradoxically, food restriction is associated with increased longevity in many animal species, but the nature, duration, and optimal time for implementation of food restriction in humans has yet to be established (6).

Animal studies and preliminary studies in small numbers of elderly human subjects suggest that hormonal regulation of appetite is altered in the older adult (7,8). Plasma concentrations of cholecystokinin are increased, and endogenous opioids are decreased (8). Firth and Prather describe multiple alterations in gastrointestinal anatomy and physiology that impair motility and contribute to complaints of dysphagia, anorexia, dyspepsia, and constipation in older adults (9) (see Table 1.1).

Poor dentition and periodontal disease affect a significant number of older adults. An average of 23% of older Americans are edentulous, with a range, by state, of 14% to 48% (1). More than 90% of edentulous older adults have both upper and lower dentures; however, 18% to 24% of those who own dentures do not wear them (1). One third of older Americans who have natural teeth have untreated root or crown caries, and 41% have periodontal

TABLE 1.1   Age-Related Changes in Gastrointestinal Physiology

Location	Alteration
Oropharynx	Xerostomia Altered protective reflexes Poor dentition, periodontal disease Altered taste perception Decreased olfactory discrimination
Esophagus	Reduced resting upper esophageal sphincter pressures Reduced lower esophageal sphincter relaxation Upward lower esophageal sphincter displacement into chest Delayed esophageal emptying with "tertiary" contractions Decreased contraction velocity and duration Reduced myenteric ganglion cells Increased amplitude of distal contractions Thickening of smooth muscle layer
Stomach	Decreased mucosal prostaglandin, sodium, bicarbonate, and mucous secretion Possible delayed emptying of liquids and solids
Pancreas	Increased gallstone formation Decreased glucose tolerance Insulin secretory defects Decreased beta-cell sensitivity to incretin hormones Impaired beta-cell compensation with glucose load
Liver	Decline in organ volume and blood flow Reduction in metabolic capacity Reduced hepatic drug clearance of rapidly cleared drugs
Small Intestine	Possible decreased small bowel transit
Colon	No significant primary changes
Ano-rectum	Reduced rectal compliance Impaired rectal sensation Decreased sphincter pressures Increased constipation Increased fecal incontinence

Source: Adapted from Firth M, Prather CM. Gastrointestinal motility problems in the elderly patient. *Gastroenterology*. 2002;122:1689, with permission from American Gastroenterological Association.

disease (10). Rates of oral cancer increase with age, and prognosis is poor (10). Poor oral health in older Americans contributes to increased pain and suffering and to impaired sensory perception, mastication, and appetite; it can also significantly alter the nature and quality of food and fluid consumed.

Although alterations in the structure and function of the gastrointestinal tract have the potential to negatively affect nutritional status, medications that impair appetite are commonly prescribed for older adults and are frequently the cause of poor food intake and poor nutritional status (see Table 1.2) (11).

TABLE 1.2　Commonly Prescribed
　　　　　　Medications With Anorexia
　　　　　　as a Major Adverse Effect

Generic Name	Brand Name
Amlodipine	Norvasc
Ciprofloxacin	Cipro
Conjugated estrogen	Premarin
Digoxin	Lanoxin
Enalapril maleate	Vasotec
Famotidine	Pepcid
Fentanyl transdermal	Duragesic
Furosemide	Lasix
Levothyroxine sodium	Synthroid
Narcotic analgesic	Lorcept
Nifedipine	Procardia XL
Nizatidine	Axid
Omeprazole	Prilosec
Paroxetine	Paxil
Phenytoin	Dilantin
Potassium chloride	K-Dur
Ranitidine HCl	Zantac
Risperidone	Risperdal
Sertraline HCl	Zoloft
Warfarin	Coumadin

Source: Reprinted with permission from Thomas DR, Morley JE, and the Council for Nutritional Clinical Strategies in Long-Term Care. Regulation of appetite in older adults. *Annals of Long-Term Care: Clinical Care and Aging.* 2002;10(7)(suppl):7. Available at: http://www.LTCnutrition.org. Accessed February 15, 2003.

ORGAN FUNCTION

In addition to alterations in gastrointestinal function and physiology, age-related changes in almost every body system may alter nutritional requirements and contribute to poor health outcomes (12). Table 1.3 gives a summary of the impact of aging processes on organ systems (12).

Many controlled clinical trials have demonstrated that topical retinoids improve the appearance of aging skin, possibly because of its effect on collagen metabolism (13). The effect of increased consumption of retinoids on aging skin has not been evaluated.

Increased consumption of antioxidants (vitamins C, E, and beta carotene) and zinc appears able to delay age-related macular degeneration (AMD) and visual acuity loss (14). Only persons at high risk

of AMD (as diagnosed by an ophthalmologist) are candidates for supplementation (14).

Changes in taste perception and olfactory impairment vary widely with age. These senses seem to be generally preserved, despite age-related declines in taste and smell receptors (15). Self-reported olfactory impairment in older adults is low and becomes less accurate as age advances (15). Objective assessment of olfactory impairment in people aged 53 years and older was approximately 24%, with prevalence increasing to approximately 62% in those older than 80 years (16). Cigarette smoking, stroke, epilepsy, nasal congestion, and upper respiratory infection also contributed to a diminished sense of smell (15,16). The implications of these findings on the nutritional health and safety of older Americans has yet to be determined.

Inflammatory processes and vascular dysfunction appear to be associated with the pathogenesis of age-associated neurodegenerative diseases, such as Alzheimer's and Parkinson's disease, and with diminished cognitive performance (17). Both vitamins C and E appear to exert a protective effect on age-related behavioral deficits, possibly through their role as antioxidants or modulators of cellular function (17). Diets rich in these nutrients and supplements for those unable to consume adequate diets are suggested (17).

Table 1.4 lists the estimated prevalence of nutrient deficiencies in healthy older adults based on composite results of surveys of older adults living in India, Europe, Canada, and the United States (18). In many cases, it is not possible to diagnose a nutritional deficiency by clinical history and physical exam. However, increased rates of infection in the respiratory, urinary, and genital tracts and impaired cognition, demonstrated by deficits in short-term memory, reduced ability for abstract tasks, and limited attention span, suggest that subtle, subclinical deficits may be present. Impaired function has also been observed at excessive levels of nutrient intake (18). Thus, recommendations regarding supplements of single nutrients or nutrient combinations, with few exceptions, are difficult to make at this time.

BODY COMPOSITION AND BODY MASS INDEX

Body weight and lean body mass decrease as age advances. Older adults exhibit an increase in percent body fat and greater visceral fat stores, even though total weight declines (12). Consensus regarding optimal weight for older adults is lacking. The standard

TABLE 1.3 Aging Effects on Organ Systems Other Than the Gastrointestinal Tract

Organ System	Aging Effect
Skin	Dryness, wrinkling, mottled pigmentation, loss of elasticity, dilation of capillaries
Head and neck	Macular degeneration, hearing loss
Cardiovascular	Thickening heart wall and valves, increased collagen, increased collagen rigidity, alterations in heart size, decreased elasticity of blood vessels with calcification
Pulmonary	Stiffening of tissue, decreased vital capacity, decreased maximum oxygen consumption, decreased breathing capacity, decreased propulsive effectiveness of cough reflex
Renal	Decreased size, decreased GFR, decreased renal blood flow, decreased active tubular secretion and reabsorption, decreased renal concentrating ability
Endocrine	Altered circulating hormone levels and actions
Nervous	Decreased sensory perception, decreased muscle response to stimuli, decreased cognition and memory, loss of brain cells
Musculoskeletal	Progressive loss of skeletal muscle, degeneration of joints, decalcification of bone

Abbreviation: GFR, glomerular filtration rate.

Source: Reprinted from Jensen GL, McGee M, Binkley J. Nutrition in the elderly. *Gastroenterol Clin North Am.* 2001;30:314, with permission from Elsevier.

TABLE 1.4 Prevalence of Nutrient Deficiencies in Apparently Healthy Elderly

Nutrient	Prevalence (%)
Vitamin A	8
Beta carotene	11
Thiamin	3
Riboflavin	4
Pyridoxine	7
Folic acid	8
Vitamin B-12	11
Vitamin C	16
Vitamin D	12
Vitamin E	10
Iron	14
Zinc	19
Selenium	7
Copper	3
Iodine	3

Source: Reprinted with permission from Chandra RK. Nutrition and the immune system from birth to old age. *Eur J Clin Nutr.* 2002;56(suppl 3):S75.

definitions for optimal body mass index (BMI) for US adults (18.5 to 24.9) are not supported by the weight of evidence in populations 65 years and older (19). Recent studies suggest that BMIs of up to 32 are associated with improved morbidity and mortality in older adults (20,21), whereas even small amounts of intentional or unintentional generalized weight loss in the older adult are associated with poor health outcomes (22). Visceral fat loss in older adults may be of benefit, but data to support this opinion are scarce. Weight maintenance as age advances, increased physical activity, and movement designed to promote improved strength, flexibility, balance, and maintenance of muscle mass are the best recommendations regarding body weight in older adults that can be offered at this time (23).

NUTRIENT REQUIREMENTS

The dietary reference intakes offer recommended dietary allowances (RDAs) or adequate intakes (AIs) when no RDA has been formulated, with specific guidelines for older adults. Recommendations are offered for two categories of older adults: those ages 51 to 70 years and those older than 70 years (12,24). Table 1.5 lists nutrient recommendations for men and women specific to these age groups (24).

TABLE 1.5 Nutrient Recommendations for Older Americans

Nutrient	Men 51-70 y	Men > 70 y	Women 51-70 y	Women > 70 y
Vitamins				
Vitamin A (μg/d)	900	900	700	700
Vitamin C (mg/d)	90	90	75	75
Vitamin D (μg/d)	10	15	10	15
Vitamin E (mg/d)	15	15	15	15
Vitamin K (μg/d)	120	120	90	90
Thiamin (mg/d)	1.2	1.2	1.1	1.1
Riboflavin (mg/d)	1.3	1.3	1.1	1.1
Niacin (mg/d)	16	16	14	14
Vitamin B-6 (mg/d)	1.7	1.7	1.5	1.5
Folate (μg/d)	400	400	400	400
Vitamin B-12 (μg/d)	2.4	2.4	2.4	2.4
Pantothenic acid (mg/d)	5	5	5	5
Biotin (μg/d)	30	30	30	30
Choline (mg/d)	550	550	425	425
Minerals				
Calcium (mg/d)	1200	1200	1200	1200
Chromium (μg/d)	30	30	20	20
Copper (μg/d)	900	900	900	900
Fluoride (mg/d)	4	4	3	3
Iodine (μg/d)	150	150	150	150
Iron (mg/d)	8	8	8	8
Magnesium (mg/d)	420	420	320	320
Manganese (mg/d)	2.3	2.3	1.8	1.8
Molybdenum (μg/d)	45	45	45	45
Phosphorus (mg/d)	700	700	700	700
Selenium (μg/d)	55	55	55	55
Zinc (mg/d)	11	11	8	8
Macronutrients				
Carbohydrate (g/d)	130	130	130	130
Total fiber (g/d)	30	30	21	21
Fat (g/d)	ND	ND	ND	ND
Linoleic acid (g/d)	14	14	11	11
α-Linolenic acid (g/d)	1.6	1.6	1.1	1.1
Protein (g/d)	56	56	46	46

Source: Adapted from Trumbo P, Schlicker S, Yates AA, Poos M. Dietary reference intakes for energy, carbohydrate, fiber, fat, fatty acids, cholesterol, protein, and amino acids. *J Am Diet Assoc.* 2002;102:1623-1625, with permission from American Dietetic Association.

Recommendations regarding Estimated Energy Requirement (EER) are based on height, weight, BMI, and activity level (24) and are derived from the following regression equations, based on data using the doubly labeled water method (25):

Men: EER = 662 − 9.53 x Age (y) x PA x (15.91 x Wt [kg] + 539.6 x Ht [m])

Women: EER = 354 − 6.91 x Age (y) x PA x (9.36 x Wt [kg] + 762 x Ht [m])

Where: PA refers to coefficient for Physical Activity levels (PAL)

PA = 1.0 if PAL ≥ 1.0 < 1.4 (sedentary)
PA = 1.12 if PAL ≥ 1.4 < 1.6 (low active)
PA = 1.27 if PAL ≥ 1.6 < 1.9 (active)
PA = 1.45 if PAL ≥ 1.9 < 2.5 (very active)

For vitamin D, it is suggested that individual needs be met by the use of fortified foods and/or supplements in cases where adequate exposure to sunlight is absent (26). Supplements are also recommended, to ensure adequate intakes of folic acid, vitamin B-12, and calcium (27). It may be difficult for older adults to consume the recommended amounts of these nutrients from food; and in the case of vitamin B-12, because 10% to 30% of older adults may malabsorb food-bound sources of this vitamin, they may not consume enough (27).

Martin et al suggest that additional supplementation with vitamins C and E may be advisable for older adults, because their recent review of the available scientific evidence suggests that 45% of the older population consume no fruit or juice and 22% consume no vegetables daily (17). They recommend daily supplements containing 200 to 400 µg of alpha-tocopherol acerate/day and 200 to 500 mg vitamin C, in combination with anti-inflammatory medication, to provide protection against the neurodegenerative changes associated with cognitive impairment and aging (17).

ALTERATIONS IN NUTRIENT REQUIREMENTS DUE TO USE OF MEDICATIONS

Drug consumption increases as people age (1). Most older Americans have one chronic disease, and 50% have two or more (1). Sixty-one percent of those aged 65 years use one or more prescription drugs daily (1). This percentage increases to more than 90% by age 85 years (28). Older Americans consume 30% of all prescription drugs and 70% of nonprescription drugs (1). The potential for impact on nutritional status is staggering. A recent review by Schumann (29) suggests the following factors that contribute to poor nutritional status in older adults taking medications regularly:

- Decreased appetite (see Table 1.2).

- Anticholinergic effects or side effects from drugs such as α- and β-sympathomimetics, codeine, and opiates, as well as tricyclic antidepressants, slow gastric emptying and peristalsis, which in turn reduce intestinal absorption of nutrients.

- Cholestyramine and sterol/stanol esters may bind bile salts and reduce absorption of the lipid soluble vitamins and carotenoid compounds.

- H2-receptor antagonists and proton pump inhibitors reduce gastric acid production, peptic digestion, and the bactericidal function of gastric secretions leading to gastrointestinal distress.

- Oral, broad-spectrum antibiotics (chloramphenicol, tetracyclines, ampicillins, and sulfonamides) destroy the intestinal flora and contribute to diarrhea and reduced food intake.

- Colchicine and methotrexate are mitotic agents, reducing intestinal villi proliferation resulting in impaired nutrient absorption.

- Drugs that are weak acids or bases, such as vitamin C, may enhance or diminish nutrient absorption.

- Antiepileptic agents, such as barbiturates, phenytoin, and primidone, induce hepatic microsomal enzymes that accelerate the metabolism of vitamin D and its renal metabolites. Rifampin and glutethimide produce similar microsomal enzyme effects. Impaired calcium metabolism and osteoporosis may result.

- Thiazide diuretics may cause hypercalcemia and hyperglycemia.

- Acid-inhibiting agents accentuate hypochlorhydria, a common condition in older adults, which may lead to impaired absorption of vitamin B-12.

- Cholestyramine and neomycin reduce vitamin B-12 absorption by inhibition of intrinsic factor, and biguanides (metformin and phenformin) reduce its intestinal absorption by up to 40%.

- High doses of vitamin C (≥ 500 mg) increase destruction of vitamin B-12 in the gut lumen.

- Thiamin may decompose in the stomach when administered with antacids, whereas diuretics (furosemide) increase its renal tubular excretion.

- Isoniazid, hydralazine, and D-penicillamine form a complex with vitamin B-6 limiting its absorption.

- Vitamin B-6 reduces the effectiveness of L-dopa by accelerating its excretion and may reduce the plasma concentration of phenytoin and phenobarbital by up to 50%.

These are but a few examples of the impact of drug use on nutritional status. This topic will be covered more extensively in Chapter 18.

SUMMARY

Nutrient requirements tend to increase with age because of poor food intake; increased requirements; and altered or reduced rates of digestion, absorption, metabolism, and excretion. It is imperative that health care providers are aware of these issues and that optimal achievable nutritional status is maintained, to ensure the health, well-being, and quality of life for our aging population.

REFERENCES

1. Greenberg S. A profile of older Americans: 2001. US Department of Health and Human Services, Administration on Aging. Available at: http://www.aoa.gov/aoa/stats/profile/2001/2001profile.pdf. Accessed January 10, 2003.

2. Wakimoto P, Block G. Dietary intake, dietary patterns, and changes with age: an epidemiological perspective. *J Gerontol A Biol Sci Med Sci*. 2001;56(special issue 2):65-80.

3. Gaston NW, Mardis A, Gerrior S, Sahyoun N, Anand RS. A focus on nutrition for the elderly: it's time to take a closer look. *Nutrition Insights*. Issue 14. Washington, DC: USDA Center for Nutrition Policy and Promotion; July 1999.

4. Guthrie JF, Lin BH. Overview of the diets of lower- and higher-income elderly and their food assistance options. *J Nutr Educ Behav*. 2002;34(suppl 1):S31-S41.

5. Vitolins MZ, Quandt SA, Bell RA, Arcury TA, Case LD. Quality of diets consumed by older rural adults. *J Rural Health*. 2002;18:49-56.

6. Meydani M. Nutrition interventions in aging and age-associated disease (Boyd Orr lecture). *Proc Nutr Soc*. 2002;61:165-171.

7. Chapman IM, MacIntosh CG, Morley JE, Horowitz M. The anorexia of aging. *Biogerontology*. 2002;3:67-71.

8. MacIntosh CG, Horowitz M, Verhagen MA, Smout AJ, Wishart J, Morris H, Goble E, Morley JE, Chapman IM. Effect of small intestinal nutrient infusion on appetite, gastrointestinal hormone release, and gastric myoelectrical activity in young and older men. *Am J Gastroenterol*. 2001;96:997-1007.

9. Firth M, Prather CM. Gastrointestinal motility problems in the elderly patient. *Gastroenterology*. 2002;122:1688-1700.

10. Vargas CM, Kramarow EA, Yellowitz JA. The oral health of older Americans. *Aging Trends*. 2001;3:1-8.

11. Thomas DR, Morley JE; Council for Nutritional Clinical Strategies in Long-Term Care. Regulation of appetite in older adults. *Ann Long-Term Care*. 2002;10(suppl):1-12. Available at: http://www.LTCnutrition.org. Accessed February 15, 2003.

12. Jensen GL, McGee M, Binkley J. Nutrition in the elderly. *Gastroenterol Clin North Am*. 2001;30:313-324.

13. Fisher GJ, Kang S, Varani J, Bata-Csorgo Z, Wan Y, Datta S, Voorhees JJ. Mechanisms of photoaging and chronological skin aging. *Arch Dermatol*. 2002;138:1462-1470.

14. Gottlieb JL. Age-related macular degeneration. *JAMA*. 2002;288:2233-2236.

15. Mattes RD. The chemical senses and nutrition in aging: challenging old assumptions. *J Am Diet Assoc*. 2002;102:192-196.

16. Murphy C, Schubert CR, Cruickshanks KJ, Klein BE, Klein R, Nondahl DM. Prevalence of olfactory impairment in older adults. *JAMA*. 2002;288:2307-2312.

17. Martin A, Youdim K, Szprengiel A, Shukitt-Hale B, Joseph J. Roles of vitamins E and C on neurodegenerative and cognitive performance. *Nutr Rev*. 2002;60:308-334.

18. Chandra RK. Nutrition and the immune system from birth to old age. *Eur J Clin Nutr*. 2002;56 (suppl 3):S73-S76.

19. Heiat A, Vaccarino V, Krumholz HM. An evidence-based assessment of federal guidelines for overweight and obesity as they apply to elderly persons. *Arch Intern Med*. 2001;161:1194-1203.

20. White JV, Parham JS. In pursuit of a healthy weight: what should we recommend for older adults? *Healthy Weight J*. 2002;16:72-75.

21. Bender R, Jockel KH, Richter B, Spraul M, Berger M. Body weight, blood pressure, and mortality in a cohort of obese patients. *Am J Epidemiol*. 2002;156:239-245.

22. White JV, Brewer DE, Stockton MD, Keeble DS, Keenum AJ, Rogers ES, Lennon ES. Nutrition in chronic disease management in the elderly. *Nutr Clin Pract*. 2003;18:3-11.

23. Drewnowski A, Evans WJ. Nutrition, physical activity and quality of life in older adults: summary. *J Gerontol*. 2001;56(special issue 2):89-94.

24. Trumbo P, Schlicker S, Yates AA, Poos M. Dietary reference intakes for energy, carbohydrate, fiber, fat, fatty acids, cholesterol, protein, and amino acids. *J Am Diet Assoc*. 2002;102:1621-1630.

25. Dietary Reference Intakes for Energy, Carbohydrate, Fiber, Fat, Fatty Acids, Cholesterol, Protein , and Amino Acids (2002). Available at http://www.nap.edu. Accessed: June 15, 2003.

26. Food and Nutrition Board. Institute of Medicine. *Dietary Reference Intakes for Calcium, Phosphorus, Magnesium, Vitamin D, and Fluoride*. Washington, DC: National Academy Press; 1999.

27. Food and Nutrition Board. Institute of Medicine. *Dietary Reference Intakes for Thiamin, Riboflavin, Niacin, Vitamin B-6, Folate, Vitamin B-12, Pantothenic Acid, Biotin, and Choline*. Washington, DC: National Academy Press; 2000.

28. Rogowski JR, Lillard LL, Kington R. The financial burden of prescription drug use among elderly persons. *Gerontology*. 1997;37:475-482.

29. Schumann K. Interactions between drugs and vitamins at advanced age. *Int J Vitam Nutr Res*. 1999;69:173-178.

CHAPTER 2

Risk Factors Associated With Poor Nutritional Status

Individuals in the United States are living longer. The estimated number of Americans 65 years and older on Census Day 2000 comprised about one in every eight Americans; this included 14.5 million men and 20.4 million women (1); this is a 12% increase from Census Day 1990. The dramatic increase in life expectancy in the past 10 to 15 years demands that clinicians be aware of the various physiologic and clinically relevant changes that occur with age (2).

Aging is a complex process, defined by the interplay of numerous and diverse life events experienced over time (3). Genetic makeup and human response are unique to each person, and poor nutrition affects the health of older adults (4). Although it is apparent that physiologic systems wear out at different rates, it remains unclear how much of this variability relates to the aging process vs attitudes and behaviors that have negatively affected health (5). A recent study by the Alliance for Aging Research found that baby boomers (ages 38 to 56 years) would rather eat what they want and die 10 years sooner than change their eating habits to live longer (6). This attitude can persist into older years, where an individual may choose not to change eating habits in spite of known or diagnosed health risks and consequences.

Oxidative stress is believed to be an important factor in aging and in many degenerative diseases (3). Regular consumption of foods rich in phytochemicals and the antioxidants vitamins C and E will enhance immune response, delay onset of Alzheimer's disease, increase resistance to tumor growth, and perhaps reduce the risk of cardiovascular disease (3,7). In addition, recent findings have begun to reveal mechanisms where folate counteracts age-related disease. Increased homocysteine levels may have adverse effects on organ systems and on the neurological system during aging (8-10). Therefore,

careful assessment of usual and recent nutrient intake is important (11).

Although aging research indicates a role for energy restriction in maintaining longevity and reducing onset of chronic disease (12), sufficient intake of nutrients and energy is essential. A body mass index (BMI) below 21 and weight loss are indicators of risk for malnutrition (13). According to the Administration on Aging, about 50% of older adults in hospitals and nursing homes are malnourished and may be discharged malnourished back into the community (1). Where available, Older Americans Act (OAA) Nutrition Programs should be contacted for the following reasons (1):

- To provide congregate and home-delivered meals
- To link older adults to supportive services
- To decrease social isolation
- To provide nutrition education and counseling to help decrease or manage chronic health conditions
- To yield higher nutrient intakes by participants
- To prevent, delay, or manage chronic health conditions through improved nutrition services

These available programs may keep a person healthy at home in the community.

When nutrition interventions are instituted early, a substantial reduction in health care expenditures may result from a decrease in the incidence or the delayed onset of many chronic conditions (14). Regardless of the setting, the identification of all nutrition risk factors, followed by in-depth nutrition assessment and intervention, can make a difference when appropriate and individualized attention is provided.

NUTRITIONAL RISK FACTORS

A risk factor is a characteristic or occurrence that increases the likelihood that a person will have or already has one or more nutrition problems (4). The greater the number of characteristics or problems that a client experiences, and the longer they persist, the greater the likelihood that poor nutritional status will result (4).

A variety of medical and psychosocial stressors have the potential to impact nutritional status. Many authors in the United States and other countries have identified factors that increase risk of poor nutritional status in older adults (3,4). Recognition of their presence often serves as an "early warning sign" of impending malnutrition.

Mowe and Bohmer cite reduced appetite and taste, dental problems, and difficulties in shopping and cooking as factors prevalent in an older population during their last month before hospital admission when compared with a reference group of older adults living at home (15). Inadequate energy intake is common in older adults and is a major cause of unexplained weight loss (16). Older adults with unintentional weight loss are at higher risk for infection, depression, and death (13). In addition, unrecognized dysphagia may lead to dehydration, malnutrition, aspiration pneumonia, and weight loss (13). Because of the potential for a reduced ability to regulate energy intake, decreased variety in the diet, functional limitations, social isolation, and depression, inadequate energy intake may lead to weight loss and health decline (16). Finally, changes in body composition may indicate loss of lean body mass and protein stores that may be difficult to correct in older adults (3,4).

Altered biochemical factors, including low serum albumin, transthyretin, and retinol-binding protein, may reflect poor protein status that should be corrected (17). Low blood urea nitrogen, hemoglobin, and hematocrit are often correlated with low protein intake (18). Serum homocysteine levels may be elevated, a possible signal of chronically low intake of folic acid and other B-complex vitamins (8,10,19). Many older Americans demonstrate metabolic evidence of low B-12 status; levels tend to vary with ethnicity and renal function (19).

A variety of tools may be used to identify nutrition risk factors. A Mini Nutrition Assessment (MNA) tool identifies 18 relevant factors (20). This tool requires further validation before widespread use (4). The Subjective Global Assessment (SGA) reviews weight change, gastrointestinal symptoms, functional capacity, and physical examination findings to identify mild-, moderate-, or high-risk levels of malnutrition. The SGA is a simple, cost-effective tool for identifying nutritional risks and for identifying older adults with increased risk of nutrition-associated complications (21). Nutritional risks from a variety of causes should be identified and addressed early, to allow interventions to have an impact. The SGA is found in Appendix A and the MNA is found in Appendix B.

One last instrument that is useful is the SCALE instrument (22), which identifies the following factors for risk of malnutrition in the elderly, especially in long-term care settings:

- **Sadness** (use available Geriatric Depression Scale)
- **Cholesterol** (less than 160 mg/dL)
- **Albumin** (less than 3.5 mg/dL)
- **Loss** of 5% of body weight
- **Eating problems** (physical or cognitive causes)

INAPPROPRIATE FOOD AND FLUID INTAKE

Inappropriate intake involves the inadequate or excessive consumption of food and fluid and their accompanying nutrients.

Reason for Concern

To maintain optimal nutritional status, a person must have access to and the ability to consume an appropriate food and fluid intake. People who are unable or unwilling to eat will die unless fed via some other modality. A study by Frisoni et al, of 72 relatively healthy older adults, showed that low intake of protein, carbohydrate, fat, and total energy were strong predictors of mortality, even after adjustment for age, gender, BMI, functional status, emotional status, energy, and nutritional status (23).

Older adults tend to eat earlier in the day, to eat smaller meals, and to eat more slowly than do younger individuals; they also tend to choose a limited variety of foods (24). Rolls demonstrated that sensory-specific satiety changes with age; this finding is proposed as a partial explanation for the habitual consumption of monotonous diets by older adults (25). A narrow range of food choices may lead to dietary inadequacies (26).

In a study of the relationship between the effects of aging on appetite and gastrointestinal transit in humans, Clarkston et al concluded that aging is associated with a diminished desire to eat, with reduced hunger, with slowing of solid and liquid gastric emptying, and with autonomic nerve dysfunction (27).

In the United States, the problem of overconsumption of food and fluid is of equal, if not greater, concern. In a study of 120 free-living older women, approximately 50% had olfactory dysfunction, which manifested itself as lower preference for foods with a sour/bitter taste and for pungent foods (fruits/vegetables), higher intake of sweets, reduced intake of low-fat milk products, and a nutrient intake profile indicative of increased risk of cardiovascular disease (28).

Interventions

The frequency with which food is eaten, the quantity and quality of the food consumed, and other factors that contribute to excessive or inadequate food or fluid intake must be routinely and systematically assessed. Questions regarding programs that provide money for food; food itself; meals for the bedridden or infirm; or broader levels of economic, medical, or social support should be included. Direct observation of food intake, dietary recall or records of food intake, and careful questioning of both older adults and caregivers or family members are additional ways in which information can be gathered. Mistaken health beliefs, distorted body image, and excessively self-imposed dietary modifications or restrictions should also be questioned. Box 2.1 describes potential nutrition interventions that can be provided for older adults.

Olfactory dysfunction is associated with decreased enjoyment of food. When chemosensory impairments are combined with changes in food intake regulatory mechanisms, the risk for nutritional deficiencies increases (24). It has been found that adding more spices and stronger odors to foods can increase intake in some older adults (25,29). Because of this impairment, it is reasonable to use a liberalized diet to improve intake, rather than always adhering to strict diets for diabetes, cardiovascular disease, and many other chronic conditions (30,31).

Documentation of the data and its availability to appropriate members of the health care team is essential. Longitudinal monitoring and appropriate adjustment of care plans developed are integral to this process. Once specific problem areas are identified, appropriate nutrition, medical, social, and/or economic interventions can be implemented.

Box 2.1   Potential Nutrition Interventions

Interventions may include but are not limited to

- Allowing adequate time for the consumption of meals and snacks
- Alterations in the flavor, texture, and temperature of foods served
- Fortification of foods or beverages
- Frequent oral feeding
- Individualized dietary counseling
- Nutrition education
- Participation in community nutrition programs
- Specialized feeding programs

POVERTY

Poverty is defined as having insufficient economic and other resources to meet basic needs. The Food Security Act of 1985 amended the Agriculture and Consumer Protection Act of 1973 to address hunger among the elderly (32). Measured in dollars, 130% of the federally designated "poverty level" is frequently used as the cutoff point for eligibility for participation in the commodity supplemental food program for the elderly and for participation in the federal food stamps program (32,33).

Reason for Concern

The poverty rate dropped in 1999 for people 65 years and older, and was the lowest for this group ever measured by the Census Bureau (1). The Census Bureau also reported that 3.2 million people in this age group were poor in 1999, down from 3.4 million in 1998 (1). A high percentage of these individuals were minorities, those living alone, and those living in rural areas (34). Low-income older adults often have limited access to food and limited food choices, particularly when utility and phone bills, medication, and similar expenses compete with already scant funds. Surveys of food consumption patterns often show that low-income adults have consistently low intakes of most nutrients (35).

Interventions

Questions regarding level and sources of income and adequacy of present income to meet basic needs must be asked whenever nutritional status is assessed.

Questions regarding the specific amount of money or other resources available specifically for food may also yield significant information about the ability of older adults to obtain the food needed to maintain health. Reliance on any type of economic assistance program to meet basic needs (eg, food, housing, medical) should trigger an awareness that funds are limited and that risk of poor nutrition may be increased.

When a person's income is insufficient to meet basic needs, economic assistance can be sought on either an emergent or continuing basis. Food assistance (eg, food stamps, home-delivered meals, congregate meals) and other similar services differ in availability and acceptability to the individual client. These resources are used less often than would be desired by a significant percentage of those eligible to receive them (33). Awareness of the full range of options available and of the patterns of use within the community may increase the likelihood that needs will be met.

SOCIAL ISOLATION

The Institute of Medicine defines social isolation as "the absence of social interactions, contacts, and relationships with family and friends, with neighbors on an individual level and with `society at large' on a broader level" (36). Social isolation is usually measured by evaluating the type and strength of a person's social support network and how they use it.

Reason for Concern

It is well documented that social ties and interaction have a positive impact on health, quality of life, and food intake (37,38). Even the oldest old tend to maintain important relationships with friends and family members, which indicates that socialization is important (39). In addition, immigrants who receive health services need culturally sensitive social interactions (40). Social integration seems to have a particularly positive impact on the postmyocardial infarction prognosis (38,41).

As age increases, losses of family and friends are inevitable. Declines in independence, self-esteem, and income are often experienced. Feelings of apathy, denial, depression, grief, and loneliness, as well as suicidal rumination, may be overwhelming. Each of these has the potential to negatively affect food intake and nutritional status.

Interventions

Attempts must be made to identify socially isolated people and to provide or to increase their opportunity for social interaction. It is particularly impor-

tant for dietetics professionals to assess individual use of senior citizen centers, congregate feeding sites, meals-on-wheels programs, and similar community resources that supply food, promote social contact, and provide opportunity to use and maintain interpersonal skills. Participation in such programs should be encouraged, when appropriate.

Deficient intakes in older adults might be ameliorated by altering environmental factors, such as the number of other people present at meals, the palatability of meals, and the time of day and location of meals (24). In institutional settings, congregate dining should be encouraged, even as self-feeding skills decline. Alternative table shapes, positioning those who require feeding assistance so that food intake in a group setting is facilitated, and the use of music at mealtime that is appropriate to the generation are minor modifications that can have a significant impact on food intake and nutritional status (42).

PHYSICAL INACTIVITY OR IMPAIRED FUNCTIONAL STATUS

Physical inactivity or impaired functional status is defined as an inadequate level of aerobic fitness or an inability to perform those activities necessary for routine self-care.

Reason for Concern

Decreased food intake and a sedentary lifestyle in older adults increase the risk for malnutrition, decline of bodily functions, and developing chronic diseases (3). Functional status is often an indicator of the ability to care for oneself. In one study, clients in whom functional status declined during hospital stay, on admission had lower left handgrip strength, had a worse Subjective Global Assessment (SGA) classification, were older, and had lower fat mass (43).

Many US adults do not achieve the recommended amount of regular physical activity. In 2000, only 26% of adults engaged in activities consistent with the physical activity recommendations (44). Physical inactivity is more prevalent among women, minorities, older adults, and the poor (45). Physical activity is important to protect health; for example, regular walking is associated with substantially lower risk of hip fracture in postmenopausal women (46).

Maintaining or improving the capacity to function, prevention or delay in the onset of the chronic diet-related diseases, and the potential to delay institutionalization may be the best reasons to encourage regular physical activity in older adults.

The prevalence of functional limitations in older adults living in the community increases with advancing age and is well described (4,47). Difficulty in performing activities of daily living (ADL) or the instrumental activities of daily living (IADL) are often cited as factors in the decision to place individuals in alternate care settings.

Interventions

A general indication of functional status is often useful in determining increased nutritional risk (47) and risk of an adverse hospital outcome (48). Tools most often used to accomplish this task are the ADL and IADL assessment protocols (49,50). Clearly, the assessment of eating behaviors and factors that contribute to eating dependency are also important (51).

Interventions targeted at inadequate nutrition offer opportunities to reduce functional disability (52). Difficulties related to eating, food preparation, or food procurement must be identified and documented early, and appropriate community, social services, or therapeutic modalities must be implemented.

SELECTED ACUTE AND CHRONIC DISEASES OR CONDITIONS

The presence of any acute or chronic disease or condition, depending on the prior health and nutritional status of the person afflicted and the nature and extent of the effects of the disease or condition, has the potential to negatively affect nutritional status. It is well documented that hospitalization, trauma, surgery, and infection often have a negative impact on nutritional health (4,42,53).

Hypertension, dyslipidemia, impaired glucose tolerance, and obesity remain the major modifiable risk factors for coronary disease afflicting older adults; fortunately, the relative risk associated with these factors diminishes with advancing age (54). Box 2.2 lists some of the more common conditions that affect older adults. Warning signs of increased nutritional risk are symptoms of diet-related diseases and conditions and decline in the ability to eat, prepare, or purchase food.

In 1997, the Nutrition Screening Initiative (NSI) published a landmark resource addressing the role of nutrition in 10 disease states commonly seen in older persons. An electronic version was made available to physicians recently (55). This document includes tips for managing nutritional concerns in cancer, chronic obstructive pulmonary disease, congestive heart failure, coronary heart disease, diabetes mellitus, and osteoporosis.

Box 2.2   Disease States Commonly Seen in Older Adults

- Arthritis
- Cancer
- Chronic obstructive pulmonary disease
- Congestive heart failure
- Coronary heart disease
- Dementia
- Diabetes mellitus
- Failure to thrive
- Hypertension
- Osteoporosis
- Pneumonia and other respiratory infections
- Renal insufficiency or failure

Nursing facility residents have chronic medical conditions that gradually lead to declining functional status, nutritional status, and pulmonary clearance. For example, nutrition-related precursors of pneumonia include presence of feeding tube, weight loss, swallowing problems, use of a mechanically altered diet, dependence for eating, and age (56). Prevention and treatment of aspiration pneumonia and dehydration are important aspects of care.

Osteoporosis and falls are also common problems. There is an important role for protein in bone health, especially in elderly frail patients; total lymphocyte count and serum albumin are suitable markers (57). Undernutrition and lack of dietary protein contribute both to impaired bone mineral conservation and increased propensity to fall (58). Persons who are at risk for falls should be closely monitored for intake of calcium, vitamin D, and other bone-building nutrients.

Almost 21 million Americans have osteoarthritis (59). Physical limitations and problems with self-feeding can occur (see functional decline). Hypertension is prevalent in approximately 40% of osteoarthritis patients; 11% have diabetes; 32% have high total cholesterol; 37% have renal impairment (60). All these factors must be considered in this population.

Hypertension is common among the aging population. Use of the Dietary Approaches to Stop Hypertension (DASH diet should be considered as a ready alternative to chronic medications, especially in mild cases and for those older adults living independently. The DASH diet encourages use of fruits, vegetables, and dairy products in proportions that yield a higher intake of potassium, calcium, and magnesium than a typical American diet. The complexity and lower caloric density of the DASH diet may not be appropriate for institutionalized older adults. Maintaining or achieving a healthier weight, improving overall activity level, and reducing alcohol intake are also steps to include. More information is available from the National Heart, Lung, and Blood Institute (61).

In renal insufficiency or failure, malnutrition is common. A recent study by Pifer et al confirmed that several nutritional indicators predict mortality among hemodialysis patients and that changes in indicator values over 6 months provide additional important prognostic information (62). Interventions that modify these indicators of nutritional status may have an important impact on the survival of hemodialysis patients and can be addressed by using nutritional supplementation between meals (63).

Adequate protein and energy intakes are essential for maintaining skin integrity. The American Medical Directors Association (AMDA), starting with a prior Agency for Health Care Policy and Research (AHCPR, 1996) document, has published clinical practice guidelines regarding the prevention and treatment of pressure ulcers (64).

Gastrointestinal motility changes associated with age are relatively subtle (2). Gastroparesis, a slowing down of the emptying rate of the stomach contents, can occur in persons with long-term diabetes mellitus and can cause altered responses to insulin therapy or early satiety with meals. Anemias can occur in aging persons when there is a decline in intrinsic factor in the stomach. Indeed, vitamin B-12 deficiency is a common finding in this population (65). In addition, hidden blood losses from the gastrointestinal tract should be questioned if hemoglobin and hematocrit are chronically lower than normal despite adequate diet and intake of related nutrients (66).

Recent gastrointestinal surgery, significant infections, or trauma will increase energy and protein needs, at least temporarily. Weight changes should be carefully monitored in this population subset, and available biochemical data evaluated regularly for signs of covert or overt malnutrition. Use of the minimum data set (MDS) findings for detection of residents at risk for malnutrition can dramatically improve quality of life (67).

Alcohol Abuse

According to the *Diagnostic and Statistical Manual of Mental Disorders* (1994), the essential feature of alcohol abuse is a pattern of potentially reversible, maladaptive behavioral changes leading to clinically significant impairment or distress due to the ingestion of alcohol (68). The symptoms are not due to a general medical condition and are not better accounted for by another mental disorder. Three main patterns of alcohol abuse or dependence include regular or daily intake of large amounts of alcohol, regular heavy drinking limited to weekends, and long periods of sobriety interspersed with binges of daily drinking lasting weeks or months. Alcohol dependence and depression often co-exist (69).

Reason for Concern

Alcohol-related problems manifest themselves in a variety of physical and psychosocial forms, including alcoholic liver disease, alcoholic dementia, peripheral neuropathy, depression, insomnia, loss of libido, late-onset seizure disorder, confusion, poor nutrition, involuntary weight loss, macrocytosis, incontinence, diarrhea, heart failure, hypertension, myopathy, falls, fractures, inadequate self-care, and adverse drug reactions.

There is a strong, specific association between prior alcohol dependence and current or recent major depression (70). With older adults, substance abuse is often invisible, masked and complicated by lack of awareness or other health problems; and signs of substance abuse may be mistaken for common signs of aging or dementia. Alcohol-related hospitalizations offer an opportunity to identify the disorder and to provide effective follow-up (71). The cost to the health care system exceeds more than $230 million annually (72).

Interventions

It is important to evaluate how often alcohol is consumed and whether this level of consumption represents a health hazard. Older adults may show a different pattern of alcohol abuse from that of younger people. Differences in body composition and changes in metabolism that occur as part of the aging process increase risk at all levels of consumption for medical and psychological problems (72).

The screening process used in assessing alcohol intake and its significance involves the use of easily administered, standardized questionnaires that are fairly sensitive when used appropriately. Box 2.3 describes the CAGE questions that can be used to identify a problem with alcohol (73,74). Other tools are also available (73).

Box 2.3   "CAGE" Questionnaire

C: Have you ever felt you ought to **Cut Down** on drinking?

A: Have people **Annoyed** you by criticizing your drinking?

G: Have you ever felt bad or **Guilty** about your drinking?

E: Have you ever had a drink first thing in the morning to steady your nerves or get rid of a hangover **(Eye-opener)**?

Source: Data are from reference 74.

Older adults are more compliant with treatment and have treatment outcomes as good as or better than younger people; age-specific treatment often improves older adult compliance outcomes (75). Once a problem has been identified, the dietetics professional should work with other members of the health care team who are involved in the treatment process, to assess the vitamin, mineral, and caloric status of the older person who is drinking; to recommend provision of critical nutrients to prevent the nutrition-related effects of alcohol withdrawal; and to correct any identified nutrient deficits.

Constipation

Constipation is the infrequent or difficult evacuation of feces. People often subjectively define constipation as the passage of fewer than "normal" bowel movements, failure to have a daily bowel movement, and/or increased difficulty in defecation.

Reason for Concern

Constipation is not an inevitable part of the aging process, but physiological alterations that sometimes accompany aging, such as decreased intestinal motility, increased transit time, and a decreased urge to defecate, may contribute to its prevalence.

About 3 million people in the United States, many of them 65 years or older, complain of chronic constipation. Constipation is the most common gastrointestinal complaint in the United States, resulting in about 2 million physician visits annually (76).

Irritable bowel syndrome (IBS) can yield intermittent bouts of either diarrhea or constipation, usually with an onset before age 50, but this may persist later in life as well. In the United States, IBS has been reported to account for up to 3.5 million physician visits annually, at an estimated cost of $8 billion (77).

Laxative use is high among older adults. Americans have spent about $725 billion annually on over-the-counter laxatives (78). The Food and Drug Administration (FDA) has banned all over-the-counter laxatives that contain phenolphthalein, because its use may increase cancer risk. Otherwise, many products are available for over-the-counter and for prescription use.

In extended care settings, factors associated with regular laxative use (30 or more doses per month) include immobility; Parkinson's disease; diabetes mellitus; and the use of iron supplements, calcium channel blockers, and antidepressants with strong to moderate anticholinergic properties (79). Changes in bowel habits often occur with diverticular disease and colon cancer. Fecal impaction, overflow incontinence, obstruction, and terminal reservoir syndrome are potential outcomes of chronic, extreme constipation.

Interventions

Systemic disease should, of course, be identified and treated. Medication protocols should be reviewed and alternatives recommended when appropriate.

Dietary modifications can be effective in the prevention or treatment of primary constipation. Increased intake of insoluble and soluble dietary fibers, fluid, and physical activity are recommended (80). Clients should be encouraged to consume diets containing 20 to 35 g of fiber daily (81,82). Coarse wheat bran provides the fecal bulking capacity; bulking agents such as psyllium, guar gum, methylcellulose, carboxymethylcellulose, and polycarbophil produce laxative effects due to their water-holding properties and the mechanical distention of the gastrointestinal tract. These bulking agents are sometimes more acceptable to clients than is coarse wheat bran.

Because the mechanism in the brain that detects dehydration is less sensitive than in younger persons, older adults do not feel thirst and tend to drink less water. In addition, many older adults intentionally restrict their water intake because of incontinence. Insufficient water intake can also lead to constipation. An adequate fluid intake (minimum 1 mL/kcal ingested, 30 mL/kg/day or 1,500 to 2,000 mL) is essential to the maintenance of healthy bowel function (83).

The gradual introduction of high-fiber diets and fiber supplements over several weeks and in slowly increasing amounts helps to minimize flatulence, distention, and the abdominal discomfort that sometimes accompanies the introduction of a high-fiber regimen. Consumption of a variety of food sources of dietary fiber is the preferred method for increasing the fiber content of the diet (84). Supplements can be used to augment the diet if the food sources fail to produce the desired effect when given an adequate trial.

People who have neuromuscular damage, adhesions due to prior surgery, chronic disability, or chronic laxative abuse do not always respond to fiber therapy. However, these circumstances do not automatically preclude a trial of fiber therapy, bowel training, and other rehabilitative efforts.

Depression

According to the American Psychiatric Association, essential features of depression include either a depressed mood or loss of interest/pleasure in all or most activities for a period of 2 weeks or longer, accompanied by four or more of the following items daily or almost every day (85):

- Significant involuntary weight change
- Insomnia or hyposomnia
- Psychomotor agitation or retardation
- Fatigue or lack of energy
- Feelings of worthlessness or excessive guilt
- Decreased ability to think or concentrate
- Recurrent thoughts of death or suicide

The altered mood should represent a change from the previous level of functioning and if it persists for longer than 2 months, it may signal a major depressive disorder or risk for suicide (86). Associated features of depression include tearfulness, anxiety, irritability, brooding or excessive rumination, and excessive concern with physical health.

Reason for Concern

Insomnia and depressive symptoms are often correlated in older individuals (87). In a study related to depression, the DETERMINE checklist was used and a score of at least 4 was associated with more symptoms of depression and lower functional ability (88). This checklist may be beneficial to target clients likely to have related problems in order to provide effective treatment (89).

Rates of major or minor depression among older adults range from 1 in 6 in primary care settings, with higher numbers among those who reside in long-term care facilities (90). Rates of new cases of depression in extended care facilities are startling:

13% of clients develop a new episode of major depression during the course of 1 year; another 18% develop new depressive symptoms (90). Older adults who need psychiatric treatment seldom receive it, but would benefit greatly (90). Major risk factors for depression in older adults include being female, unmarried, widowed; having stressful life events or lack of social support; or having concomitant physical conditions such as stroke, cancer, or dementia (91). Up to 40% of people continue to experience depression over time and risk for suicide is serious (85,92).

Depression or depressive symptoms significantly affect quality of life. Level of function, productivity, and perceived physical and emotional health are also impaired. Nutritional status is in jeopardy, because associated diagnostic symptoms of depression relate to changes in appetite and weight and to lack of interest in food (85). Indeed, depression has been shown to be a leading cause of unexplained weight loss in older adults (20).

Many of the psychotropic drugs commonly used to treat depression, such as antidepressants, antipsychotics, antianxiety agents, and anticholinergic agents, have significant side-effect profiles and may negatively affect ability to eat and, in turn, nutritional status. Oversedation, cognitive impairment, delirium, increased or decreased appetite, dry mouth, nausea, anorexia, and constipation—all common adverse effects of many of these drugs—may contribute to increased nutritional risk (20,85).

Interventions

Numerous screening tools are available to assess emotional status (47). Although dietetics professionals do not routinely administer these instruments, they should be able to recognize their content, use, and implications. Changes in mood, attitude, or level of performance should alert all professionals to the potential for depression. Discussion of this possibility with other members of the health care team is appropriate, as is regular inquiry into the client's emotional status. A useful resource on depression in aging is available from the American Society on Aging (93).

A routine review of medications prescribed to treat depression is indicated in light of their significant potential to negatively affect nutritional status. Drug-free periods or reductions in dosages should be recommended, particularly if these agents are shown to be a significant source of nutritional impairment. Dietetics professionals should also be familiar with numerous drugs (growth hormone, megestrol, cyproheptadine, tetrahydrocannabinol, anabolic steroids, and prokinetic agents) that may be used in the treatment of anorexia of aging with limited success (20). It is important to note any side effects that occur, such as gastrointestinal upset.

Oral Health Problems

Tooth loss, dental caries, lack of or poorly fitting dentures, periodontal disease, pathologies of the oral tissues, dry mouth, and orofacial pain are considered oral health problems (47,94).

Reason for Concern

Problems with the oral cavity often impair one's ability to eat. Local as well as systemic morbidity may result, and decreased life satisfaction is common. Although recent data from national surveys suggest that older adults retain their teeth for a longer period of time, of those older than 65 years, 40% are edentulous and only 2% have all 28 teeth (94). Edentulism is more common among those individuals who live in rural areas where dental care is less available (95). Keeping one's own teeth or use of adequate prostheses generally helps with intake of a better variety of foods and overall nutritional status (96).

Root caries, gingivitis, periodontal pockets, and loss of periodontal attachment are more common among older adults (94). Risk factors for the development of periodontal disease include diabetes mellitus, advanced age, osteoporosis, HIV infection, genetic susceptibility, smoking, and stress, as well as plaque accumulation and infrequent dental examinations (97,98).

Oral squamous cell carcinomas comprise 2% to 3% of all new malignancies diagnosed in the United States (99). Risk factors for the development of oral cancer include advanced age, tobacco and/or alcohol use, chronic sun exposure, and a previous diagnosis of cancer (100). Premalignant lesions (leukoplakia and erythroplakia) should be addressed early. Most deaths from oral cancer occur in older individuals (101).

A major cause of unexplained weight loss in older adults is poor oral health. As the number of dental problems increases, so does the rate of weight loss (102). Systemic diseases and their treatments frequently affect salivary, oral motor, and oral sensory function (103). Diminished or altered taste perceptions are often experienced by people with complete dentures; less saliva is available to mix with foods. Oral pathogens, due to bacteremia or aspiration of oral contents, may also lead to serious systemic infections.

Interventions

Periodic examination of the oral cavity, with documentation of specific findings, is an essential component of nutrition assessment. Appropriate intervention has the potential to significantly improve food intake, nutritional status, and quality of life.

Use of saliva substitutes may be especially beneficial in dry mouth (xerostomia). Use of medications, such as pilocarpine, may prove to be beneficial; studies are ongoing (104).

Sensory Impairment

Sensory impairment involves the abnormal, diminished, delayed, or absence of perception or response to stimuli.

Reason for Concern

Functional declines in sensory organs occur with advancing age and are associated with increased risk of poor nutritional status. Declines in hearing and vision are among the 10 most common conditions reported by persons 65 years and older (105). Marked alterations in taste, smell, and trigeminal nerve sensation may also occur, with a decline in appetite and intake.

Aging diminishes chemosensory functioning, in particular the sense of smell, thus possibly decreasing the enjoyment from food; strong flavor in an appropriate context can improve the hedonic quality (106). Taste threshold sensitivity declines with age; perception of flavor intensity decreases with age, with perceptions of salty and sweet flavors diminishing the most (107).

Olfaction is significantly impaired with age, particularly in clients with Alzheimer's disease. Older adults with and without Alzheimer's show impairments in odor memory. Flavor preference changes as age increases, with higher concentrations of sugar, salt, and casein hydrolysate needed to elicit a favorable food preference rating (108). Arthritis, peripheral neuropathies, and other tactile impairments may also negatively affect nutritional status. Food preparation becomes more difficult, increasing the likelihood of burns and other injuries; even the ability to access food appropriately becomes more difficult (47,105).

Interventions

The use of flavor and odor enhancers for older adults is becoming more widespread (109). Bright contrasting colors in food, plates, and eating utensils, as well as dining areas that are well lit, may also contribute to increased food intake. Hearing-impaired adults may be reluctant to eat in noisy, crowded dining rooms or at large tables, because they are unable to hear mealtime conversations and feel increasingly isolated. The appearance, crispness, or crunchiness of a food can often make up for some of the taste or smell deficits.

If all the senses are diminished, however, food intake often declines and social contact dwindles.

Caffeine, a natural ingredient in tea, coffee, and chocolate, enhances the sensory appeal of beverages (110). This may have implications for older adults, especially for including favorite beverages on a regular basis with meals.

Recognition of these factors and modification of the eating environments of older adults may facilitate improved food intake. The use of a simple multivitamin-mineral supplement to replace zinc and other appetite-enhancing nutrients may be useful to boost immune function (111), and to stimulate appetite.

Chronic or Inappropriate Medication or Supplement Use

Chronic medication use is the long-term use of prescribed or over-the-counter (OTC) medication. Inappropriate medication use refers to medications prescribed or consumed in such a manner that dosage, type, or other characteristics are incompatible with the physiology (including the nutritional status) or psychology of the aging person (47). In addition, more individuals are purchasing and using supplements, such as herbs and botanical products (112), some of which are not known to provide beneficial effects and may actually have untoward effects.

Reason for Concern

In older adults, the potential is high for inappropriate use of medications, causing drug-nutrient or drug-drug interactions, with negative effects on nutritional status (113). In a community setting, many older adults report taking at least one drug daily, and some take five or more. Inappropriate use may also occur; this often involves gastric, cardiovascular, and central nervous system drugs (114). Having a single prescribing physician and a single dispensing pharmacy seems to reduce the potential for inappropriate drug combinations (115).

With dietary supplements, the guidelines are changing constantly. Even the supplement facts labels on the bottles are often misleading and out-of-date, lacking details about possible drug interactions, maximum safe dosages, and specific recommendations about who should and should not take the supplement.

Interventions

The potential for both prescribed and OTC drugs to negatively impact nutritional status is well documented (42). Dietetics professionals must be constantly alert to the possibility of adverse drug events. They must also be well versed in the effect that drugs have on nutritional status and be prepared to intervene early in the course of treatment. Drug-alcohol incompatibilities are also recognizable and preventable in most instances.

Drugs available for the treatment of weight loss include megestrol acetate, dronabinol, testosterone, oxandrolone, and recombinant human growth hormone (116). The use of these medications continues to be evaluated for effectiveness in older adults.

Until more is known about dietary supplements, a cautious approach and rigorous self-education are recommended by the following groups: the National Institutes of Health, the Food and Drug Administration, the National Academy of Sciences (NAS), the Federal Trade Commission, the US Department of Health and Human Services, the Council for Responsible Nutrition (a Washington-based trade association representing more than 100 nutritional supplement companies), and the Center for Science in the Public Interest (6). More information about use of supplements is available from the National Institutes of Health (117).

SUMMARY

It is important to view each older adult as a unique individual with a singular set of nutritional needs and concerns (4,47). Although functional impairment and progressive disability tend to increase with age, generalizations regarding the care of specific clients are, for the most part, inappropriate. Familiarity with each client's individual circumstances and requirements, as well as routine surveillance and continuity of care, offers the most promise for prompt identification of increased risk and timely, appropriate nutrition intervention. Through such practices, optimal achievable nutritional health will be maintained, and quality of life will be maximized.

REFERENCES

1. Administration on Aging. Fact for Features from the Census Bureau. Available at: http://www.census.gov/population/estimates/nation/intfile2-1.txt. Accessed March 11, 2004.
2. Orr WC, Chen CL. Aging and neural control of the GI tract: IV. Clinical and physiological aspects of gastrointestinal motility and aging. *Am J Physiol Gastrointest Liver Physiol.* 2002;283:G1226-G1231.
3. Meydani M. Nutrition interventions in aging and age-associated disease (Boyd Orr lecture). *Proc Nutr Soc.* 2002;61:165-171.

4. Institute of Medicine. The Role of Nutrition in Maintaining Health in the Nation's Elderly: Evaluating Coverage of Nutrition Services for the Medicare Population, 2000. Available at: http://www.nap.edu/books/0309068460/html. Accessed March 15, 2004.

5. American Institute for Cancer Research. *Food, Nutrition and the Prevention of Cancer: A Global Perspective.* Washington, DC: American Institute for Cancer Research; 1997.

6. Alliance for Aging Research Web site. Available at: http://www.agingresearch.org/living_longer/spring_00/feature/feature_body.htm. Accessed December 3, 2002.

7. Engelhart MJ, Geerlings MI, Ruitenberg A, van Swieten JC, Hofman A, Witteman JC, Breteler MM. Dietary intake of antioxidants and risk of Alzheimer disease. *JAMA.* 2002;287:3223-3229.

8. Duthie SJ, Whalley LJ, Collins AR, Leaper S, Berger K, Deary IJ. Homocysteine, B vitamin status, and cognitive function in the elderly. *Am J Clin Nutr.* 2002;75:908-913.

9. Mattson MP, Kruman II, Duan W. Folic acid and homocysteine in age-related disease. *Ageing Res Rev.* 2002;1:95-111.

10. Morris MS. Folate, homocysteine, and neurological function. *Nutr Clin Care.* 2002;5:124-132.

11. Gallagher FA, Leif BJ, Niedert K, Robinson, G. *Nutrition Risk Assessment.* Chicago, Ill: American Dietetic Association; 1999.

12. Kirkland JL. The biology of senescence: potential for prevention of disease. *Clin Geriatr Med.* 2002;18:383-405.

13. Huffman GB. Evaluating and treating unintentional weight loss in the elderly. *Am Fam Physician.* 2002;65:640-650.

14. Chernoff R. Nutrition and health promotion in older adults. *J Gerontol A Biol Sci Med Sci.* 2001;56(special issue 2):47-53.

15. Mowe M, Bohmer T. Nutrition problems among home-living elderly people may lead to disease and hospitalization. *Nutr Rev.* 1996;54:S22-S24.

16. Roberts SB. Regulation of energy intake in older adults: recent findings and implications. *J Nutr Health Aging.* 2000;4:170-171.

17. Vanitallie TB. Frailty in the elderly: contributions of sarcopenia and visceral protein depletion. *Metabolism.* 2003;52(10 Suppl 2):22-26.

18. Carlson TH. Laboratory data in nutrition assessment. In: Mahan LK, Escott-Stump S, eds. *Krause's Food, Nutrition and Diet Therapy.* 11th ed. Philadelphia, Pa: WB Saunders; 2004:439-442.

19. Morris MS, Jacques PF, Rosenberg IH, Selhub J. Elevated serum methylmalonic acid concentrations are common among elderly Americans. *J Nutr.* 2002;32:2799-2803.

20. Morley JE, Miller DK, Perry HM III, Patrick P, Guigoz Y, Vellas B. Anorexia of aging, leptin, and the Mini Nutritional Assessment. *Nestle Nutrition Workshop Series Clinical Performance Programme.* 1999;1:67-76.

21. Sacks GS, Dearman K, Replogle WH, Cora VL, Meeks M, Canada T. Use of subjective global assessment to identify nutrition-associated complications and death in geriatric long-term care facility residents. *J Am Coll Nutr.* 2000;19:570-577.

22. Morley JE. Why do physicians fail to recognize and treat malnutrition in older persons? *J Am Geriatr Soc.* 1991;39:1139.

23. Frisoni GB, Franzoni S, Rozzini R, Ferrucci L, Boffelli S, Trabucchi M. Food intake and mortality in the frail elderly. *J Gerontol A Biol Sci Med Sci.* 1995;50:M203-M210.

24. de Castro JM. Age-related changes in the social, psychological, and temporal influences on food intake in free-living, healthy, adult humans. *J Gerontol A Biol Sci Med Sci.* 2002;57:M368-M377.

25. Rolls BJ. Do chemosensory changes influence food intake in the elderly? *Physiol Behav.* 1999;66:193-197.

26. Bernstein MA, Tucker KL, Ryan ND, O'Neill EF, Clements KM, Nelson ME, Evans WJ, Fiatarone Singh MA. Higher dietary variety is associated with better nutritional status in frail elderly people. *J Am Diet Assoc* 2002;102:1096-1104.

27. Clarkston WK, Pantano MM, Morley JE, Horowitz M, Littlefield JM, Burton FR. Evidence for the anorexia of aging: gastrointestinal transit and hunger in healthy elderly vs. young adults. *Am J Physiol.* 1997;272:R243-R248.

28. Duffy VB, Backstrand JR, Ferris AM. Olfactory dysfunction and related nutritional risk in free-living, elderly women. *J Am Diet Assoc.* 1995;95:879-884.

29. Murphy C, Schubert CR, Cruickshanks KJ, Klein BE, Klein R, Nondahl DM. Prevalence of olfactory impairment in older adults. *JAMA.* 2002;288:2307-2312.

30. Dorner B, Niedert KC, Welch PK. Liberalized diets for older adults in long-term care (American Dietetic Association position paper). *J Am Diet Assoc.* 2002;102:1316-1323.

31. Aldrich JK, Massey LK. A liberalized geriatric diet fits most dietary prescriptions for long-term-care residents. *J Am Diet Assoc.* 1999;99:478-480.

32. Food and Nutrition Service. Commodity Supplemental Food Program: elderly income guidelines (notice). *Federal Register.* 2000;65:20799. Available at: http://www.fns.usda.gov/cga/Federal-Register/2000/041800.pdf. Accessed March 15, 2004.

33. Guthrie JF, Lin BH. Overview of the diets of lower- and higher-income elderly and their food assistance options. *J Nutr Educ Behav.* 2002;34(Suppl 1):S31-S41.

34. Vitolins MZ, Quandt SA, Bell RA, Arcury TA, Case LD. Quality of diets consumed by older rural adults. *J Rural Health.* 2002;18:49-56.

35. Fey-Yensan N, English C, Pacheco HE, Belyea M, Schuler D. Elderly food stamp participants are different from eligible nonparticipants by level of nutrition risk but not nutrient intake. *J Am Diet Assoc.* 2003;103:103-107.

36. Institute of Medicine. *The Second Fifty Years: Promoting Health and Preventing Disability.* Washington, DC: National Academy Press; 1990.

37. Krause N. Church-based social support and health in old age: exploring variations by race. *J Gerontol B Psychol Sci Soc Sci.* 2002;57:S332-S347.

38. Eng PM, Rimm EB, Fitzmaurice G, Kawachi I. Social ties and change in social ties in relation to subsequent total and cause-specific mortality and coronary heart disease incidence in men. *Am J Epidemiol.* 2002;155:700-709.

39. Field D, Gueldner SH. The oldest-old: how do they differ from the old-old? *J Gerontol Nurs*. 2001;27:20-27.

40. Strumpf NE, Glicksman A, Goldberg-Glen RS, Fox RC, Logue EH. Caregiver and elder experiences of Cambodian, Vietnamese, Soviet Jewish, and Ukrainian refugees. *Int J Aging Hum Dev*. 2001;53:233-252.

41. Seeman TE. Social ties and health: the benefits of social integration. *Ann Epidemol*. 1996:6:442-451.

42. Nutrition screening initiative. In: White JV, ed. *The Role of Nutrition in Chronic Disease*. Washington, DC: American Academy of Family Physicians; 1997. Available at: http://www.aafp.org/x16093.xml. Accessed 15 March 2004.

43. Humphreys J, de la Maza P, Hirsch S, Barrera G, Gattas V, Bunout D. Muscle strength as a predictor of loss of functional status in hospitalized patients. *Nutrition*. 2002;18:616-620.

44. Prevalence of physical activity, including lifestyle activities among adults—United States, 2000–2001. *CDC MMWR*. 2003;52:764-769. Available at: http://www.cdc.gov/mmwr/preview/mmwrhtml/mm5232a2.htm. Accessed March 15, 2004.

45. *Surgeon General's Report on Physical Activity and Health*. Washington, DC: Centers for Disease Control; 1996.

46. Feskanich D, Willett W, Colditz G. Walking and leisure-time activity and risk of hip fracture in postmenopausal women. *JAMA*. 2002;288:2300-2306.

47. White JV. Risk factors for poor nutritional status. *Prim Care Clin*. 1994;21:19-32.

48. Sager MA, Rudberg MA. Functional decline associated with hospitalization for acute illness. *Clin Geriatr Med*. 1998;14:669-679.

49. Katz S, Downs TD, Cash HR. Progress in the development of the index of ADL. *Gerontology*. 1970;10:20-30.

50. Whittle H, Goldenberg D. Functional health status and instrumental activities of daily living performance in noninstitutionalized elderly people. *J Adv Nurse*. 1996;23:220-227.

51. Consultant Dietitians in Health Care Facilities. *Dining Skills: Practical Interventions for the Caregiver of Eating Disabled Older Adults*. Chicago, Ill. American Dietetic Association; 2001.

52. Bryant LL, Shetterly SM, Baxter J, Hamman RF. Modifiable risks of incident functional dependence in Hispanic and non-Hispanic white elders: the San Luis Valley Health and Aging Study. *Gerontology*. 2002;42:690-697.

53. American Medical Directors Association. *Pressure Ulcers: Clinical Practice Guideline*. Columbia, Md: American Medical Directors Association; 1996.

54. Kannel WB. Coronary heart disease risk factors in the elderly. *Am J Geriatr Cardiol*. 2002;11:101-107.

55. American Academy of Family Physicians. A Physician's Guide to Nutrition in Chronic Disease Management for Older Adults. Available at: http://www.aafp.org/x16105.xml. Accessed March 15, 2004.

56. Langmore SE, Skarupski KA, Park PS, Fries BE. Predictors of aspiration pneumonia in nursing home residents. *Dysphagia*. 2002;17:298-307.

57. Di Monaco M, Vallero F, Di Monaco R, Mautino F, Cavanna A. Biochemical markers of nutrition and bone mineral density in the elderly. *Gerontology*. 2003;49:50-54.

58. Eastell R, Lambert H. Strategies for skeletal health in the elderly. *Proc Nutr Soc*. 2002;61:173-180.

59. National Institute of Arthritis and Muscoloskeletal and Skin Disorders Web site. Available at: http://www.niams.nih.gov/hi/topics/arthritis/artrheu.htm. Accessed March 15, 2004.

60. Singh G, Miller JD, Lee FH, Pettitt D, Russell MW. Prevalence of cardiovascular disease risk factors among US adults with self-reported osteoarthritis: data from the Third National Health and Nutrition Examination Survey. *Am J Managed Care*. 2002;8 (15 suppl):S383-S391.

61. National Heart, Lung and Blood Institute. DASH diet. Available at: http://www.nhlbi.nih.gov/hbp/prevent/h_eating/h_eating.htm. Accessed March 15, 2004.

62. Pifer TB, McCullough KP, Port FK, Goodkin DA, Maroni BJ, Held PJ, Young EW. Mortality risk in hemodialysis patients and changes in nutritional indicators: DOPPS. *Kidney Int*. 2002;62:2238-2245.

63. Caglar K, Fedje L, Dimmitt R, Hakim RM, Shyr Y, Ikizler TA. Therapeutic effects of oral nutritional supplementation during hemodialysis. *Kidney Int*. 2002;62:1054-1059.

64. American Medical Directors Association. Pressure Ulcer Guidelines. Available at: http://www.amda.com/info/cpg/pressureulcer.htm. Accessed March 15, 2004.

65. Dharmarajan TS, Adiga GU, Norkus EP. Vitamin B12 deficiency. Recognizing subtle symptoms in older adults. *Geriatrics*. 2003;58:30-38.

66. Solomon DH, Glynn RJ, Bohn R, Levin R, Avorn J. The hidden cost of nonselective nonsteroidal anti-inflammatory drugs in older patients. *J Rheumatol*. 2003;30:792-798.

67. Crogan NL, Corbett CF. Predicting malnutrition in nursing home residents using the minimum data set. *Geriatr Nurs*. 2002;23:224-226.

68. *Diagnostic and Statistical Manual of Mental Disorders, 4th ed. (DSM-IV)* (abbreviated version). Washington, DC: American Psychiatric Association; 1994. Available at: http://www.psychologynet.org/dsm.html. Accessed March 15, 2004.

69. National Institute of Mental Health. Older adults and depression. Available at: http://alcoholism.about.com/library/blnimh13.htm. Accessed March 15, 2004.

70. Hasin DS, Grant BF. Major depression in 6050 former drinkers: association with past alcohol dependence. *Arch Gen Psychiatry*. 2002;59:794-800.

71. Smothers BA, Yahr HT, Sinclair MD. Prevalence of current DSM-IV alcohol use disorders in short-stay, general hospital admissions, United States, 1994. *Arch Intern Med*. 2003;163:713-719.

72. Fink A, Hays RD, Moore AA, Beck JC. Alcohol-related problems in older persons. Determinants, consequences, and screening. *Arch Intern Med*. 1996;156:1150-1156.

73. McCusker MT, Basquille J, Khwaja M, Murray-Lyon IM, Catalan J. Hazardous and harmful drinking: a comparison of the AUDIT and CAGE screening questionnaires. *QJM*. 2002;95:591-595.

74. Mayfield D, McLeod G, Hall P. The CAGE questionnaire: validation of a new alcoholism screening instrument. *Am J Psychiatry*. 1974;131:1121-1123.

75. American Society on Aging. Alcohol medications and other drugs. Available at: http://www.asaging.org/aod/facts.cfm. Accessed December 3, 2002.

76. National Institute of Digestive Diseases Information Clearinghouse. Available at: http://digestive.niddk.nih.gov/ddiseases/pubs/constipation/index.htm. Accessed March 15, 2004.

77. American Academy of Family Physicians Web site. Available at: http://www.aafp.org. Accessed December 3, 2002.

78. Sweeney M. Constipation: diagnosis and treatment. *Home Care Provid.* 1997;2:250-255.

79. Harari D, Gurwitz JH, Avorn J, Choodnovskiy I, Minaker KL. Correlates of regular laxative use by frail elderly persons. *Am J Med.* 1995;513-518.

80. Lembo A, Camilleri M. Chronic constipation. *N Engl J Med.* 2003;349:1360-1368.

81. Slavin JL, Greenberg NA. Partially hydrolyzed guar gum: clinical nutrition uses. *Nutrition.* 2003;19:549-552.

82. Marlett JA, McBurney MI, Slavin JL; American Dietetic Association. Position of the American Dietetic Association: health implications of dietary fiber. *J Am Diet Assoc.* 2002;102:993-1000.

83. Harris N. Nutrition in aging. In: Mahan LK, Escott-Stump S, eds. *Krause's Food, Nutrition and Diet Therapy.* 11th ed. Philadelphia, Pa: WB Saunders; 2004:331.

84. Beyer P. Medical nutrition therapy for lower gastrointestinal disorders. In: Mahan LK, Escott-Stump S, eds. *Krause's Food, Nutrition and Diet Therapy.* 11th ed. Philadelphia, Pa: WB Saunders; 2004:707-709.

85. American Psychiatric Association. *Diagnostic and Statistical Manual of Mental Disorders, 4th ed (DSM-IV).* Washington, DC: American Psychiatric Association; 1994.

86. Bruce ML, Ten Have TR, Reynolds CF 3rd, Katz II, Schulberg HC, Mulsant BH, Brown GK, McAvay GJ, Pearson JL, Alexopoulos GS. Reducing suicidal ideation and depressive symptoms in depressed older primary care patients: a randomized controlled trial. *JAMA.* 2004;291:1081-1091.

87. Buysse DJ. Insomnia, depression and aging. Assessing sleep and mood interactions in older adults. *Geriatrics.* 2004;59:47-51.

88. Boult C, Krinke UB, Urdangarin CF, Skarin V. The validity of nutritional status as a marker for future disability and depressive symptoms among high-risk older adults. *J Am Geriatr Soc.* 1999;47:995-999.

89. Fischer LR, Wei F, Solberg LI, Rush WA, Heinrich RL. Treatment of elderly and other adult patients for depression in primary care. *J Am Geriatr Soc.* 2003;51:1554-1562.

90. Reynolds CF 3rd, Kupfer DJ. Depression and aging: a look to the future. *Psychiatr Serv.* 1999;50:1167-1172.

91. National Institutes of Mental Health. Depression. Available at: http://www.nimh.nih.gov/publicat/depression.cfm#ptdep2. Accessed March 15, 2004.

92. Diagnosis and treatment of depression in late life. NIH Consensus Statement Online. November 4-6, 1991. 9(3):1-27. Available at: http://consensus.nih.gov/cons/086/086_statement.htm. Accessed January 25, 1998.

93. American Society on Aging. Clinical depression. Available at: http://www.asaging.org/blues/about.html. Accessed December 3, 2002.

94. Caplan DJ, Weintraub JA. The oral health burden in the United States: a summary of recent epidemiologic studies. *J Dent Educ.* 1993;57:853-862.

95. Vargas CM, Yellowitz JA, Hayes KL. Oral health status of older rural adults in the United States. *J Am Dent Assoc.* 2003;134:479-486.

96. Marshall TA, Warren JJ, Hand JS, Xie XJ, Stumbo PJ. Oral health, nutrient intake and dietary quality in the very old. *J Am Dent Assoc.* 2002;133:1369-1379.

97. Iacopino AM. Periodontitis and diabetes interrelationships: role of inflammation. *Ann Periodontol.* 2001;6:125-137.

98. Krejci CB, Bissada NF. Periodontitis—the risks for its development. *Gen Dent.* 2000;48:430-436.

99. Casiglia J, Woo SB. A comprehensive review of oral cancer. *Gen Dent.* 2001;49:72-82.

100. Shugars DC, Patton LL. Detecting, diagnosing, and preventing oral cancer. *Nurse Pract.* 1997;22:105, 109-110,113-115.

101. Davidson BJ, Root WA, Trock BJ. Age and survival from squamous cell carcinoma of the oral tongue. *Head Neck.* 2001;23:273-279.

102. Sullivan DH, Martin W, Flaxman N, Hagen JE. Oral health problems and involuntary weight loss in a population of frail elderly. *J Am Geriatr Soc.* 1993;41:725-731.

103. Shay K, Ship JA. The importance of oral health in the older patient. *J Am Geriatr Soc.* 1995;43:1414-1422.

104. Porter SR, Scully C, Hegarty AM. An update of the etiology and management of xerostomia. *Oral Surg Oral Med Oral Pathol Oral Radiol Endod.* 2004;97:28-46.

105. Callahan LF, Rao J, Boutaugh M. Arthritis and women's health: prevalence, impact, and prevention. *Am J Prev Med.* 1996;12:401-409.

106. Tuorila H, Niskanen N, Maunuksela E. Perception and pleasantness of a food with varying odor and flavor among the elderly and young. *J Nutr Health Aging.* 2001;5:266-268.

107. Mojet J, Heidema J, Christ-Hazelhof E. Taste perception with age: generic or specific losses in suprathreshold intensities of five taste qualities? *Chem Senses.* 2003;28:397-413.

108. Lassila HC, Stoehr GP, Ganguli M, Seaberg EC, Gilby JE, Belle SH, Echement DA. Use of prescription medications in an elderly rural population: the Movies project. *Ann Pharmacotherapy.* 1996;30:589-595.

109. Mathey MF, Siebelink E, de Graaf C, Van Staveren WA. Flavor enhancement of food improves dietary intake and nutritional status of elderly nursing home residents. *J Gerontol.* 2001;56:200-205.

110. Drewnowski A. The science and complexity of bitter taste. *Nutr Rev.* 2001;59:163-169.

111. Ahluwalia N. Flavor enhancement of food improves dietary intake and nutritional status of elderly nursing home residents. *J Gerontol.* 2001;5:200-205.

112. Tyler VE. Herbal medicine: from the past to the future. *Public Health Nutr.* 2000;3:447-452.

113. Routledge PA, O'Mahony MS, Woodhouse KW. Adverse drug reactions in elderly patients. *Br J Clin Pharmacol*. 2004;57:121-126.

114. Hanlon JT, Artz MB, Pieper CF, Lindblad CI, Sloane RJ, Ruby CM, Schmader KE. Inappropriate medication use among frail elderly inpatients. *Ann Pharmacother*. 2004;38:9-14.

115. Tamblyn RM, McLeod PJ, Abrahamowicz M, Laprise R. Do too many cooks spoil the broth? Multiple physician involvement in medical management of elderly patients and potentially inappropriate drug combinations. *Can Med Assoc J*. 1996;154:1177-1184.

116. Thomas DR, Kamel HK, Morye JE. Management of protein energy malnutrition and dehydration. In: *Supplement to Annals of Long-Term Care*. St. Louis, Mo: Council for Nutritional Clinical Strategies in Long-Term Care. February 2004. Available at: http://www.LTCnutrition.org. Accessed March 15, 2004.

117. National Institutes of Health. Facts About Dietary Supplements. Available at: http://www.cc.nih.gov/ccc/supplements/intro.html. Accessed March 15, 2004.

CHAPTER 3

Housing Options

A time arrives in the lives of many older adults when circumstances dictate the need for a different housing arrangement (1-3). These circumstances may be spurred by illness or death of a spouse or by physical changes occurring with age, and are generally based on one or more of the following:

- Need or desire for security
- Need for some degree of assistance with activities of daily living (ADLs)
- Health concerns

SECURITY
Many otherwise independent older adults enjoy the security of living in an arrangement in which they can be around others in their age group and know someone can check on them on a daily basis. They may also seek companionship and the social opportunities that come with living in a community setting with other older adults, while maintaining a high degree of independence and privacy.

ASSISTANCE
Need for assistance varies widely. Some older adults require minimal assistance with bathing and dressing or just reminders to take medications at appointed times. Assistance with meals, laundry, and transportation may also be a tremendous benefit. At the opposite end of the spectrum, other older adults require extensive assistance with ADLs and may be totally dependent on others for nutrition and hydration. Requirements in this category are very individual and need to be matched carefully with the availability of services furnished by the different types of housing arrangements.

HEALTH
Choice of housing may also be driven by health concerns. The degree of need for nursing care and physician intervention will dictate the type of living arrangement necessary to meet individual needs. Requirements may be as simple as assistance in monitoring blood glucose or blood pressure or as complex as caring for those with multiple health problems and compromised immune systems.

Fortunately, there are a number of housing options available that offer varying degrees of security, personal assistance, and health care, and that can be matched to the individual. The most common housing options can be divided into two groups—those catering to independent older adults and those designed to meet the needs of older adults who require some degree of assistance or health care services.

OPTIONS FOR INDEPENDENT OLDER ADULTS

Home Modification
"Home modification" is the term used when the family home is modified to accommodate physical changes in the aging or disabled individual. These modifications allow independent older adults to remain home longer by incorporating simple changes in the home environment.

Installing grab bars in the tub, adding a shower chair, changing door knobs to handles, and increasing light-bulb wattage are examples of actions that can be taken to make the house more "senior friendly." These relatively inexpensive changes may allow individuals to remain in a familiar environment longer and more safely while still preserving independence and privacy. This option is also relatively inexpensive and does not require separation from a familiar home or from long-term neighbors and friends.

Retirement Communities

Retirement communities may also be referred to as congregate living, senior apartments, or independent living (4). The retirement community may be an independent operation or part of a continuing care retirement community (CCRC).

Retirement communities are developed for older adults who can live independently and who require no assistance with ADLs. They are designed for those who want the security and convenience of community living but wish to maintain the privacy of independent housing.

In addition to housing, many retirement communities offer educational, social, and recreational activities. Meal plans and housekeeping services may be available at an additional cost. Retirement communities may also offer amenities, such as a swimming pool, fitness center, or clubhouse, to enhance social interaction and opportunities for companionship.

Retirement communities run the gamut from economical basic housing to high-end "club style" living, depending on what the customer can afford or wishes to spend and the types of amenities desired. Although health care services are not routinely furnished, some communities allow the person to contract privately with home health services to meet individual needs for assistance with medicines or personal care.

Retirement communities are not subject to formal regulation and receive no state or federal funding; residents pay privately. Cost depends on the type of housing chosen, the level of assistance provided, and the need for health care services.

CCRCs are designed to allow older adults to "age in place," within the same community, as physical and health needs change (5). In a typical arrangement, the community may offer independent housing, assisted living, and a nursing facility. Residents move from one type of residence to another, as health needs demand. Some housing options may be equipped with features such as grab bars and emergency call service, to prolong the ability to live independently. CCRCs are designed to provide services along the entire continuum of health care needs and to allow residents to remain at the same location, by eliminating the need to move from one community setting to another as needs change.

Accessory Apartments

Accessory apartments are apartments developed within single-family homes. Examples include basements, attics, or garages that have been remodeled to provide a separate, private living space within the home.

This arrangement could work one of several ways. An adult child could provide space for an elderly parent within his/her home, or an independent senior could build the apartment within his/her own home for lease and perhaps in exchange for services such as cooking or housekeeping. Benefits of this arrangement include additional revenue (with the lease arrangement) and the security of having someone near without sacrificing privacy. Drawbacks include building costs and possible conflict with local zoning restrictions. Persons considering this option should first check with local zoning authorities.

Elder Cottages Housing Opportunities

Similar to the accessory apartment concept, elder cottages housing opportunities (ECHOs) involve the purchase of a small, portable cottage that can be placed in the yard of a single-family home, perhaps that of an adult child (6). Again, the advantages include a private living space but one close to a family member who can check on the occupant frequently. Because the unit is portable, it can be removed when it is no longer needed. Zoning laws may prohibit use of this type of housing.

OPTIONS FOR OLDER ADULTS NEEDING ASSISTANCE

Older adults who are unable to function independently have a number of options as well. The amount of assistance needed and the need for medical care will determine which type of housing is most suitable when independence is no longer an option.

Assisted Living

Assisted-living facilities have gained immense popularity in the last decade (7,8). Residents of these facilities generally do not require a high level of care but may be unable to live alone safely. Seen as an alternative to "institutional" living, the number of assisted-living facilities has proliferated across the country. Access to assisted living is widely available.

Most assisted-living arrangements include support services, such as housekeeping, meals, and transportation. In addition, they usually offer recreational and social activities as well. Some health care services may be provided, and there are staff members available around the clock.

Assisted-living facilities are usually residential in character and focus on maximizing the independence of residents. Arrangements vary widely—some may offer a choice of studio or one- or two-bedroom apartments that may include a limited kitchen area. Meal plans may include two or three meals per day and, at some facilities, restaurant-style dining. Fees may be based on the level of services desired. As in retirement communities, assisted-living facilities can be very basic or quite upscale. Some may also contain a separate unit designed to meet the unique needs of residents with Alzheimer's dementia. In general, this type of housing provides some combination of housing, support services, and health care tailored to meet individual needs.

Board and Care Homes

Board and care homes are also referred to as adult family homes, group homes, and adult foster care. These facilities are generally smaller than assisted-living facilities or may be private homes.

Services available usually include such basics as meals and assistance with ADLs. Although there are exceptions in some states, medical care is usually not provided. As in assisted living, this type of housing is residential in character and allows the senior the opportunity to live in a home-like environment with security, companionship, and support as needed. Licensure requirements vary by state, and residents may be able to apply social security income (SSI).

Foster Care

"Foster care" is the term given to arrangements in which individual families take in an older adult and provide meals, laundry service, and some assistance with ADLs. Again, SSI may be applied to the payment. As with board and care, those older adults who choose this option remain in a home-like environment and are given support, as needed, with encouragement to remain independent as long as possible.

Nursing Facilities

Nursing facilities, or long-term care facilities, are the housing of choice for older adults who need skilled nursing care or long-term assistance (9). Nursing facilities residents may be admitted directly from the hospital after an acute health episode or may be transferred from home or other settings.

Nursing facilities provide round-the-clock medical care and employ licensed nurses who care for the residents under the supervision of a physician. Some facilities also provide short-term rehabilitation services.

Residents of these facilities often have complex medical conditions that require a high level of care provided by an onsite medical staff. Admission may often be based on need rather than personal choice.

Most nursing facilities offer semiprivate, furnished rooms, with bathrooms shared by two people (similar to many hospital rooms). Private rooms may also be available at additional expense. Some facilities allow residents to bring some furnishings from home. Like other housing options mentioned, nursing home environments vary widely, from basic to very upscale, but are generally considered institutional in character.

Nursing facilities are heavily regulated by state and federal agencies and are subject to inspections, to ensure compliance with laws applicable to the industry. Payment options depend on access to Medicare and Medicaid and availability of private insurance.

Hospice Care

Hospice care is a specialty service provided for those who are terminally ill (10). Hospice provides both medical and support services, including social workers, counselors, and home health aides. Care may be provided in the home setting, in a hospice facility, in a hospital, or in a nursing facility, depending on the needs of the individual and the availability of particular facilities within the region. Medicare will pay for hospice for persons who qualify, but the amount of coverage may vary depending on where care is provided.

Respite Care

Respite care is typically a short-term stay in a facility, to allow caregivers the opportunity to rest from the daily demands of caring for an individual or to take a vacation without worrying about a loved one. Length of stay may be anywhere from a few days to a month (11). Respite care may be offered by assisted living facilities or by nursing homes and may be covered by Medicaid or private insurance.

SUMMARY

Housing options for older adults vary by degree and type of assistance and support required by each individual. As the number of older adults increases, so too are housing options likely to multiply to meet the demands of this expanding market. Those considering a change of housing should investigate types of facilities available within the local community and match services offered by those facilities to the particular needs of the individual.

REFERENCES

1. Housing options for seniors. Senior Site. Available at: http://www.seniorsite.com/jodee/jodee_meddy_housing_options_for_seniors_1.asp. Accessed November 6, 2003.

2. Housing options for seniors. Available at: http://allsands.com/Lifestyles/Seniors/housingforseni_ymi_gn.htm. Accessed November 6, 2003.

3. Housing information for seniors and their families. First Gov for Seniors Web site. Available at: http://www.seniors.gov/retirementplanner/housing.html. Accessed November 6, 2003.

4. Find your ideal community. Retirement Net Web site. Available at: http://www.retirenet.com. Accessed November 6, 2003.

5. Selecting a continuing care retirement community. Continuing Care Accreditation Commission Web site. Available at: http://www.ccaconline.org/ccrc.htm. Accessed November 6, 2003.

6. ECHO cottage housing: helping families stay closer. AARP Web site. Available at: http://www.aarp.org/confacts/housing/echo.html. Accessed November 6, 2003.

7. Assisted Living Federation of America Web site. Available at: http://www.alfa.org. Accessed November 6, 2003.

8. Assisted Living INFO Web site. Available at: http://www.assistedlivinginfo.com. Accessed November 6, 2003.

9. Valuing the experience of the end of life. National Hospice and Palliative Care Organization Web site. Available at: http://www.nhpco.org/templates/1/homepage.cfm. Accessed November 6, 2003.

10. Nursing home compare. Medicare Web site. Available at: http://www.medicare.gov/NHCompare/home.asp. Accessed November 6, 2003.

11. Ingram D. Respite care. The Arc Web site. Available at: http://www.thearc.org/faqs/respite.html. Accessed November 6, 2003.

CHAPTER 4
Community-Based Nutrition Services

An increase in demand for community-based nutrition services has resulted from the ever-growing numbers of older adults and their desire to remain independent, living in their own homes (1). Changes in the health care system and in public policy that have resulted in earlier discharge of ill older adults from hospitals to community-based care have also increased the need for these services (2). The increase in home- and community-based care is reflected in a shifting from congregate meals to larger numbers of home-delivered meals (3).

Home- and community-based services, including nutrition services, are administered and/or funded by several federal agencies (4), including the following agencies and programs discussed in this chapter:

- Administration on Aging
  - Older Americans Nutrition Program
  - Eldercare Locator
- US Department of Agriculture
  - Child and Adult Care Food Program
  - Seniors Farmers' Market Nutrition Pilot Program
  - Food Stamp Program
  - Food Stamp Nutrition Education
  - Commodity Supplemental Food Program
  - Emergency Food Assistance Program
- Medicare and Medicaid Services
  - Centers for Medicare & Medicaid Services
  - Medicaid Home and Community-Based Service (HCBS) Waiver Program

FOOD INSUFFICIENCY
Older adults who report food insufficiency (defined as an inadequate amount of food intake due to lack of resources) experience lower mean intake of sev-

eral nutrients, lower intake of the vegetable and meat groups, lower dietary variety, lower mean serum levels of certain nutrients, and higher risk of being underweight. In addition, they are generally in poor or fair health (5).

Food insufficiency is linked to poverty. In the NHANES III survey by the National Center for Health Statistics of the Centers for Disease Control and Prevention, 79% of those surveyed with food insufficiency had an income below the cutoff for food stamp eligibility (130% of poverty level). Other causes of food insufficiency among older adults may include decreased mobility, lack of ability for self care, and limited availability of help with daily activities. These contribute to the inability to buy and prepare food, and, therefore, food insufficiency may be the result (5).

Older adults with food insufficiency have reported a notably lower intake of calories and nutrients and are particularly at risk of malnutrition. Vitamin and mineral deficiencies can weaken immune systems and may increase risk of cognitive dysfunctions. The dietetics professional has a role in helping the food-insecure older adult access food programs to maintain or acquire a healthy diet (5,6). The nutrition programs discussed below may provide a safety net for older adults.

OLDER AMERICANS NUTRITION PROGRAM
The most visible community-based nutrition programs for older adults stem from the US Department of Health and Human Services, Administration on Aging's (AoA's) Older Americans Nutrition Program (OANP). This federally funded program, under the Older American Act (OAA), provides for congregate and home-delivered meals, along with other services, through the Aging Network, which includes 57 State Units on Aging, 655 Area Agencies on Aging, and thousands of local providers (7).

Meals served under the OANP must provide at least one third of the daily recommended dietary allowances established by the Food and Nutrition Board of the National Academy of Sciences National Research Council. As amended in 2000, the OAA requires the incorporation of the reference daily intakes (RDIs) and adequate intakes (AIs). As well as meeting nutrient requirements, menus need to reflect the food preferences and needs of participants and must be planned with the advice of a registered dietitian or individual with comparable expertise (8). OANP meal participants are better nourished than matched nonparticipants (9). OANP meals often constitute 30% to 50% of the daily nutrient intake of older adults (9). Additionally, participation is associated with higher levels of socialization in both ambulatory and homebound elderly adults. This is key, because of the relationship between social isolation and poor nutritional status (10).

Eligibility for program participation is not based on income status. Individuals are given the opportunity to make a donation toward the cost of the meals and other services. Services are targeted to people aged 60 years and older having the greatest economic or social need. Special attention is given to low-income minorities. In addition, the following individuals may receive services: a spouse of any age; disabled persons younger than age 60 who reside in housing facilities occupied primarily by the elderly, where congregate meals are served; disabled persons who reside at home and accompany older adults to meals; and nutrition service volunteers (8).

CONGREGATE NUTRITION SERVICES

Congregate meals are served 5 or more days per week, where feasible. The meal can be breakfast, lunch, or dinner, or any combination of these meals that meets the needs of participants. These meals are offered in a variety of settings, such as in senior centers, community and faith-based facilities, schools, and adult day-care facilities. Some communities have even offered congregate meals in local restaurants, in the absence of senior centers or as a way of providing ethnic foods (11).

In more traditional senior center settings, participants are provided access to other services. A variety of nutrition services may be provided, such as nutrition screening, assessment, education, and counseling. Supportive services, such as transportation, shopping assistance, physical activity programs, health screening, health promotion, and other services, are also often available (12).

The number of congregate participants and meals served has been steadily declining nationwide (13). Meal participants tend to have greater health and nutritional risk than the general older adult population and have an average age of 76 years (13).

HOME-DELIVERED MEALS

In contrast with congregate meals, the number of home-delivered meals (HDMs) has steadily increased each year (14). Because older adults are being discharged earlier from hospitals and nursing homes, many require a care plan that includes HDMs and other nutrition services (eg, nutrition screening, assessment, education, and counseling).

A case manager often plays an integral role in the cross-referral and coordination of service delivery of home and community-based care services. For more information about these services, see Home- and Community-Based Care section, below.

HDMs (also known as "meals on wheels") are a valuable asset for increasing the nutrient intake of older adults who are at nutritional risk. Participants may have more health problems than participants at congregate meal sites. These programs can decrease length and frequency of hospital stays and help to allow participants to continue to live in their homes. OAA regulations allow for a wide range of HDMs that can be provided to older adults. Meals may be delivered hot, cold, frozen, dried, canned, or as supplemental foods. Breakfast, lunch, dinner, or a mixture of two or three meals may be provided 5 or 7 days per week (8). Many programs provide participants with shelf-stable meals to be used when emergency conditions prevent the regular meal delivery (14,15).

ELDERCARE LOCATOR

Community-based services available in any community in the nation can be located by contacting the Eldercare Locator (16). This is helpful to families living great distances from aging relatives in need of care. Since 1991, this nationwide toll-free service provided by the AoA has helped older adults connect with information and referral (I&R) services of their state and area agencies on aging. These I&R programs help identify appropriate services in a specific area. The toll-free Eldercare Locator service operates Monday through Friday, 9:00 a.m. to 8:00 p.m., Eastern Time, and can be reached at 800/677-1116. Information can also be accessed from the Eldercare Web site (16).

CHILD AND ADULT CARE FOOD PROGRAM

The Child and Adult Care Food Program (CACFP) provides healthy meals and snacks to eligible children and adults who are enrolled in participating care centers. The program provides meals and snacks to 86,000 low-income adults annually who receive care in nonresidential adult day-care centers (17). The Food and Nutrition Service (FNS), which administers USDA's food assistance programs including CACFP, provides grants to states. In most states, the program is managed by the state educational agency. However, governors may decide to have the childcare component and the adult day care run by different state agencies. The Web site offers additional program information and meal requirements (18).

SENIORS FARMERS' MARKET NUTRITION PROGRAM

The Seniors Farmers' Market Nutrition Program (SFMNP) is a new program established by USDA's Commodity Credit Corporation (CCC). Under the program, CCC makes grants to states and Indian tribal governments to provide coupons to low-income older adults. These coupons may be exchanged for eligible foods at farmers' markets, roadside stands, and community-supported agriculture programs (19).

SFMNP's primary goals are to provide consumers with locally grown, healthful fruits, vegetables, and herbs; increase consumption of agricultural produce; and support the establishment and expansion of farmers' markets, roadside stands, and community-supported agriculture programs. More information about the program may be obtained from the SFMNP Web site (19).

The SFMNP varies by state for the dollar allotment to each participant and for the length of the program. A survey of participants of the Iowa SFMNP (20) revealed that the program promoted healthy eating habits, as evidenced by older adults in the program reporting that they ate more fruits and vegetables and bought fruits and vegetables they had never tried before. Purchasing fresh fruits and vegetables directly from the farmer was a new experience to about one third of the older adults. Once introduced to the farmers' market, 73.9% of the older adults continued buying produce at the farmers' market, even when they had used all their SFMNP checks. The SFMNP provides the opportunity for older adults to obtain fresh fruits and vegetables and expand the variety of their diets (20).

FOOD STAMP PROGRAM

The Food Stamp Program is a USDA food assistance program, providing monthly benefits for eligible participants to purchase approved food items at approved stores. The purpose of the Food Stamp Program is to end hunger and to improve nutrition and health. It helps low-income households buy the food they need for a nutritionally adequate diet. The amount of food stamps provided is based on the USDA's Thrifty Food Plan, which is an estimate of how much it costs to buy food to prepare nutritious, low-cost meals. This estimate is changed every year to keep pace with food prices (21).

Approximately 3.4 million older adults (10.2%) were below the poverty level in 2000. This poverty rate was not statistically different from the historic low reached in 1999. Another 2.2 million older adults (6.7%) were classified as "near-poor" (income between the poverty level and 125% of this level). One of every 12 older whites (8.9%) was poor in 2000, compared with 22.3% of older African Americans and 18.8% of elderly Hispanics. Higher than average poverty rates for older adults were found among those who lived in central cities (12.4%), outside metropolitan areas (ie, rural areas) (13.2%), and in the South (12.7%). Older women had a higher poverty rate (12.2%) than older men (7.5%) in 2000. Older adults living alone or with nonrelatives were much more likely to be poor (20.8%) than were older adults living with families (5.1%). The highest poverty rates (38.3%) were experienced by older Hispanic women who lived alone or with nonrelatives (22).

Nationally, 30% of eligible older adults participate in the Food Stamp Program (23). They commonly cite pride and the perceived stigma of Food Stamp Program participation as barriers to taking part in the program. Older adults also report low benefits and the burdens of the application process as reasons for nonparticipation (24). States now have options for improving the application process for older adults. The Electronic Benefits Transfer (EBT) debit-type card has replaced the traditional paper check system, making the use of food stamps less noticeable and removing some of the stigma of participating in the program. Older recipients can use their benefits to buy eligible food in authorized retail food stores, purchase food at Senior Farmers' Markets, or make donations for meals at senior meal programs (23). The numbers of potential older food stamp participants will increase especially after 2005, when the oldest of the baby boom generation reaches age 60 (25).

For the older adults who participated in 2000, the average monthly benefits were $59 (24). Income and resources affect benefits. Older adults must meet the "net income test," which requires that monthly cash income after certain deductions be no higher than 100% of the federal poverty guideline. In 2003, the federal poverty level was $1,010 per month for a two-person household. The deductions include a standard deduction for certain housing, utility, and out-of-pocket medical expenses above $35. Participants may own $3,000 in assets, not including the family home. The receipt of Supplemental Security Income (SSI) automatically qualifies an older adult for food stamps. For more information, call the Food Stamp hotline, 800/221-5689, or visit the Food Stamp Program Web site (26).

FOOD STAMP NUTRITION EDUCATION PROGRAM

The Food Stamp Program plays a pivotal role in improving nutrition in the United States, especially among low-income individuals. The objective of this USDA program is to provide educational programs to aid recipients in making healthful food choices. These programs use the most recent dietary advice found in government publications, such as the Food Guide Pyramid and Dietary Guidelines for Americans (27). FNS encourages states to provide nutrition education messages that focus on strengthening and reinforcing the link between food security and a healthy diet. Fifty percent of eligible administrative costs to operate Food Stamp Nutrition Education activities are reimbursed by USDA (27).

The Cooperative Extension System (CES) is the principal state agency that develops and presents food stamp nutrition education programs. Other participating agencies may include public health departments, welfare agencies, and other university academic centers (27). Nutrition materials appropriate for older adults are available at the Food Stamp Nutrition Connection Web site (28).

COMMODITY SUPPLEMENTAL FOOD PROGRAM

The Commodity Supplemental Food Program (CSFP) works to improve the health of low-income women, new mothers, infants, children, and people at least 60 years of age, by supplementing their diets with commodity foods supplied by the USDA. The food packages are not intended to supply a complete diet but are good sources of many important nutrients (29). Food packages include a variety of foods, such as nonfat dry and evaporated milk, juice, farina, oats, ready-to-eat cereal, rice, pasta, egg mix, peanut butter, dry beans or peas, canned meat or poultry or tuna, cheese, and canned fruits and vegetables. Local agencies determine the eligibility, distribute foods, and provide nutrition education. Older adults must have income at or below 130% of the Federal Poverty Income Guidelines ($15,522 for a family of two, April 2002). States may require that participants be at nutritional risk. The program is not available in every state. Additional information can be obtained at the FNS Web site (29).

EMERGENCY FOOD ASSISTANCE PROGRAM

The Emergency Food Assistance Program (TEFAP) is a federal program (administered by FNS) that helps supplement the diets of low-income Americans, including older adults, by providing them with emergency food and nutrition assistance at no cost (30). Through TEFAP, commodity foods are made available to states, which distribute these commodities to local agencies such as food banks. The food then goes to programs that directly serve the public (31).

MEDICARE AND MEDICAID SERVICES

Centers for Medicare & Medicaid Services (CMS) is a federal agency within the US Department of Health and Human Services. CMS administers the Medicare and Medicaid programs—two national health care programs that benefit about 75 million Americans (32).

Participation in the Medicaid program by states is optional (currently, all states except Arizona, which has developed an alternative program, operate a Medicaid program) (32). The federal government provides broad national Medicaid guidelines for each state. The states, in turn, establish their own eligibility standards, determine the type, amount, duration, and scope of services, set the rate of payment for services, and administer the program. As a result, Medicaid programs vary considerably from state to state (32). States can also apply for "Medicaid waivers," which provide states with additional flexibility to modify eligibility requirements as well as the spectrum of covered services in a state's basic benefits package (14).

MEDICAID HOME AND COMMUNITY-BASED SERVICE WAIVER PROGRAM

Home and community-based service (HCBS) waivers give states the flexibility to develop and implement creative alternatives to placing Medicaid-eligible individuals in hospitals, nursing facilities, and intermediate care facilities. This program can be an effective framework for the delivery of services to older adults, with an emphasis on prevention and providing alternatives to costly institutional service delivered to the older population (33).

The HCBS waiver program provides the option for many older adults to remain in their own homes instead of moving to a nursing facility. With the assistance of this program, individuals can be cared for in their homes and communities while preserving their independence and ties to family and friends. HCBS provides a cost-effective option for states when compared with providing similar care in nursing facilities. The services vary by state, and provision of services is determined after an assessment of the individual's needs and willingness to accept service (33-35). Examples of services available include the following (34):

- Adult day care
- Assistive devices
- Chore services
- Emergency response system
- Home-delivered meals
- Homemaker services
- Home/vehicle modification
- Mental health outreach
- Nursing
- Nutrition counseling
- Respite care
- Senior companion
- Transportation

HOMEMAKER AND PERSONAL SERVICE

Most older adults have at least one chronic condition and many have multiple conditions. The most frequently occurring condition is arthritis (36). Disability takes a much heavier toll on the very old. According to the 2000 Census, 41% of people 65 years or older have some disability (37). Among homebound Elderly Nutrition Program participants, 77% need assistance with or have considerable difficulty performing one or more ADLs, including shopping for food or preparing meals. About 43% of the homebound participants have been hospitalized or have stayed in a long-term-care facility during the past year (10). Among homebound participants, 39% receive personal care, 66% use homemakers, and 16% have home health aides (10).

Many older adults use the services of homemakers and personal service aides to assist with shopping, meal preparation, bathing, housekeeping, transportation, and information sources. These homemakers and aides can be trained to use the nutrition screening initiative DETERMINE Your Nutritional Health Checklist, to make referrals to dietetics professionals (see Chapter 16) (38). They can also provide referrals to other support staff, such as nurses, therapists, and social services.

ADULT DAY CARE/ADULT DAY HEALTH

Adult day care provides personal care for dependent adults in a nonresidential, supervised, protective, congregate setting during some portion of a 24-hour day, 5 to 7 days a week. By supporting families and caregivers, an adult day-care program enables persons served to remain in their home. There are two types of adult day-care programs: (a) programs that offer participants the opportunity to socialize, to enjoy peer support, and to receive nutrition, health, and social services in a safe, familiar environment; and (b) programs that provide intensive health, therapeutic, and social services to individuals with severe medical problems and to those at risk of nursing home placement (39).

Depending on the assessed needs of the clients served, the interdisciplinary team providing care may include the dietetics professional. The environment of care of an adult day-services program is designed to maximize the functional levels of the persons served (40).

Participants may receive a meal and two snacks while at adult day care, thus obtaining a significant portion of their daily nutritional requirements. Meal programs, such as the Congregate Meal Program or the USDA Child and Adult Day Care Food Program, may be applicable for the adult day care program participants. The dietetics professional can help with menu development and identification of meal programs, to maximize nutrition as well as positive budget considerations.

CORRECTIONAL FACILITIES

The aging trends are also reflected in the incarcerated population. In addition to the aging trends, the total number of persons incarcerated is increasing (41). The increase is due in part to the fact that many inmates have been sentenced to life imprisonment without parole. Between 1995 and 2002, the incarcerated population increased 3.6% annually, with the federal prison population increasing 7% (41). The US

Department of Justice estimates that, by 2005, 16% of inmates will be 50 years of age or older (41).

This aging population will need more health care services, including medical nutrition therapy (MNT). Many states already have specialized geriatric facilities that provide assisted living and nursing facility level of care. Along with this level of care come the requirements of nutrition care and the involvement of the dietetics professional.

Good nutrition care for aging incarcerated older adults can be part of a cost-effective health plan designed to avoid costly complications of chronic illnesses such as heart disease, cancer, and diabetes. The difficulty in providing a healthy low-fat or other therapeutic diet is that financial resources are restricted in this setting; however, balanced against the cost of a later illness, preventive MNT is an important part of a total program. Some correctional institutions use the services of the dietetics professional to assist in healthy menu writing, therapeutic diets, and in some cases, nutrition counseling for diabetic or cardiac inmates (42).

Religious preferences of the prisoners may pose a challenge for the dietetics professional in correctional food service. To avoid lawsuits, inmates must have access to religious foods and medical care, including the availability of medically necessary diets. Therapeutic diets in correctional facilities typically include fat-controlled, cholesterol-controlled, diabetic, sodium-controlled, high-fiber, renal, and dysphagia diets. Menus are developed with the Food Guide Pyramid as a guide, averaging 2,800 to 3,200 kcal per day (42).

Many food service operations in correctional institutions use inmate labor in food preparation. The dietetics professional can help to set up training programs and develop creative ways to use older workers.

HOME CARE

Home care includes many services delivered to individuals who require help with ADLs or need medical, nursing, social, or therapeutic services. Home care can compliment care given by family and friends and allows the older adult to maintain some independence while remaining at home (16).

An increasing number of older adults are using home care services. Because the length of hospital stays is decreasing, more patients require skilled services at home after hospitalization. In other cases, home care allows individuals to avoid being hospitalized (43). The 1998 Home and Hospice Care Survey findings indicate that approximately 3% of the US population received formal home care services. Of

these recipients, 68.6% were older than 65 years and 62.3% were women (44).

Since the Balanced Budget Act of 1997 instituted changes in Medicare home health reimbursement, there has been a 31% decline in home care agencies (44). In contrast, hospital-based and freestanding agencies have notably increased in number (45).

As the client population continues to shift from acute care to home care, dietetics professionals are taking a more active role in home health. Nutrition services can help to market a home health agency by giving it a competitive advantage. Generally, nutrition therapy services are not included in the list of reimbursable services. They are, however, an allowable administrative cost (45). Home intravenous and enteral companies need the expertise of registered dietitians. Dietitians can assist in preventing complications as a result of weight loss and malnutrition, can work with providers and caregivers on cost-effective nutrition interventions, and can work with insurance companies on reimbursement issues. Other important roles for dietitians in home care include educating clients and caregivers, developing nutrition care maps and protocols (such as nutrition screening and referral procedures), and securing reimbursement for nutrition services.

Knowledge of regulations for home care, visibility with direct care staff, and public relations with administrative personnel are essential in home care work. To be successful, dietitians must be knowledgeable in nutrition care, equipment use, education, and marketing, and they should be politically savvy. To work in home care, dietitians also need training in how to make a successful home visit, because this area of practice is unique in dietetics practice.

Referrals to see a client in their own home, in assisted living, or in retirement communities provide an excellent opportunity for the dietitians to assess the client and then negotiate interventions to achieve mutually agreed upon client-centered goals. Communication of the nutrition interventions to other home care team members is essential for ongoing education and for reinforcement, because the extent to which the dietitian is involved will depend on reimbursement, agency policy, and the number of hours the dietitian is employed.

HOME THERAPY AND HOME INFUSION SERVICES

Most home health agencies have therapy services available for home-bound clients. Physical therapists, physical therapy assistants, occupational therapists and assistants, and speech language pathologists visit clients in the home to assess and provide therapies as needed. Dietetics professionals can work jointly with speech language pathologists to provide information on appropriate food consistencies and suggestions for dysphagia diets. Home infusion companies and home health agencies provide home intravenous therapy, including antibiotic therapy, total parenteral nutrition (TPN), peripheral parenteral nutrition (PPN), and hydration therapy. There are opportunities for registered dietitians to be part of the home care nutrition support team for TPN and PPN clients (46).

OUTPATIENT CLINICS AND INTERDISCIPLINARY ASSESSMENT CLINICS

Ambulatory care centers are becoming multiple service providers, offering services such as physician and specialist care, outpatient surgery, wound care, diabetes education, wellness classes, rehabilitation, mental health care, and even fitness services. These centers provide assessment, treatment, counseling, and education. Clients come from home, nursing homes, group homes, adult-care centers, or assisted living facilities to receive treatment or preventive care.

Because older adults have special needs, they may have difficulty understanding education provided under stressful situations and will need more assistance in their home after procedures than do younger individuals. Dietetics professionals need to provide additional follow-up on educational sessions provided to older adults, to ensure comprehension. Older adults may have special nutritional considerations if NPO for tests that make them too weak to prepare their own meals when they return home. The dietetics professional should make appropriate referrals to improve the nutritional outcomes of the outpatient clinics for older adults.

REFERENCES ———————————●

1. HHS/AoA Long-term Care Initiatives. Available at: http://www.ncsl.org/programs/health/ASAspeech. Accessed February 26, 2004.
2. Statistics: a profile of older Americans, 2002. Dept of Health and Human Services, Administration on Aging Web site. Available at: http://www.aoa.gov/prof/Statistics/profile/12.asp. Accessed February 26, 2004.
3. Final Annual GPRA Performance Plan for Fiscal Year 2003 and Revised Annual Performance Plan for Fiscal Year 2002 and Annual Performance Report for Fiscal Year 2001 (February 2002). Dept of Health and Human Services, Administration on Aging Web site.

4. Available at: http://www.aoa.gov/about/legbudg/performance/03gpra.pdf. Accessed February 26, 2004.
4. National Policy and Resource Center on Nutrition And Aging. Older Americans Act Aging Services Network. Available at: http://www.fiu.edu/-nutreldr/Aging_Network/aging_network.htm. Accessed February 7, 2004.
5. Food insufficiency and the nutritional status of the elderly population. *Nutrition Insights* (May 2000). US Dept of Agriculture, Center for Nutrition Policy and Promotion Web site. Available at: http://www.usda.gov/cnpp/Insights/Insight18.pdf. Accessed April 24, 2004.
6. Olson CM, Holben DH. Position of the American Dietetic Association: domestic food and nutrition security. *J Am Diet Assoc.* 2002; 102:1840-1847.
7. Fact sheet. Dept of Health and Human Services, Administration on Aging Web site. Available at: http://www.aoa.gov/eldfam/How_To_Find/Agencies/Agencies.asp. Accessed February 26, 2004.
8. Older Americans Act. Dept of Health and Human Services, Administration on Aging Web site. Available at: http://www.aoa.gov/about/legbudg/oaa/legbudg_oaa.asp. Accessed February 26, 2004.
9. The Elderly Nutrition Program fact sheet. Dept of Health and Human Services, Administration on Aging Web site. Available at: http://www.aoa.dhhs.gov/press/fact/alpha/fact_elderly_nutrition.asp. Accessed February 26, 2004.
10. Millen B, Ohls J, Ponza, M, McCool A. The Elderly Nutrition Program: an effective national framework for preventive nutrition interventions. *J Am Diet Assoc.* 2002;102:234-240.
11. Restaurant-based congregate nutrition sites and restaurant voucher programs. National Policy and Resource Center on Nutrition and Aging Web site. Available at: http://www.fiu.edu/%7Enutreldr/Ask_the_Expert/Congregate_nutrition_sites/congregate_nutrition_sites.htm. Accessed February 26, 2004.
12. Wellness activities for older adults. National Policy and Resource Center on Nutrition and Aging Web site. Available at: http://www.fiu.edu/%7Enutreldr/Ask_the_Expert/Wellness/Wellness_Programs.htm. Accessed February 26, 2004.
13. Increasing participation at Older Americans Act Title III funded congregate meal sites. National Policy and Resource Center on Nutrition and Aging Web site. Available at: http://www.fiu.edu/%7Enutreldr/Ask_the_Expert/Participation/Participation_in_AOA_Act.htm. Accessed February 26, 2004.
14. Reppas S, Rosenzweig L, Silver H. Older Americans nutrition program toolkit. National Policy and Resource Center on Nutrition and Aging Web site. Available at: http://www.fiu.edu/-nutreldr/OANP_Toolkit/OANP_Toolkit_homepage.htm. Accessed February 26, 2004.
15. Emergency preparedness. National Policy and Resource Center on Nutrition and Aging Web site. Available at: http://www.fiu.edu/%7Enutreldr/Ask_the_Expert/Emerg_Prep/emergency_prep_8.23.htm. Accessed February 26, 2004.

16. Eldercare Locator Web site. Available at: http://eldercare.gov. Accessed February 26, 2004.

17. Facts about the Child and Adult Care Food Program. Child and Adult Care Food Program Web site. Available at: http://www.fns.usda.gov/cnd/care/cacfp/cacfpfaqs.htm. Accessed February 26, 2004.

18. Why is CACFP important? Child and Adult Care Food Program Web site. Available at: http://www.fns.usda.gov/cnd/care/CACFP/aboutcacfp.htm. Accessed February 26, 2004.

19. Senior Farmers' Market Nutrition Program. Available at: http://www.fns.usda.gov/wic/SeniorFMNP/SeniorFMNPoverview.htm. Accessed February 26, 2004.

20. Russell C. Iowa Seniors Farmers Market Nutrition Program Survey Report. 2002. Available at: http://www.state.ia.us/elderaffairs/Documents/Nutrition/srfarmersmarket.pdf. Accessed February 7, 2004.

21. Thrift Food Plan administrative report. Available at: http://www.usda.gov/cnpp/FoodPlans/TFP99/Index.html. Accessed February 26, 2004.

22. US Census Bureau. Poverty in the United States: 2000. *Current Population Reports.* September 2001. Available at: http://www.census.gov/prod/2001pubs/p60-214.pdf. Accessed March 3, 2004.

23. Wilde P, Cook P, Gundersen C, Nord M, Tiehen L. The Decline in Food Stamp Program Participation in the 1990s. *Food Assistance and Nutrition Research Reports.* No. 7 (June 2000). Available at: http://www.ers.usda.gov/publications/fanrr7. Accessed February 26, 2004.

24. Wilde P, Dagata E. Food stamp participation by eligible older Americans remains low. *Food Review.* 2002;(Summer-Fall):25-29. Available at: http://www.ers.usda.gov/publications/FoodReview/Sep2002/frvol25i2e.pdf. Accessed April 19, 2004.

25. US Dept of Agriculture, Food and Nutrition Services. Elderly participants in minimum benefit. November 2002. Available at: http://www.fns.usda.gov. Accessed February 7, 2004.

26. Food stamp program. Food and Nutrition Service Web site. Available at: http://www.fns.usda.gov/fsp. Accessed February 26, 2004.

27. Nutrition program facts: food stamp nutrition education. Food and Nutrition Service Web site. Available at: http://www.fns.usda.gov/fsp/nutrition_education/factsheet.htm. Accessed March 4, 2004.

28. Food Stamp Nutrition Connection Web site. Available at: http://www.nal.usda.gov/fnic/foodstamp/index.html. Accessed February 26, 2004.

29. About CSFP. Food and Nutrition Service Web site. Available at: http://www.fns.usda.gov/fdd. Accessed February 26, 2004.

30. Food, Nutrition, and Consumer Services. Available at: http://www.usda.gov/news/pubs/fbook97/08nutr.pdf. Accessed February 26, 2004.

31. About TEFAP. Food and Nutrition Service Web site. Available at: http://www.fns.usda.gov/fdd/programs/tefap/about-tefap.htm. Accessed March 4, 2004.

32. Centers for Medicare and Medicaid Services Web site. Available at: http://cms.gov. Accessed February 26, 2004.

33. HCBS Workbook. Centers for Medicare and Medicaid Services Web site. Available at: http://www.cms.hhs.gov/medicaid/waivers/hcbsworkbook.asp. Accessed February 26, 2004.

34. Iowa Department of Human Services. Medicaid home- and community-based services/elderly waiver. Available at: http://www.dhs.state.ia.us/medical services/waiverdocs/elderly%20packet112102.doc. Accessed February 7, 2004.

35. Quality in home and community based services. Centers for Medicare & Medicaid Services Web site. Available at: http://www.cms.hhs.gov/medicaid/waivers/quality.asp. Accessed February 26, 2004.

36. Arthritis Foundation Web site. Available at: http://www.arthritis.org. Accessed February 26, 2004.

37. US Census Bureau Web site. Available at http://www.census.gov. Accessed February 7, 2004.

38. Nutrition Screening Initiative. DETERMINE Your Nutritional Health Checklist. Washington, DC: Nutrition Screening Initiative; 1991. Available at: http://www.aafp.org/x17367.xml. Accessed April 14, 2004.

39. National Adult Day Services Organization Web site. Available at: http://www.nadsa.org. Accessed February 26, 2004.

40. *Standards Manual: Adult Day Services, June 2002-2003.* Tucson, Ariz: Commission on Accreditation of Rehabilitation of Rehabilitation Facilities; 2002.

41. US Dept of Justice. Corrections Statistics. October 2003. Available at: http://www.ojp.usdoj.gov/bjs/correct.htm#Programs. Accessed February 7, 2004.

42. Wakeen B, Roper J. *Correctional Foodservice and Nutrition Manual.* Chicago, Ill: Consultant Dietitians in Healthcare Facilities; 2001.

43. Highlights: national health expenditures 2002. Centers for Medicaid and Medicare Services Web site. Available at: http://www.cms.hhs.gov/statistics/nhe/historical/highlights.asp. Accessed February 26, 2004.

44. National Association for Home Care. Basic statistics about home care. November 2001. Available at: http://www.nahc.org/Consumer/hcstats.html. Accessed February 7, 2004.

45. *CD-HCF Practice Guide for Nutrition in Home Care.* Chicago, Ill: Consultant Dietitians in Health Care Facilities; 1995:11B-3.

46. *CD-HCF Home Care Manual.* Chicago, Ill: Consultant Dietitians in Health Care Facilities; 1995:11F-6.

CHAPTER 5

Cardiovascular Disease

ATHEROSCLEROTIC HEART DISEASE

Cardiovascular disease often involves atherosclerosis, the development of plaque within the walls of arteries. Identification of occluded coronary arteries by cardiac catheterization indicates the need for angioplasty or coronary artery bypass grafts (CABG). The combination of severe plaques and formation of blood clots can block arterial flow. If coronary arteries are blocked, a myocardial infarction may occur. If the blockage is in arteries to the brain, a cerebral vascular accident (CVA, or stroke) may occur. Blockage in peripheral arteries, or peripheral vascular disease, results in intermittent claudication (cramp-like pain in the lower legs due to lack of circulation) (1,2).

In healthy older adults, the focus is on prevention of cardiovascular disease through reduction of modifiable risks. Such risks include elevated low-density lipoprotein cholesterol, (LDL-C), low high-density lipoprotein cholesterol (HDL-C), hypertension, obesity, and smoking. In compromised or infirm older adults, optimizing serum lipid levels can still be of value. However, the dietetics professional must ensure that modifications in diet and physical activities do not limit provision of adequate nutrition. If an older adult has symptomatic disease or has had surgical intervention, dietary modifications and pharmacologic intervention may be indicated (3).

Nutrition Recommendations

The American Heart Association has guidelines for prevention of heart disease (4). The Adult Treatment Panel III (ATP III) guidelines of the National Cholesterol Education Program (NCEP) serve as the standard for treatment of high blood cholesterol (3). ATP III guidelines identify LDL-C goals of 100 mg/dL for those with coronary artery disease (CAD). A goal of less than 130 mg/dL for those with two or more risk factors is suggested. Although significant observational studies and clinical trials support cholesterol-lowering approaches (diet, exercise, and medication) to reduce coronary heart disease (CHD), there is less evidence about these approaches for the older population (3). Studies indicate that those in their 60s with a risk greater than 20% can benefit from initiation of lipid-lowering medications (3). Clinical judgment must be used to determine how aggressive an approach to take in lowering LDL-C in the 65- to 80-year-old population (3).

The indicated medical nutrition therapy (MNT) focuses on the principles of therapeutic lifestyle changes (TLC) set forth in ATP III. TLC is also appropriate for well-nourished, hyperlipidemic clients without evidence of heart disease. TLC centers on the following four tenets (3):

1. Keeping LDL-C–raising nutrients (eg, saturated fat and cholesterol) low

2. Adding therapeutic options of stanol/sterol esters and soluble fiber

3. Maintaining a healthy weight

4. Including physical activity

For some older adults, it is appropriate to modify saturated fat and cholesterol. This can be achieved by the use of low-fat and nonfat dairy products, low-fat meat in limited portions, dried beans, egg whites, peanut butter, poultry, and fish (3). Inclusion of two daily servings of margarine that contains plant stanol or sterol esters can provide for an additional 10% to 15% lowering of LDL-C (5). Inclusion of 10 to 20 g of soluble fiber can also lower cholesterol by 5% to 10% (3). *Trans* fatty acids prevalent in stick margarine and commercially prepared bakery goods should be limited (3).

The dietetics professional should be alert to clients in whom use of cholesterol-lowering diets could compromise nutritional status. Liberalization of the principles of TLC is indicated for clients unable to maintain good nutritional status. Clients who have followed a cholesterol-lowering diet for decades may need to liberalize their diets. In these cases, diet should be liberalized to foster calorie and protein intake to meet individual needs. For example, although TLC indicates no more than two egg yolks per week to keep dietary cholesterol below 200 mg daily, this allowance may be adjusted to one egg per day, to provide a soft and inexpensive source of protein for the older adult (3,6).

METABOLIC SYNDROME

Metabolic syndrome is a constellation of factors, including hypertension, hyperglycemia, dyslipidemia, and prothrombotic and proinflammatory state. Individuals with at least three of five criteria listed in Table 5.1 are identified as having metabolic syndrome and are at greater risk for cardiovascular disease (3). Weight management and physical activity are important features of prevention and treatment of metabolic syndrome. Intervention to prevent metabolic syndrome in a 50- or 60-year-old person can eliminate or forestall the need for medication to treat hypertension and diabetes. A weight loss of only 10% body weight in an overweight client can produce beneficial effects on blood pressure, serum lipids, and glucose. Elevated triglyceride and depressed HDL-C levels can be improved by several lifestyle changes (3). See Table 5.2 (3).

Although the older adult may not be a candidate for an intensive aerobic exercise program, numerous means of increasing physical activity are available and should be encouraged in conjunction with advice from the client's physician (3). Walking, participating in water aerobics, and even chair exercises can provide physical activity to treat metabolic syndrome.

Nutrition Recommendations

The dietetics professional should be aware of the lipid-elevating characteristics of some medications. Most notable is prednisone, but other medications, including some diuretics, can increase serum

TABLE 5.1. Clinical Identification of Metabolic Syndrome

Risk Factor	Defining Level
Abdominal obesity	Waist circumference
Men	> 40 in
Women	> 35 in
Triglycerides	$\geq$ 150 mg/dL
High-density lipoprotein cholesterol	
Men	< 40 mg/dL
Women	< 50 mg/dL
Blood pressure	$\geq$ 130/$\geq$ 85 mm Hg
Fasting glucose	$\geq$ 110 mg/dL

Source: Expert Panel on Detection, Evaluation, and Treatment of High Blood Cholesterol in Adults. Executive summary of the third report of the National Cholesterol Education Program (NCEP) expert panel on detection, evaluation, and treatment of high blood cholesterol in adults (Adult Treatment Panel III). *JAMA.* 2001;285:2486-2497. Complete report available at: http://www.nhlbi.nih.gov. Accessed March 11, 2004.

TABLE 5.2. Lifestyle Modifications to Improve Serum Lipids

Goal	Lifestyle Changes
To lower triglycerides	• Include monounsaturated fats, such as olive oil and canola oil.
	• Include n-3 fatty acids, such as those found in salmon, tuna, mackerel.
	• Avoid high-carbohydrate diets.
	• Eliminate alcohol.
	• Lose weight if overweight.
To raise high-density lipoprotein cholesterol	• Use monounsaturated fat in place of polyunsaturated fat.
	• Lose weight if overweight.
	• Limit *trans* fatty acid intake.
	• Avoid high-carbohydrate diets.
	• Increase physical activity.

Source: Data are from reference 3.

lipids (3,7). Recognition of the effect of medication on serum lipids can help clients appreciate changes that are not due to dietary effects. In addition, in some situations, a client's medication regimen may be changed for more optimal serum lipid management.

When working with older adults, the dietetics professional must be aware of the many alternative approaches for cardiovascular disease. Healthy older adults may benefit from incorporating into the diet soy and n-3 fatty acids in the form of fatty fish (3,8), and/or 25 grams of soy protein daily (9). The evidence is mixed as to any benefit from garlic (3,10), because the advantage of it in food would require daily intake of two to three raw cloves of garlic. Natural alpha-tocopherol (a form of vitamin E supplementation) in amounts of 400 to 800 mg/day does not appear to be harmful and can reduce LDL oxidation, an early step in atherogenesis (11,12). However, only one (13) of several recent clinical trials (14,15) has found reduction in cardiovascular events with supplementation of vitamin E over several years. Given a slight increase in hemorrhagic stroke in one study, vitamin E supplementation is not advised when a client is on a blood thinning agent such as Coumadin (13). Clients with hypertension should consult with their physician before starting vitamin E or any other supplement. Supplementation of folic acid and vitamins B-12 and B-6 can lower elevated homocysteine, an independent risk factor for CHD (16).

HYPERTENSION

Hypertension is a major risk factor for the development of CHD, cardiomyopathy, and CVA. The Joint National Committee on Prevention, Detection, Evaluation and Treatment of High Blood Pressure (JNC 7) provides national guidelines for the diagnosis and treatment of hypertension (17). Because blood pressure will rise as elasticity of the blood vessels decreases, hypertension is common and present in more than half of Americans older than 60 years (18). Controlling weight and sodium intake are the most important principles for control of hypertension among older adults (19). The Trial of Nonpharmacologic Interventions in the Elderly (TONE) recently provided support for emphasizing sodium reduction (less than 2 g/day) and weight loss if overweight for the control of blood pressure among a population aged 60 to 80 years (19). Lifestyle modifications lowered blood pressure, reduced the need to resume blood pressure medications, and reduced the number of cardiovascular events (19).

Nutrition Recommendations

JNC7 (17) recommends weight loss if overweight, limiting sodium intake, and the Dietary Approaches to Stop Hypertension (DASH) diet (20), which provides an overall dietary pattern high in potassium, calcium, and magnesium and relatively low in sodium. The diet includes eight to ten servings of fruits and vegetables, two to three servings of low-fat dairy products, limited amounts of lean meat, and whole grains and nuts. Although it is effective in controlling hypertension (21), the complexity and lower caloric density of the DASH diet may not be appropriate for some older adults.

CHRONIC HEART FAILURE

Chronic heart failure (CHF; previously known as congestive heart failure) can result from compromised pulmonary function or significant atherosclerotic heart disease. Classic symptoms include enlarged heart, shortness of breath, fatigue, edema, and congestion. Heart failure is classified into Classes I to IV, with IV representing an inability to perform physical activities without discomfort and symptoms of cardiac insufficiency even at rest (22).

In assessing nutritional status of heart failure patients, dietetics professionals should be aware of inadequate intake of protein and calories. Intake may be reduced by early satiety as a result of lower functional gastric volume, hepatomegaly and ascites, dyspnea and fatigue, and reduced palatability of lower sodium diets. Body weight and serum albumin are poor indicators of nutritional status, given the potential for excessive fluids and dilution of blood levels (23).

Nutrition Recommendations

MNT for CHF includes limiting sodium to 2 to 3 g/day for healthy older adults (22). Fluid intake is generally limited to 1.5 to 2 L, especially when hyponatremia is present (22). Adherence to sodium and fluid restrictions can prevent worsening of heart failure and may reduce hospitalizations (24). Clients living independently should be educated on the recommended level of dietary sodium, on use of the nutrition label, and on how to distinguish between very high and very low sources of sodium (25). For older adults with compromised health, a more liberal approach to sodium in the diet may be needed to maintain adequate nutritional status (6).

CHRONIC OBSTRUCTIVE PULMONARY DISEASE

Airflow obstruction during expiration is the defining characteristic of chronic obstructive pulmonary disease (COPD). However, physiologic manifestations and nutritional implications differ significantly between the two primary presentations of the disease: chronic bronchitis and emphysema. A common physical finding in both chronic bronchitis and emphysema is dyspnea on exertion. Chronic bronchitis clients are likely to be overweight, whereas emphysemic clients are thin and wasted in appearance. During exacerbation of chronic bronchitis, the physical examination often indicates cyanosis (hypoxia) and dependent edema due to right ventricular failure. Diagnostic features of chronic bronchitis include chronic cough for more than 3 months of the year, mucous hypersecretion, sputum production, and bronchial gland hypertrophy (26).

Those with emphysema often prefer to sit leaning forward and may adopt "pursed lip" breathing to prevent premature airway closure during expiration (hypercarbic). With mild to moderate emphysema, dyspnea is present only during significant exertion. Since emphysema worsens with age, effort dyspnea is often attributed to aging or deconditioning until the disease is quite advanced. The pathology of emphysema is loss of elasticity and destruction of lung tissue, with resultant collapse of unsupported airways (26).

COPD is the fourth leading cause of death in the United States, with a 57% higher death rate for males than for females (27). COPD rates increase with age, and the impact of COPD on morbidity is severe, because clients with even moderate disease are frequently limited in their abilities to perform activities of daily living (27).

The prevalence of malnutrition in those with COPD varies from 20% to 70%, with the higher prevalence reported in those with emphysema (28). Malnutrition decreases ventilatory muscle strength, skeletal muscle, exercise tolerance, and immunocompetence (28). Mortality risk is higher among those who are malnourished and those with a low body mass index than among well-nourished clients (29-31). Recent reports indicate that pulmonary inflammation is detected in the systemic circulation (32). That begins the vicious cycle of loss of skeletal mass that limits exercise capacity and has a negative impact on prognosis (32).

A high dietary intake of n-3 fatty acids may have anti-inflammatory benefits in COPD clients (33,34).

Protein energy malnutrition (PEM) is associated with an imbalance between energy intake and expenditure. Results of studies on energy expenditure and metabolic rate in COPD clients have been mixed. Baarends et al found that the basal metabolic rate was not higher in COPD clients than in matched controls, but their total energy expenditure was 20% higher (35). A recent study indicated COPD clients required 140% of estimated basal energy expenditure (BEE) to achieve energy balance (36). Basal metabolic rate of COPD clients in a stable phase has been found to be related to plasma concentrations of tumor necrosis factor but not to respiratory function (26).

Energy intake may be impaired in COPD clients by the following (37):

- Shortness of breath while preparing or eating food

- Altered taste perceptions due to aerophagia, altered bicarbonate, and pH levels

- Early satiety caused by flattened diaphragm or aerophagia

- Gastrointestinal (GI) disturbances from lack of oxygen to the GI tract

- Anorexia and nausea due to medications

- Depression due to chronic disease

- Medication side effects

Factors that affect diet adequacy in persons with COPD are included in Box 5.1

Nutrition Recommendations

MNT for those with pulmonary disease should be based on individual assessment. A useful screening tool has been developed that identifies the need for further assessment and treatment of adult COPD clients (38) (see Figure 5.1). For malnourished clients, a high-calorie, high-protein, moderate-carbohydrate diet is indicated, with estimated energy needs of 1.5 to 1.7 x BEE and 1.5 to 2.0 grams protein per kilogram of body weight (39). Significant evidence exists that protein needs of healthy older adults may exceed the current RDA of 0.8 g/kg and are likely to be in the 1.0 to 1.2 g/kg range for nitrogen balance (40). Small concentrated feedings to minimize fatigue and adequate fluid to liquefy secretions are important components of the diet. A meta-analysis of nine studies did not find any evidence that nutritional supplementation (oral, enteral, or parenteral) significantly influenced measurements of lung function or exercise capacity in clients with stable COPD (41).

Box 5.1   Drug-Nutrient Interactions of Common Medications

The following medications commonly used with pulmonary-compromised or ventilator-dependent clients have drug-nutrient interactions (DNIs) that must be addressed during the nutrition assessment phase and in the client's provided DNI education.

1. Prednisone
   - Increases appetite
   - Increases potassium and vitamin C loss
   - Worsens intolerance to glucose
   - Increases sodium retention
   - Decreases calcium absorption
2. Theophylline
   - Avoid caffeine—increases the incidence of adverse effects.
   - Avoid charbroiled foods—increases elimination of the drug and reduces its half-life by as much as 50%.
   - High-protein foods increase elimination. Eat the same amount of protein foods each day.
   - Food may slow absorption of drug but prevent gastrointestinal distress.
3. Albuterol, Terbutaline, Metaproterenol, Pirbuterol (fast-acting bronchodilators)
   - Limit caffeine and xanthine intake.
   - May cause high blood glucose levels in individuals with diabetes.
4. Ipratropium Bromide (anticholinergics)
   - Adverse effects may include dry mouth, stomach upset, metallic/bitter taste, and/or excessive thirst.
5. Acetylcysteine (mucolytic)
   - Side effects may include nausea, metallic odor/taste, dry mouth.
   - Provide 30 minutes to 1 hour before meals to decrease nausea.
   - Give with cola or soft drink to disguise taste.

ASTHMA

Asthma is defined as airflow obstruction that is at least partially reversible. It is characterized by hyperresponsiveness of the airways to a variety of stimuli resulting in spasm of the bronchial tubes or swelling of their mucous membranes. Asthma can be allergic or nonallergic and can be exacerbated by exercise, cold air, or infections. Environmental control is key to prevention of exacerbations (26). In older adults, quality of life issues, including encouraging a health-maintenance program with attention to resistance against infection and disease, are especially important (42).

Commonly used treatments include short-acting β-2 agonists, such as Albuterol combined with inhaled corticosteroids. When β-2 agonists are combined with K-Loop diuretics, they may significantly deplete potassium and magnesium, leading to cardiac arrhythmias. Inhaled corticosteroids promote dermal thinning, with increased potential for bruising. Other adverse effects, especially in older women, include bone mineral density loss and acceleration of osteoporosis (42).

Nutrition Recommendations

For those with asthma, ensure adequate hydration to liquefy secretions and provide small, balanced meals to prevent distention of the stomach. Nutrient-dense meals rich in foods that may support immunocompetence are encouraged. Calcium and vitamin D supplementation is recommended in some cases (39).

PNEUMONIA

Pneumonia involves acute inflammation of the alveolar spaces of the lung. Bacterial pneumonia is the most common form in adults, but other pathogens include anaerobic bacteria and other Gram-negative bacilli. Combined, pneumonia and influenza are ranked as the seventh leading cause of death in the United States. For those persons aged 65 years and older, they are the fifth leading cause of death. In bedridden older individuals, hypostatic pneumonia is more common, as is aspiration pneumonia from the aspiration of food or foreign substance into the lungs (43). LaCroix et al found that older adults in the United States with reduced body cell mass and

FIGURE 5.1

Screening form for malnutrition. Reprinted from Thorsdottir I, Gunnarsdottier I, Eriksen B. Screening method evaluated by nutritional status measurements can be used to detect malnourishment in chronic obstructive pulmonary disease. *J Am Diet Assoc.* 2001;101:648-654, with permission from American Dietetic Association.

NATIONAL UNIVERSITY HOSPITAL
Department of Clinical Nutrition   **SCREENING FOR MALNUTRITION**

This screening sheet should be used to assess adult patients'
need for nutritional therapy.

PATIENT'S I.D.

Answer the following questions and assess scores accord-
ingly. If the sum of a patient's scores is 5 or more, a referral
should be sent to the Department of Clinical Nutrition.

QUESTION	ANSWER	ASSESSMENT	SCORES
1. Height: _____ m	BMI: kg/m²	> 20: 0 points 18-20: 2 points < 18: 4 points	
Weight: _____ kg	_____		_____
2. Recent unintentional weight loss?	☐ Yes ☐ No	<u>Unintentional weight loss:</u> > 5% past month or > 10% previous 6 mo.: 4 points 5-10% previous 1-6 mo. 2 points Other 0 points	
If yes, how much? _____ kg	% of weight loss		
Over what period? _____ months	_____		_____
		<u>Questions 3 to 6:</u> Yes: 1 point No: 0 points	
3. Is patient over age 65?	☐ Yes ☐ No		_____
4. Problems last weeks or months?			
A. Vomiting lasting more than 3 days?	☐ Yes ☐ No		_____
B. Daily diarrhoea (more than 3 liquid stools per day)?	☐ Yes ☐ No		_____
C. Continuous loss of appetite or nausea?	☐ Yes ☐ No		_____
D. Difficulty in chewing or swallowing?	☐ Yes ☐ No		_____
5. Hospitalized for 5 days or more during previous 2 months?	☐ Yes ☐ No		_____
6. Major surgery in the past month? If yes, list type _____	☐ Yes ☐ No		_____
7. Diseases—5 points Burn > 15% Malnutrition Multiple trauma	☐ Yes ☐ No		_____

Completed by _____   Date _____   Sum scores _____

low albumin are two to three times more likely to die from pneumonia than well-nourished older adults with pneumonia (44).

Predisposing factors to pneumonia in older adults include the following (43):

- Age greater than 65 years
- Underlying comorbid illness, such as COPD, CHF, and neurological disorders
- Malnutrition, macro- or microaspiration
- Institutionalization or recent hospitalization
- Endotracheal or nasogastric intubation

Atypical presentation of pneumonia in older adults may delay diagnosis and initiation of antibiotic therapy.

Nutrition Recommendations

A soft diet progressing to a regular diet is recommended, with adequate hydration, to address increased fluid needs from fever. In nursing facility clients, attention to possible swallowing deficits, especially in cognitively impaired individuals, may help prevent the development of aspiration pneumonia.

SUMMARY

Nutritional considerations for cardiopulmonary disease cover a wide range of approaches, from lifestyle modifications to careful control of sodium and fluid intake. Among older adults, to avoid malnutrition, it is important to balance the need for dietary modifications with provision of adequate protein and energy. For older adults with pulmonary disease, the focus is on getting adequate protein and energy intake. For those in the early stages of aging, MNT, such as antihypertensive diets, may reduce the need for some medications.

REFERENCES ●

1. Stern S, Behar S, Gottlieb S. Aging and diseases of the heart. *Circulation*. 2003;108:E99-E101.
2. Peripheral Vascular Disease. Available at: www.americanheart.org/presenter .jhtml?identifier=4692. Accessed March 20, 2004.
3. National Institutes of Health. *Third Report of the National Cholesterol Education Program Expert Panel on Detection, Evaluation, and Treatment of High Blood Cholesterol in Adults (Adult Treatment Panel III)*. Bethesda, Md: National Institutes of Health; 2001. NIH Publication 01-3670.
4. Krauss RM, Eckel RH, Howard B, Appel LJ, Daniels SR, Deckelbaum RJ, Erdman JW, Kris-Etherton P, Goldberg IJ, Kotchen TA, Lichtenstein AH, Mitch WE, Mullis R, Robinson K, Wylie-Rosett J, St. Jeor S, Suttie J, Tribble DL, Bazzarre TL. AHA dietary guidelines: revision 2000: a statement for healthcare professionals from the nutrition committee of the American Heart Association. *Circulation*. 2000;102:2284-2299.
5. Cater NB. Plant stanol ester. Review of cholesterol-lowering efficacy and implications for CHD risk reduction. *Prev Cardiol*. 2000;3:121-130.
6. Dorner B, Niedert KC, Welch PK. American Dietetic Association. Liberalized diets for older adults in long-term care (position paper). *J Am Diet Assoc*. 2002;102:1316-1323.
7. Pronsky ZM. *Food Medication Interactions*. 12th ed. Birchrunville, Pa: Food-Medication Interactions; 2002.
8. Hu FB, Bronner L, Willett WC, Stampfer MJ, Rexrode KM, Albert CM, Hunter D, Manson JE. Fish and omega-3 fatty acid intake and risk of coronary heart disease in women. *JAMA*. 2002;287:1815-1821.
9. Food and Drug Administration. Regulations for unqualified health claims described in Food Labeling Guide, Appendix C. Available at: http:// www.cfsan.fda.gov/ ~dms/flg-6c.html. Accessed December 10, 2003.
10. Thompson CA. Dietary supplements in the prevention and treatment of cardiovascular disease. *Cutting Edge*. 2002;23:23-27.
11. Fuller C, Huet B, Jialal I. Effects of increasing doses of alpha-tocopherol in providing protection of low-density lipoprotein from oxidation. *Am J Cardiol*. 1998;81:231-233.
12. Jialal I, Traber M, Devaraj S. Is there a vitamin E paradox? *Curr Opin Lipidol*. 2001;12:49-53.
13. Stephens NG, Parsons A, Schofield PM, Kelly F, Cheeseman K, Mitchinson MJ. Randomized controlled trial of vitamin E in patients with coronary disease: Cambridge Heart Antioxidant Study (CHAOS). *Lancet*. 1996;347:781-786.
14. GISSI-Prevenzione Investigators. Dietary supplementation with n-3 polyunsaturated fatty acids and vitamin E after myocardial infarction: results of the GISSI-Prevenzione trial. *Lancet*. 1999;354:447-455.
15. Heart Outcomes Prevention Evaluation Study Investigators. Vitamin E supplementation and cardiovascular events in high-risk patients. *N Engl J Med*. 2000;342:154-160.
16. Lobo A, Naso A, Arheart K, Kruger WD, Abou-Ghazala T, Alsous F, Nahlawi M, Gupta A, Moustapha A, van Lente F, Jacobsen DW, Robinson K. Reduction of homocysteine levels in coronary artery disease by low-dose folic acid combined with vitamins B6 and B12. *Am J Cardiol*. 1999;83:821-823.
17. National Institutes of Health. The Seventh Report of the Joint National Committee on the Detection, Evaluation, and Treatment of High Blood Pressure. Bethesda, Md: National Institutes of Health; 2003. Available at: http://www.nhlbi.nih.gov/guidelines/ hypertension/jncintro.htm. Accessed March 24, 2004.
18. Burt VL, Cutler JA, Higgins M, Horan MJ, Labarthe D, Whelton P, Brown C, Roccella EJ. Prevalence of hypertension in the US adult population: results from the Third National Health and Nutrition Examination Survey, 1988-1991. *Hypertension*. 1995;25:305-313.

19. Appel LJ, Espeland MA, Easter L, Wilson AC, Folmar S, Lacy CR. Effects of reduced sodium intake on hypertension control in older individuals. *Arch Intern Med.* 2001;161:685-693.

20. The DASH diet. Available at: http://www.nhlbi.nih .gov/health/public/heart/hbp/dash/newdash2.pdf. Accessed February 17, 2003.

21. Sacks FM, Svetkey LP, Vollmer WM, Appel LJ, Bray GA, Harsha D, Obarzanek E, Conlin PR, Miller ER III, Simons-Morton DG, Karanja N, Lin PH. Effects on blood pressure of reduced dietary sodium and the Dietary Approaches to Stop Hypertension (DASH) Diet. *N Engl J Med.* 2001;344:3-10.

22. Hunt SA, Baker DW, Chin MH, Cinquegrani MP, Feldman AM, Francis GS, Ganiats TG, Goldstein S, Gregoratos G, Jessup ML, Noble RJ, Packer M, Silver MA, Stevenson LW. ACC/AHA guidelines for the evaluation and management of chronic heart failure in the adult: executive summary: a report of the American College of Cardiology/American Heart Association Task Force on Practice Guidelines (Committee to revise the 1995 guidelines for the evaluation and management of heart failure). *Circulation.* 2001;104:2996-3007.

23. Carson JA, Grundy SM. Cardiovascular disease. In: Hark L, Morrison G, eds. *Medical Nutrition and Disease.* 3rd ed. Malden, Mass: Blackwell Science; 2003:201-218.

24. Drazner M. Heart failure. Clinical Nutrition B Lecture; University of Texas Southwestern Medical Center at Dallas; January 26, 2004; Dallas, Texas.

25. Neily JB, Toto KH, Gardner EB, Rame JE, Yancy CW, Sheffield MA, Dries DL, Drazner MH. Potential contributing factors to noncompliance with dietary sodium restriction in patients with heart failure. *Am Heart J.* 2002;143:29-33.

26. Johnson MM, Chin R, Haponik EF. Nutrition, respiratory function, and disease. In: Shils M, Olson J, Shike M, Ross CA, eds. *Modern Nutrition in Health and Disease.* 9th ed. Philadelphia, Pa: Williams & Wilkins; 1999:1473-1490.

27. American Lung Association—COPD Lung Profiler. Available at: http://www.lungusa.org. Accessed January 15, 2003.

28. Akner G, Cederholm T. Treatment of protein-energy malnutrition in chronic nonmalignant disorders. *Am J Clin Nutr.* 2001;74:6-24.

29. Pouw EM, Ten Velde GP, Croonen BH, Kester AD, Schols AM, Wouters EF. Early non-elective readmission for chronic obstructive pulmonary disease is associated with weight loss. *Clin Nutr.* 2000;19:95-99.

30. Gosker H, Wouters EF, van der Vusse GJ, Schols AM. Skeletal muscle dysfunction in chronic obstructive pulmonary disease and chronic heart failure: underlying mechanisms and therapy perspectives. *Am J Clin Nutr.* 2000;71:1033-1047.

31. Landbo C, Prescott EA, Lange P, Vestbo J, Almdal TP. Prognostic value of nutritional status in chronic obstructive pulmonary disease. *Am J Respir Crit Care Med.* 1999;160:1856-1861.

32. Agusti A. Systemic effects of chronic obstructive pulmonary disease. *Novartis Found Sym.* 2001;234:242.

33. Schwartz J. Role of Polyunsaturated fatty acids in lung disease. *Am J Clin Nutr.* 2000;71(suppl):393S-396S.

34. Tabak C, Feskens EJ, Heederik D, Kromhout D, Menotti A, Blackburn HW. Fruit and fish consumption: a possible explanation for population differences in COPD mortality (The Seven Countries Study). *Eur J Clin Nutr.* 1998;52:819-825.

35. Baarends EM, Schols AMWJ, Pannemans DLE, Westerterp KR, Wouters EFM. Total free living energy expenditure in patients with severe chronic obstructive pulmonary disease. *Am J Respir Crit Care Med.* 1997;155:549-554.

36. Thorsdottir I, Gunnarsdottir I. Energy intake must be increased among recently hospitalized patients with chronic obstructive pulmonary disease to improve nutritional status. *J Am Diet Assoc.* 2002;102:247-249.

37. Mueller DH. Medical nutrition therapy for pulmonary disease. In: Mahan LK, Escott-Stump S, eds. *Krause's Food Nutrition and Diet Therapy.* 10th ed. Philadelphia, Pa: WB Saunders Co; 2000:945-948.

38. Thorsdottir I, Gunnarsdottier I, Eriksen B. Screening method evaluated by nutritional status measurements can be used to detect malnourishment in chronic obstructive pulmonary disease. *J Am Diet Assoc.* 2001;101:648-654.

39. Escott-Stump S. *Nutrition and Diagnosis-Related Care.* 5th ed. Philadelphia, Pa: Lippincott Williams & Wilkins; 2002

40. Campbell WW, Trappe TA, Wolfe RR, Evans NJ. The recommended dietary allowance for protein may not be adequate for older people to maintain skeletal muscle. *J Gerontol A Biol Sci Med Sci.* 2001;56:M373-M380.

41. Ferreira IM, Brooks D, Lacasse Y, Goldstein RS. Nutritional support for individuals with COPD: a meta-analysis. *Chest.* 2000;117:672-678.

42. NAEPP Working Group Report. Considerations for diagnosing and managing asthma in the elderly. National Institutes of Health Pub. No. 96-3662. Available at: http://www.nhlbi.nih.gov/health/prof/lung/asthma/as_elder.htm. Accessed March 24, 2004.

43. Feldman C. Pneumonia in the elderly. *Med Clin North Am.* 2001;85:1441-1459.

44. LaCroix AZ, Lipson S, Miles TP, White L. Prospective study of pneumonia hospitalizations and mortality of US older people: the role of chronic conditions, health behaviors, and nutritional status. *Public Health Rep.* 1989;104:350-360.

CHAPTER

6 Diabetes

In 2001, the prevalence of those diagnosed with diabetes increased to 7.9% among US adults, an increase of 61% since 1990, when the prevalence was 4.9% (1). An estimated 16.7 million adults have diagnosed diabetes (6.9 million men; 9.8 million women), and if undiagnosed diabetes is included, it is likely that approximately 10% of US adults have diabetes (2). In no population is the increase in diabetes more dramatic than among older adults. In 2001, 18.4% of US adults aged 65 years or older had diagnosed diabetes (2). Nearly 45% of all people diagnosed with diabetes are older adults (1).

Type 2 diabetes accounts for 90% to 95% of all diagnosed cases of diabetes and is associated with older age, obesity, family history of diabetes, physical inactivity, impaired glucose tolerance, and race/ethnicity (eg, African Americans, Hispanics, American Indians, Asian Americans, and Pacific Islanders are at greater risk). However, type 2 diabetes is becoming increasingly common in children, adolescents, and younger adults (2).

AGING AND DIABETES

The recognition of diabetes in older adults is often a problem. Because of the normal physiologic changes associated with aging, older adults may not present with the typical symptoms of diabetes (3). The renal threshold for glucose increases with advanced age, and therefore glycosuria is not seen at usual levels. Polydipsia may be absent because of decreased thirst associated with advanced age. Dehydration is often more common with hyperglycemia because of older adults' altered thirst perception and delayed fluid supplementation. More often, changes such as confusion or incontinence and complications relating to diabetes are the presenting symptoms (3).

Older adults are more likely to be diagnosed with type 2 diabetes, but type 1 diabetes can occur at any age, even in the eighth and ninth decades of life (2). In the development of type 2 diabetes, both insulin resistance and insulin deficiency are factors. Insulin resistance is associated with an increased waist circumference, hypertension, elevated triglycerides, and low high-density lipoprotein (HDL) cholesterol. In the presence of insulin resistance, greater amounts of insulin must be provided to compensate for the loss of tissue sensitivity to insulin. Even though insulin levels may be relatively high, they are still inadequate to compensate for the high glucose levels that are the result of decreased glucose uptake by muscle and other insulin-sensitive tissues. With increasing severity over time, beta cells of the pancreas may fail to meet the additional needs for insulin in response to hyperglycemia, particularly in those who are obese. Therefore, as the disease progresses, insulin deficiency becomes the prominent defect (3).

Insulin release occurs in two phases—an initial surge in postprandial insulin in response to rapidly rising blood glucose and a second-phase insulin release. Insulin deficiency in older adults includes loss of the first-phase insulin release. Deficient first-phase insulin release results in elevations of glucose that are much greater after meals than when fasting (3). This postprandial hyperglycemia increases with age and typically is more extreme in older individuals than in younger persons with comparable fasting glucose concentrations (4). As a result of this postprandial hyperglycemia, in those persons 70 years of age and older, more than half will have fasting glucose levels within the normal range, and the diagnosis of type 2 diabetes may be missed if fasting glucose values are used for diagnosis (5). In contrast with lean older adults and younger adults with diabetes, there is no impairment in the second-phase insulin release among obese older adults (6).

The term *latent autoimmune diabetes in adults* (LADA) is used to describe lean older adults who may also display autoimmune changes normally attributed to younger clients with type 1 diabetes. Islet cell antibodies and marked insulin deficiency are increasingly seen in lean older adults with diabetes (6). Although many maintain good glycemic control for several years with sulfonylureas, these individuals become "insulin dependent" more rapidly than antibody-negative persons with type 2 diabetes. Hypoglycemia is often a risk of diabetes treatment in older adults. Glucose counterregulation involving glucagon, epinephrine, and growth hormone responses are diminished, which may contribute to the reduction in the usual warning symptoms for hypoglycemia (7).

Other complication aspects of the physiology of aging include changes in the pharmacokinetics of both insulin and oral medications. Treatment must take into consideration changes in drug absorption, distribution, metabolism, and clearance, and these alterations affect individual drug choices and dosing decisions (7).

DIAGNOSIS OF DIABETES

Normoglycemia is defined as a fasting plasma glucose level less than 100 mg/dL (5.5 mmol/L) and a 2-hour postglucose level less than 140 mg/dL (7.7 mmol/L) (8). Prediabetes is defined as a fasting plasma glucose level greater than 100 mg/dL (5.5 mmol/L) and less than 126 mg/dL (7 mmol/L) or a 2-hour postglucose level less than 200 mg/dL (11.1 mmol/L) (8). The current criteria for diagnosis of diabetes in older adults are the same as those for younger adults. The American Diabetes Association has the following criteria for diagnosis of diabetes (8):

- Two fasting plasma glucose (FPG) levels ≥ 126 mg/dL on two separate occasions
- A random plasma glucose ≥ 200 mg/dL with symptoms, or
- A 2-hour oral glucose tolerance test (OGTT) ≥ 200 mg/dL

Whatever test is used, it must be confirmed on a subsequent day, unless unequivocal symptoms of hyperglycemia are present. Because of the ease of use, acceptability to clients, and lower cost, the FPG is usually recommended (8). However, in older adults it may actually miss 31% of cases (5), and a 2-hour OGTT may be useful in diagnosing diabetes if there is clinical uncertainty.

COMPLICATIONS OF DIABETES IN OLDER ADULTS

Although hyperglycemia may not affect life expectancy in older adults, it can significantly impact quality of life by exaggerating symptoms already associated with older age. Common problems include malaise and weakness; osmotic diuresis with resulting nocturia, sleep disturbance, dehydration, and possible incontinence; visual disturbances and impaired mobility, which may lead to falls with serious injury and fractures; impaired driving ability due to visual impairment; undiagnosed depression; and difficult social issues (9). Cognitive functions are also affected by poor glycemic control, which may be prevented or even reversed with tight glycemic control (10).

Effective glycemic control is essential for prevention of micro- and macrovascular complications associated with diabetes. However, treatment for dyslipidemia and hypertension is also important.

Hyperosmolar hyperglycemic state (HHS) is a condition that occurs rarely, but when it does occur it is usually in persons older than 65 years with type 2 diabetes. HHS is defined as extremely high blood glucose levels, elevated serum osmolality, profound dehydration, and absence of or only small amounts of ketones. Impaired consciousness can result but not ketosis or acidosis. Glucose levels generally range from greater than 600 to 2,000 mg/dL (33.3 to 111.1 mmol/L), with an average of 1,000 mg/dL (55.5 mmol/L). Clients with this condition have sufficient insulin to prevent lipolysis but not enough to prevent hyperglycemia. Treatment of HHS consists of hydration and small doses of insulin to correct hyperglycemia (11).

INTERVENTIONS

Managing diabetes in older adults can be difficult because of complex comorbid medical conditions and because some older adults may have a lower functional status. Because most complications are preventable with good control, it is appropriate to treat diabetes aggressively, with individualized goals in older adults. Special circumstances may impact therapeutic strategies to achieve optimal control. American Diabetes Association management goals are listed in Table 6.1 (8).

Goals of therapy for older adults should include an evaluation of their functional status, life expectancy, social and financial support, and their own desires for treatment. The ideal hemoglobin A_{1c} target of < 7% may be difficult to achieve in some older adults, but it is recommended (12). Research is lacking regarding the benefit of tight control in the oldest old (80 years of

TABLE 6.1. Management Goals for Adults With Diabetes

Factor	Goal
Glycemic control	
A$_{1C}$	< 7.0%*
Preprandial plasma glucose	90-130 mg/dL (5.0-7.2 mmol/L)
Peak postprandial plasma glucose	< 180 mg/dL (< 10.0 mmol/L)
Blood pressure	< 130/80 mmHg
Lipids	
LDL cholesterol	< 100 mg/dL (< 2.6 mmol/L)
Triglycerides	< 150 mg/dL (< 1.7 mmol/L)
HDL cholesterol	> 40 mg/dL (> 1.1 mmol/L) for men
	> 50 mg/dL (> 1.4 mmol/L) for women

Abbreviations: HDL, high-density lipoprotein; LDL, low-density lipoprotein.

*Referenced to a nondiabetic range of 4.0% to 6.0%, using a Diabetes Control and Complications Trial–based assay.

Source: Adapted from American Diabetes Association. Standards of medical care for patients with diabetes mellitus. *Diabetes Care.* 2004;27(suppl 1):S15-S35, with permission from The American Diabetes Association. Copyright ©2004 American Diabetes Association.

age or older). Major trials to date have not reported data for this population. Therapy should be chosen on the basis of the individual needs and issues of each individual. Coexisting medical problems, such as dementia or psychiatric illnesses, may require a simplified approach to diabetes care.

As always, client education, particularly regarding healthy food choices and physical activity, is essential for effective care of diabetes in older adults. To be relevant and effective, educational efforts should be individualized to each client.

NUTRITION THERAPY

Aging is associated with many biological changes that may predispose older adults to nutritional deficiencies (13). Therefore, any nutritional intervention must start with a thorough assessment that includes a clinical and nutritional history and a psychosocial and environmental evaluation. There is limited research on the changing nutrition needs with aging and virtually none in aging subjects with diabetes. The most reliable indicator of poor nutritional status in an older adult is probably a change in body weight. In general, any gain or loss of more than 10 pounds or 10% of body weight in less than 6 months should be evaluated, to determine whether the cause is nutrition related (14).

The need for weight loss in overweight older adults should be carefully evaluated. Older adults with diabetes, especially those in nursing facilities, tend to be underweight rather than overweight. Low body weight is associated with greater morbidity and mortality in this age group (15).

Nutrition therapy plays a critical role in the successful management of diabetes. The recommended macronutrient composition of the diet and the individualization of carbohydrate and fat components for older adults with diabetes do not differ from the general recommendations for older adults with diabetes (16,17). Providing optimal nutrition through healthful food choices is the underlying principle of nutrition care, but the goals of nutrition therapy for older adults with diabetes are the following (14):

- Provide adequate calories and nutrient intake
- Assist in the maintenance of blood glucose levels within the target range
- Facilitate effective management of coexisting morbidities
- Prevent, delay, or treat nutrition-related complications
- Promote quality of life, safety, and overall well-being

Knowing outcomes from nutrition interventions and when to evaluate intervention outcomes is important. Medical nutrition therapy (MNT) delivered by dietetics professionals has been shown to lower A$_{1c}$ by 2% in newly diagnosed persons with type 2 diabetes and by 1% in persons with type 2 diabetes of an average 4-year duration and in newly diagnosed type 1 diabetes (18). The outcomes of nutrition therapy on glycemia and lipids will be known by 3 months (19), and at that time an evaluation of the need to combine (or adjust) medication(s) with MNT should be undertaken.

Carbohydrate

Foods containing carbohydrate (eg, grains, vegetables, fruits, low-fat milk) are important components of a healthful diet and should be included in the food/meal plan of persons with diabetes. However, with regard to the effects of total carbohydrate on glucose concentrations, the total amount of carbohydrate in meals (and snacks if desired) is more important than the source (starch or sugar) or the type (high or low glycemic index) (16,17). Numerous studies have reported that when subjects are allowed to choose from a variety of starches and sugar, the glycemic response is similar, as long as the total amount of carbohydrate is kept constant (20). Therefore, the first decision for food and meal planning is the total amount of carbohydrate that the person with diabetes chooses to have for meals or snacks. Numerous studies have shown that sucrose does not increase glucose levels more rapidly or more highly than isocaloric amounts of starch (20). Sucrose and sucrose-containing foods do not need to be restricted in people with diabetes, but they should be substituted for other carbohydrate sources or, if added, covered with insulin or other glucose-lowering medication (16,17).

Although different carbohydrates do have different glycemic responses (glycemic index), there is limited evidence to show long-term benefit when low-glycemic-index diets are implemented (21). The focus for older adults should be on total carbohydrate.

Fiber

Fiber is an important component of a healthful diet, but there is no reason to recommend that people with diabetes eat a greater amount of fiber than other Americans. Although very large amounts of fiber (50 g/day; usual intake is 15 to 20 g/day) may have beneficial effects on postprandial glycemia, insulin, and lipid levels, it is not known whether most clients will regularly consume enough dietary fiber over the long-term to see this benefit (16,17). Any increase in dietary fiber should be done cautiously in older adults, especially in those who are not ambulatory or are likely to become dehydrated.

Protein

There is no evidence to suggest that usual intake of protein (15% to 20% of energy intake) be changed in persons who do not have renal disease. There is some evidence that lowering protein intake to 0.8 to 1.0 g/kg/day in those with microalbuminuria or to 0.8 g/kg/day with overt nephropathy may slow the progression of renal disease (16,17).

Protein is probably the most misunderstood nutrient, and inaccurate advice is frequently given to persons with diabetes. Although nonessential amino acids undergo gluconeogenesis, in subjects with controlled diabetes, the glucose produced does not enter the general circulation (22,23). Protein does not slow the absorption of carbohydrate (23), and adding protein to the treatment of hypoglycemia does not prevent subsequent hypoglycemia (24). Furthermore, protein is just as potent a stimulant of insulin secretion as carbohydrate (22,23).

The long-term effects of a diet high in protein and low in carbohydrate are unknown. Although initially blood glucose levels may improve and weight may be lost, it is unknown whether long-term weight loss is maintained any better with these diets than with other low-calorie diets (16,17). In a randomized trial comparing a low-carbohydrate, high-protein diet to a low-calorie, high-carbohydrate, low-fat (conventional) diet, the low-carbohydrate diet produced a greater weight loss than the conventional diet for the first 6 months, but the difference was not significant at 1 year (25).

Fat

Limiting intake of saturated fatty acids, *trans* fatty acids, and dietary cholesterol is recommended, especially in individuals with LDL-C of 100 mg/dL or higher (16,17). To lower LDL-C, the calories from saturated fat can be reduced if weight loss is desirable. If weight loss is not a goal, calories from saturated fat may be replaced with carbohydrate or monounsaturated fat. However, increasing monounsaturated fat intake may result in increased calories and weight gain, and therefore careful attention must be paid to total energy intake. Reduced fat diets when maintained long-term contribute to modest weight loss and improvement in dyslipidemia (26).

Micronutrients

There is no evidence of benefit from vitamin or mineral supplementation in persons with diabetes who do not have underlying deficiencies. Exceptions are for folate for the prevention of birth defects and calcium for the prevention of bone disease (16,17). However, a daily multivitamin supplement may be appropriate for older adults, especially those with reduced energy intake. Routine supplementation of the diet with antioxidants has not proven beneficial, and therefore supplements are not recommended (27).

Alcohol

Because of reduced alcohol tolerance with age, alcohol ingestion by older adults should be examined carefully. Just as for the general public, individuals with diabetes who choose to drink alcohol should limit their intake to one drink for women and two drinks for men (16,17). When light-to-moderate amounts of alcohol are consumed with food, blood glucose and insulin levels are not affected (28). For individuals using insulin or insulin secretagogues (an agent that stimulates secretum), alcohol should be consumed with food to prevent hypoglycemia. Alcoholic beverages should be considered an addition to the regular food/meal plan for all those with diabetes. No food should be omitted (16,17).

Special Considerations for Type 2 Diabetes

Previously, nutrition advice focused on losing weight and avoiding sugars (13). However, current nutrition therapy focuses on lifestyle strategies that will improve control of hyperglycemia, dyslipidemia, and hypertension. Because many persons with type 2 diabetes are insulin resistant and overweight, nutrition therapy often begins with lifestyle strategies that reduce energy intake and increase energy expenditure through physical activity. Although these strategies should be implemented as soon as the diagnosis of diabetes (or impaired glucose intolerance) is made, caution should be exercised when recommending weight loss for older adults (16,17).

Reduced energy intake and moderate weight loss have been shown to improve glycemic control and insulin resistance in the short term (16,17). However, long-term data assessing the extent to which these improvements can be maintained are not available. As is true of the general population, persons with diabetes have difficulty with achieving long-term weight loss. When used alone, standard weight reduction diets providing 500 to 1,000 fewer kilocalories than estimated energy requirements are unlikely to produce long-term weight loss (16,17). Recent data from the Finnish Diabetes Prevention Program (29) and the Diabetes Prevention Program (30) demonstrate that, to sustain a 5% to 7% loss of starting weight over a period of 2 to 4 years, structured, intensive lifestyle programs are required that emphasize lifestyle changes, including education, reduced fat (< 30% of daily energy) and energy intake, regular physical activity, and regular participant contact.

Special Considerations for Insulin Users

The food/meal plan is based on the individual's appetite, preferred foods, and usual schedule of meals and physical activity. After the dietetics professional works with the individual and develops an eating plan, insulin therapy can be integrated into food and physical activity schedules (16,17).

Intensive or physiological insulin regimens, consisting of basal (background) insulin and bolus (premeal, rapid-acting) insulin or insulin pump therapy, provides increased flexibility in timing and frequency of meals, amount of carbohydrate eaten at meals, and timing of physical activity (31,32). Carbohydrate is the nutrient that most affects postprandial glucose and is the major determinant of premeal insulin doses (32). By knowing the amount of carbohydrate and the amount of insulin needed to cover it, an insulin-to-carbohydrate ratio can be determined. Adjustments in bolus insulin doses can then be made for alterations from the usual amount of carbohydrate ingested at meals (31,32).

Conventional or fixed insulin therapy usually consists of rapid-acting and intermediate-acting insulins given before breakfast and the evening meal. For this type of insulin therapy, consistency in the day-to-day carbohydrate content of meals, as well as timing of meals, is important, especially in persons who are not adjusting their premeal insulin doses (33).

MEAL PLANNING OPTIONS IN NURSING FACILITIES

In nursing facility settings, malnutrition and dehydration may develop because of lack of food choices, poor quality of food, and unnecessary restriction. Specialized diabetic diets do not appear to be superior to standard (regular) diets in such settings (34). Therefore, the imposition of dietary restrictions on older, diabetic residents in nursing facilities is not warranted (35-37). Residents with diabetes should be served regular (unrestricted) menus, with consistent distribution and timing of carbohydrates (± 15 grams for meals or snacks) (17). It is usually preferable to make medication changes to control blood glucose than to implement food restrictions (35,36).

There is absolutely no evidence to support the prescribing of diets such as "no concentrated sweets" or "no sugar added," which are often served to older adults in nursing facilities. No matter which diet is used, the carbohydrate level must be consistent from meal to meal and from day to day (36).

PHYSICAL ACTIVITY

Diabetes education of older adults must include encouragement for physical activity to the limit of ability. Regular participation in physical activity, preferably in a variety of forms, will improve not only cardiorespiratory status but also diabetes control (38). Suggestions for increasing physical activity should be individualized according to the person's interests, resources, and abilities. Regular activity programs should start slowly and gradually increase in intensity and duration with time.

Many nursing facilities now offer exercise programs for the physically challenged. Persons with diabetes who are deemed able to participate after a medical examination should be encouraged to participate to the extent of their ability.

DRUG THERAPY OPTIONS

As the disease process of diabetes progresses, it usually becomes necessary to combine oral medications with nutrition therapy. If FPG is greater than 300 mg/dL, particularly with symptoms, insulin therapy may be started instead. Blood glucose data and A_{1c} values are used to determine when therapy needs to be changed (39). Oral medications for diabetes, their site of action, advantages, and disadvantages are listed in Table 6.2 (40). The use of newer oral medications, alone or in combination, provides numerous options for the management of type 2 diabetes.

If target glucose goals are not attained by nutrition therapy alone or with nutrition therapy and oral medications, insulin either alone or in combination with oral medications is required (39).

TABLE 6.2. Oral Glucose-Lowering Medications for Type 2 Diabetes

Class and Drugs	Principal Action	Advantages	Disadvantages	Concerns in Older Adults
Sulfonylureas (second generation) Glipizide (Glucotrol and Glucotrol XL), Glyburide (Glynase Prestabs), Glimepiride (Amaryl)	Stimulate insulin action from the beta cell of the pancreas	• Inexpensive • Effective in combination • Been used for years	• Hypoglycemia • Weight gain • Loss of response with time	Some drugs or metabolites may accumulate in renal insufficiency.
Meglitinides Repaglinide (Prandin), Nateglinide (Starlix)	Stimulate insulin secretion from the beta cells of the pancreas	•Used before meals and are short-acting • Lower risk of hypoglycemia than with sulfonylureas • Can be used in renal insufficiency	• Must be taken before meals (multiple dosing) • Less effective with prior sulfonylurea failure	None
Biguanide Metformin (Glucophage and Glucophage XR)	Decrease hepatic glucose production	• No weight gain • Minimal hypoglycemia • Lipid neutral • Relatively inexpensive	• Gastrointestinal upset • Potential lactic acidosis (rare)	Contraindicated with declining renal function

(continues)

TABLE 6.2. (continued)

Class and Drugs	Principal Action	Advantages	Disadvantages	Concerns in Older Adults
Thiazolidinediones Pioglitazone (Actos), Rosigli–tazone (Avandia)	Improve peripheral insulin sensitivity	•Well tolerated • No hypoglycemia • Raise HDL-C	• Weight gain • Edema • Fall in hematocrit • Requires liver function monitoring • May increase LDL-C • Expensive	Should not be used in elderly patients with CHF due to associated edema and weight gain
Alpha glucosidase inhibitors Acarbose (Precose), Miglitol (Glyset)	Delay carbohydrate absorption	•Low systemic toxicity • Reduce postprandial glucose • No weight gain	• Poorly tolerated due to flatulence and diarrhea • Expensive	Adverse gastrointestinal effects may be especially troublesome
Combination drugs Glyburide/ metformin (Glucovance), Rosiglitazone/ metformin (Avandamet), Glipizide/ metformin (Metaglip)				

Abbreviations: CHF, congestive heart failure; HDL-C, high-density lipoprotein cholesterol; LDL-C, low-density lipoprotein cholesterol.

Source: Adapted from Franz MJ, Reader D, Monk A. *Implementing Group and Individual Medical Nutrition Therapy for Diabetes.* Alexandria, Va: American Diabetes Association; 2002:66, with permission from the American Diabetes Association.

Copyright ©2002 American Diabetes Association.

Types of insulin and their time actions are listed in Table 6.3 (40). The transition to insulin often begins with a long-acting insulin, such as glargine, or an intermediate-acting insulin, such as NPH, given at bedtime to control fasting glucose levels. In addition, oral medications (often an insulin sensitizer such as metformin), are continued during the day, to control daytime glucose levels. However, many clients with type 2 diabetes will eventually require two or more injections of insulin daily to achieve adequate glycemic control. If large doses of insulin are required, oral medications, such as an insulin sensitizer, metformin or thiazolidinedione, may be combined with the insulin regimen. Circumstances that require insulin in type 2 diabetes include failure to achieve adequate control on oral medications and during periods of acute injury, infection, or surgery (39).

All persons with type 1 diabetes need replacement of insulin that mimics normal insulin action, such as the intensive or flexible insulin regimens. Persons with type 2 diabetes usually do better

TABLE 6.3. Action Times of Human Insulin Preparations

Type of Insulin	Onset of Action	Peak Action	Usual Effective Duration	Monitor Effect in:

Rapid-acting
  Lispro (Humalog)
  Aspart (Novolog)
	< 15 min	0.5 to 1.5 h	2 to 4 h	2 h

Short-acting Regular	0.5 to 1 h	2 to 3 h	3 to 6 h	4 h (next meal)
Intermediate-acting NPH	2 to 4 h	6 to 10 h	10 to 16 h	8 to 12 h

Long-acting
  Glargine
  Ultralente
	Approximately 1 h
	6 to 10 h
		—
		10 to 16 h
			24 h
			18 to 20 h
				10 to 12 h
				10 to 12 h

Mixtures 70/30 (70% NPH, 30% regular)	0.5 to 1 h	Dual	10 to 16 h	
Humalog Mix 75/25 (75% neutral protamine lispro [NPL], 25% lispro)	< 15 min	Dual	10 to 16 h	
Novolog Mix 70/30 (70% neutral protamine aspart [NPA], 30% aspart)	< 15 min	Dual	10 to 16 h	

Source: Adapted from Franz MJ, Reader D, Monk A. *Implementing Group and Individual Medical Nutrition Therapy for Diabetes.* Alexandria, Va: American Diabetes Association; 2002:70, with permission from the American Diabetes Association. Copyright ©2002 American Diabetes Association.

with this type of regimen as well, but may be on a course that includes both insulin and oral medications (39).

SUMMARY

Matching of food intake to diabetes medications and physical activity patterns should be attempted, and the correctness of the match should be checked by the use of blood glucose monitoring. Monitoring of glucose, A_{1c}, lipids, and blood pressure is used to determine whether changes in medication(s) are necessary. Encouraging the least restrictive diet with consistent carbohydrates and mealtimes provides the client with an improved quality of life.

REFERENCES

1. Mokdad AH, Ford ES, Bowman BA, Dietz WH, Vinicor F, Bales VS, Marks JS. Prevalence of obesity, diabetes, and obesity-related health risk factors, 2001. *JAMA.* 2003;289:76-79.

2. Centers for Disease Control and Prevention. *National Diabetes Fact Sheet: General Information and National Estimates on Diabetes in the United States, 2000.* Atlanta, Ga: US Dept of Health and Human Services, Centers for Disease Control and Prevention; 2002.

3. Meneilly GS, Tessier D. Diabetes in elderly adults. *J Gerontol Med Sci.* 2001;56A:M5-M13.

4. Bando Y, Ushiogi Y, Okafuji K, Toya D, Tanaka N, Fujisawa M. The relationship of fasting plasma glucose values and other variables to 2-h postload plasma glucose in Japanese subjects. *Diabetes Care.* 2001;24:1156-1160.

5. Balkau B. Diabetes epidemiology: collaborative analysis of diagnostic criteria in Europe: the DECODE study. *Diabetes Med.* 2000;42:282-286.

6. Meneilly GS. Pathophysiology of type 2 diabetes in the elderly. *Clin Geriatr Med.* 1999;15:239-253.

7. Meneilly GS, Cheung E, Tuokko H. Altered responses to hypoglycemia of healthy elderly people. *J Clin Endocrinol Metab.* 1994;78:1341-1348.

8. American Diabetes Association. Standards of medical care for patients with diabetes mellitus. *Diabetes Care.* 2004;27(suppl 1):S15-S35.

9. Gregg EW, Yaffe K, Cauly JA, Rolka DB, Blackwell TL, Narayan KM, Cummings SR. Is diabetes associated with cognitive impairment and cognitive decline among older women? Study of the Osteoporotic Fractures Research Group. *Arch Intern Med.* 2000;160:174-180.

10. Reaven GM, Thompson LW, Nahum D. Relationship between hyperglycemic and cognitive function in older NIDDM patients. *Diabetes Care.* 1990;13:16-21.

11. Kitabchi AE, Umpierrez GE, Murphy MB, Barrett EJ, Kreisberg RA, Malone JI, Wall BM. Management of hyperglycemic crises in patients with diabetes mellitus (technical review). *Diabetes Care.* 2001;124:131-153.

12. Chau D, Edelman SV. Clinical management of diabetes in the elderly. *Clin Diabetes.* 2001;19:172-175.

13. Reed RL, Mooradian AD. Nutritional status and dietary management of elderly patients with diabetes. *Clin Geriatr Med.* 1990;6:883-901.

14. Mooradian AD, McLaughlin S, Boyer CC, Winter J. Diabetes care for older adults. *Diabetes Spectrum.* 1999;12:70-77.

15. Mooradian AD, Osterwell D, Petrasek D, Morley JE. Diabetes mellitus in elderly nursing home patients: a survey of clinical characteristics and management. *J Am Geriatr Soc.* 1988;36:391-396.

16. American Diabetes Association. Evidence-based nutrition principles and recommendations for the treatment and prevention of diabetes and related complications (position statement). *Diabetes Care.* 2004;27(suppl 1):S36-S46.

17. Franz MJ, Bantle JP, Beebe CA, Brunzell JD, Chiasson J-L, Garg A, Holzmeister LA, Hoogwerf BJ, Mayer-Davis E, Mooradian AD, Purnell JQ, Wheeler M. Evidence-based nutrition principles and recommendations for the treatment and prevention of diabetes and related complications (technical review). *Diabetes Care.* 2002;25:148-198.

18. Pastors JG, Franz MJ, Warshaw H, Daly A, Arnold M. How effective is medical nutrition therapy in diabetes care? *J Am Diet Assoc.* 2003;103:827-831.

19. Franz MJ, Monk A, Barry B, McClain K, Weaver T, Cooper N, Upham P, Bergenstal R, Mazze RS. Effectiveness of medical nutrition therapy provided by dietitians in the management of non-insulin-dependent diabetes mellitus: a randomized, controlled clinical trial. *J Am Diet Assoc.* 1995;95:1009-1017.

20. Franz MJ. Carbohydrate and diabetes: is the source or the amount of more importance? *Current Diabetes Reports.* 2001;11:177-186.

21. Franz MJ. The glycemic index. Not the most effective nutrition therapy intervention (editorial). *Diabetes Care.* 2003;26:2466-2468.

22. Gannon MC, Nuttall JA, Damberg G, Gupta V, Nuttall FQ. Effect of protein ingestion on the glucose appearance rate in people with type 2 diabetes. *J Clin Endocrinol Metab.* 2001;86:1040-1047.

23. Nuttall FQ, Mooradian AD, Gannon MC, Billington C, Krezowski P. Effect of protein ingestion on the glucose and insulin response to a standardized oral glucose load. *Diabetes Care.* 1984;7:465-470.

24. Gray RO, Butler PC, Beers TR, Kryshak EJ, Rizza RA. Comparison of the ability of bread versus bread plus meat to treat and prevent subsequent hypoglycemia in patients with insulin-dependent diabetes mellitus. *J Clin Endocrinol Metab.* 1996;81:1508-1511.

25. Foster GD, Wyatt HR, Hill JO. A randomized trial of a low-carbohydrate diet for obesity. *N Engl J Med.* 2003;348:2082-2090.

26. Lichtensein AH, Ausman LM, Carrasco W, Jenner JL, Ordovas JM, Schaefer EJ. Short-term consumption of a low fat diet beneficially affects plasma lipid concentrations only when accompanied by weight loss. *Arterioscler Thromb.* 1994;14:1751-1760.

27. Vivekananthan DP, Penn MS, Sapp SK, Hsu A, Topol EJ. Use of antioxidant vitamins for the prevention of cardiovascular disease: meta-analysis of randomized trials. *Lancet.* 2003;361:2017-2023.

28. Howard AA, Arnsten JH, Gourevitch MN. Effect of alcohol consumption on diabetes mellitus. A systematic review. *Ann Intern Med.* 2004;140:211-219.

29. Tuomilehto J, Lindstrom J, Eriksson JG, Valle TT, Hamalainen H, Ilanne-Parikka P, Keinanen-Kiukaanniemi S, Laakso M, Louheranta A, Rastas M, Salminen V, Uusitupa M, Aunola S, Cepaitis Z, Molchanov V, Hakumaki M, Mannelin M, Martikkala V, Sundvall J. Prevention of type 2 diabetes mellitus by changes in lifestyle among subjects with impaired glucose tolerance. *New Engl J Med.* 2001;344:1343-1350.

30. Diabetes Prevention Program Research Group. Reduction in the incidence of type 2 diabetes with lifestyle intervention or metformin. *N Engl J Med.* 2002;346:393-403.

31. DAFNE Study Group. Training in flexible, intensive insulin management to enable dietary freedom in people with type 1 diabetes: dose adjustment for normal eating (DAFNE) randomized trial. *BMJ.* 2002;325:746-752.

32. Rabasa-Lhoret R, Garon J, Langlier H, Poisson D, Chiasson J-L. Effects of meal carbohydrate on insulin requirements in type 1 diabetic patients treated intensively with the basal-bolus (ultralente-regular) insulin regimen. *Diabetes Care.* 1999;22:667-673.

33. Wolever TMS, Hamad S, Chiasson J-L, Josse RG, Leiter LA, Rodger NW, Ross SA, Ryan EA. Day-to-day consistency in amount and source of carbohydrate intake associated with improved glucose control in type 1 diabetes. *J Amer Coll Nutr.* 1999;18:242-247.

34. Coulston AM, Mandelbaum D, Reaven GM. Dietary management of nursing home residents with non-insulin dependent diabetes mellitus. *Am J Clin Nutr.* 1990;51:62-71.

35. American Diabetes Association. Translation of the diabetes nutrition recommendations for health care institutions (position statement). *Diabetes Care.* 2004;27(suppl 1):S55-S57.

36. Schafer R, Bohannon B, Franz MJ, Freeman J, Holmes A, McLaughlin S, Haas L, Kruger D, Lorenz R, McMahon M. Translation of the diabetes nutrition recommendations for health care institutions (technical review). *Diabetes Care.* 1997;20:96-105.

37. Dorner B, Niedert KC, Welch PK. American Dietetic Association. Liberalized diets for older adults in long-term care (position paper). *J Am Diet Assoc.* 2002;102:1316-1323.

38. Pratley H, Hagberg JM, Dengel DR. Aerobic exercise training-induced reductions in abdominal fat and glucose-stimulated insulin responses in middle-aged and older men. *J Am Geriatr Soc.* 2000;48:1055-1031.

39. Fonseca VA, Kulkarni K, Golightly L, Richard B. *Managing Type 2 Diabetes in the Elderly.* New York, NY: Postgraduate Institute of Medicine; 2001.

40. Franz MJ, Reader D, Monk A. *Implementing Group and Individual Medical Nutrition Therapy for Diabetes.* Alexandria, Va: American Diabetes Association; 2002.

CHAPTER 7

Hepatic/Liver Disease

Medical nutrition therapy (MNT) in older adults with hepatobiliary diseases focuses on the use of dietary manipulations to achieve two goals: (*a*) to maintain nutritional status and (*b*) to help manage the sequelae of liver disease. Hepatic disease may affect the metabolism of any or all nutrients, may increase nutrient losses, and/or may compromise oral intake (1-3). Although there are many liver diseases, the two most common are alcoholic liver disease and chronic hepatitis viruses (primarily hepatitis B or C). Liver diseases are chronic and progress from the initial insult to fibrosis and eventually to cirrhosis. As liver disease progresses, MNT becomes more important.

NUTRITION ASSESSMENT

Nutrition assessment in older adults with hepatic disease is complex, because of the impact of the liver's synthetic function on usual assessment parameters such as albumin and prealbumin (3,4). The incidence and severity of malnutrition depends on the definition and the assessment parameters that are used (5-7). Subjective Global Assessment (SGA) is thought to be a more valid process in hepatic disease. The individual's oral intake, physical examination, anthropometric measures, and laboratory values are viewed in a combined fashion, to assess the client's baseline nutritional status (8). The information is then used to formulate an appropriate MNT plan (see Table 7.1) (9-11). Comorbidities, such as heart and renal dysfunction and diabetes mellitus, need to be assessed in conjunction with the hepatic disease process (1,2).

NUTRITIONAL COMPLICATIONS

Muscle Wasting

A variety of studies have been done to assess energy needs in those with hepatic disease, but clear, specific results have not been forthcoming (12-14). This is because of the complexity and the variety of liver diseases, the differences in staging of the disease process, and the dependence of many calorie calculations on weight. Because many individuals have fluid retention (ascites and/or edema), their true, dry weight is often unknown. Therefore, energy estimations should be made on the basis of a dry weight (if available) or a combination of the individual's usual and ideal weights (3). Harris-Benedict basal plus 20% (or 25 to 30 kcal/kg) would be an appropriate starting point for energy requirements (15). This should be reassessed for adequacy on an individual basis (5,12-14). Individuals with significant ascites have an increased risk of being hypermetabolic and require about 10% more kilocalories per day (16).

Although not all older adults with hepatic disease are malnourished, many can become so if their energy intake is inadequate. Inadequate intake may be due to such primary reasons as anorexia, early satiety, diet restrictions, altered taste perceptions, and other related problems (eg, social, dentition). Secondary influences may include diarrhea from fat malabsorption, lactulose therapy, or increased metabolism due to ascites (1,17). A critical factor is the importance of eating on a regular schedule, to avoid catabolism induced by the fasting state. Many individuals can maintain or even improve their nutritional status by avoiding prolonged periods without food. This can be achieved by eating four to six times per day, to help ensure that adequate intake is consumed to meet nutrition needs (18,19).

Ascites/Edema

Fluid retention in the form of ascites or edema is one of the most obvious symptoms of hepatic disease. This is caused by the retention of sodium and

TABLE 7.1. Nutrition Assessment

Component	Purpose	Element
Physical assessment	• General nutrition condition	• Weight appropriate • Weight changes • Muscle wasting • Ascites or edema
	• Degree and distribution of deficiencies	• Fat and muscle loss • Physical changes • Functional capability • Psychosocial and economic issues
History	• Cause, degree, and duration of nutrient deficiencies	• Medical history • Appetite • Diet history • Gastrointestinal function • Medications • Supplements
Anthropometrics	• Objective measures to evaluate and monitor progress	• Midarm circumference • Triceps skinfold • Handgrip strength
Laboratory tests	• Selectively interpret those affected by nonnutritive factors	• Electrolytes • Albumin • Prealbumin • Renal function • Glucose • Vitamins and minerals

Source: Adapted from Hasse JM. Adult liver transplantation. In: Hasse JM, Blue LS, eds. *Comprehensive Guide to Transplant Nutrition.* Chicago Ill: American Dietetic Association; 2002:58-89, with permission from American Dietetic Association.

fluid due to altered renal function, hypoalbuminemia, and portal hypertension (20). The first line of nutrition therapy is to have the individual restrict sodium intake to 2,000 mg/day (20). Although very-low-sodium diets may be beneficial in controlling fluid retention, there is a high risk of compromised energy and nutrient intake because of the rigid restriction. For those individuals on diuretic therapy, regular monitoring of electrolytes is necessary. When hyponatremia occurs, restrictions of 1 to 1.5 liters per day of fluid intake are often used to aid in the concentration of the serum (21). The emphasis should be placed on restricting free water and other nonnutritive fluids while maintaining intake of nutrient-dense beverages, such as milk, juice, and nutritional supplements (1).

Portal Systemic Encephalopathy/ Hepatic Encephalopathy

Historically, portal systemic encephalopathy (PSE), the alteration of mental status staged from normal to comatose on a 0- to 4-point scale, was thought to be due to protein intolerance, with subsequent ammonia production in the gastrointestinal tract (22). Treatment usually included severe protein restriction of 20 to 40 grams of protein per day (23). Today, we know that very few older adults are in fact protein sensitive, and most cases of acute PSE result from factors such as gastrointestinal bleeding, dehydration, electrolyte imbalance, renal dysfunction, and infection (24). Once these medical problems are addressed and management is maximized, the PSE often resolves. In those clients with chronic PSE, most will tolerate an intake of at least 1.0 gram of protein per kilogram of dry or ideal weight without exacerbating their PSE symptoms (25). Alterations in protein intake are necessary in only a relatively small number of clients with chronic, recurrent PSE, despite maximal medical therapy, and in about 20% to 30% of those clients with a transjugular intrahepatic portosystemic shunt (TIPS) placed (26). In the latter situation (post-TIPS), protein may be better tolerated if consumed in small portions divided throughout the day (eg, limiting meat portions to no more than 2 or 3 oz per feeding) (27). The goal of providing as much protein as possible without provoking PSE requires an increased dependence on vegetable, carbohydrate, and dairy sources, as well as on nutritional supplement products (28). A very few individuals with end-stage liver disease and refractory, chronic PSE may require strict protein restrictions and/or use of specialized hepatic formulas to control their PSE (2,15,17,27). This should be tempered with a balance of quality of life and the right to make one's own end-of-life decisions.

Obesity

Many people with hepatic disease are malnourished, but there are also a considerable number of people with liver disease who are obese. Obesity alone is a major risk factor for developing nonalcoholic fatty liver disease (29). Other situations that put those with hepatic disease at risk for obesity include the chronic use of steroids to treat autoimmune liver disease, lifelong poor eating habits, psychosocial issues, and the lack of exercise due to aging and what can be overwhelming fatigue from the hepatic disease (30).

Success with assisting people to lose weight is limited. Safe weight loss may occur in motivated individuals using a program of moderate energy restriction, high fiber content, and increased activity/exercise (31,32). In addition, those programs that offer supportive counseling or close follow-up may be especially beneficial for people with a strong psychosocial component in their obesity (32). Patients who lose weight rapidly should be monitored for increased losses of lean tissue. Again, any planned weight loss in the older adult must be tempered with a need for a well-balanced diet and with quality of life issues; it should also be aligned with the older adult's advance directives.

Osteopenia

Osteopenia, the alteration in bone structure seen in hepatic disease, is commonly due to the dysmetabolism of calcium and vitamin D, long-term steroid use,

alcohol consumption, and age (33,34). Those individuals with osteopenia should consume 1,500 mg of calcium daily between their diet and their supplementation. Calcium supplements with vitamin D should be chosen in a form well tolerated (eg, gastrointestinal tolerance, pill size) (34). Management also includes the optimization of nutritional status, appropriate hormone replacement, and physical therapy, to maintain or improve overall muscle mass and to encourage appropriate body mechanics (34). Medications to stimulate bone formation may be helpful (35).

Vitamins and Minerals

The absorption, metabolism, and storage of many vitamins and minerals are often abnormal in those with hepatic diseases. Most older adults will benefit from a general multivitamin and mineral supplement. However, because of alterations in iron metabolism in a number of hepatic diseases, those products with a high iron content should be used with physician approval (36). Standard therapy for those with acute alcohol withdrawal is supplemental doses of thiamin (100 mg/day) and folic acid (1 mg/day) for at least 2 weeks. The risk of fat-soluble vitamin deficiency is quite high in those with a cholestatic liver disease and in those who are malnourished (37). Because of inadequate bile salt concentration in the bowel, supplementation is given in the water-miscible form (see Table 7.2 [37]).

Magnesium, phosphorus, and zinc requirements may be increased in hepatic disease, whereas the need for copper (Wilson's disease) and iron (hemachromatosis) are reduced (36). Zinc supplementation (220 mg zinc sulfate three times daily) may be beneficial in the treatment of PSE (11).

TABLE 7.2. Fat-Soluble Vitamin Supplementation Protocol

Vitamin	Dosage
Vitamin A (aquasol A)	25,000 IU 3 times/week
Vitamin D (ergocalciferol)	50,000 IU 3 times/week
Vitamin E (aquasol E/ alpha-tocopheryl)	400 IU/day

Source: Data are from references 10 and 11.

Glucose Intolerance

Carbohydrate metabolism is affected even in the early stages of hepatic dysfunction. Some individuals will exhibit hyperglycemia and insulin resistance or hyperinsulinemia. When those with liver disease have depleted their glycogen stores, the starvation response accelerates and leads to the catabolism of muscle and fat stores for energy (38). The consumption of frequent feedings and the minimization of episodes of fasting can eliminate this process (18,19).

NUTRITION SUPPORT

Enteral or parenteral nutrition may be necessary to support individuals with hepatic disease when their dietary intake is inadequate. The goal of nutrition support is to provide for the correction of any deficiencies while supporting hepatic regeneration. This may be especially important in the survival of those with alcoholic hepatitis (27,38). Enteral feeding via small-bore tubes is usually well tolerated even in those clients with esophageal varices (39).

LIVER TRANSPLANTATION

Liver transplantation is the only viable treatment for end-stage liver disease. Its success rate is dependent primarily on the type and severity of hepatic disease and not on the age of the recipient. Poor nutritional status before transplantation is a risk factor for survival and prolongs the recovery period (40,41). After transplantation, older adults should be able to return to their normal, healthy lifestyle (42). Individuals who have had transplants will need to be monitored for adverse effects of the transplant and the immunosuppressive medications. Adverse effects with nutrition-related components include renal insufficiency, hypertension, diabetes mellitus, hyperlipidemia, obesity, and osteopenia (43). Some older adults will not be candidates for a transplant due to comorbidities that would affect survival after transplantation (44).

END OF LIFE

For older adults at the very end stages of liver disease, it may be prudent to liberalize diet and fluid restrictions. The focus should be on comfort care and quality of life (see Chapter 25).

SUMMARY

MNT in older adults with hepatic disease is a critical aspect of their total medical management program and may be crucial in altering their morbidity and mortality. Intervention should include the optimization of energy and protein intake while imposing only those dietary restrictions necessary to manage the symptoms of the hepatic disease. Close attention to providing appropriate vitamin and mineral supplementation is also necessary.

REFERENCES

1. Hasse J, Weseman B, Fuhrman MP, Loeffler M, Francisco-Ziller N, DiCecco S. Nutrition therapy for end-stage liver disease: a practical approach. *Support Line.* 1997;19:8-15.
2. Francisco-Ziller N, DiCecco S. Nutritional care of the pretransplant patient. *Top Clin Nutr.* 1998;13:1-14.
3. Pomposelli JJ, Burns DL. Nutrition support in the liver transplant patient. *Nutr Clin Prac.* 2002;17:341-349.
4. Lochs J, Plauth M. Liver cirrhosis; rational and modalities for nutritional support—the European Society of Parenteral and Enteral Nutrition consensus and beyond. *Curr Opin Clin Nutr Metab Care.* 1999;2:345-349.
5. Ackerman PA, Jenkins RL, Bistrian BR. Preoperative nutrition assessment in liver transplantation. *Nutrition.* 1993;9:350-356.
6. Hasse JM, Blue LS, Crippen JS, Goldstein RM, Jennings LW, Gonwa TA, Husberg BS, Levy MF, Klintmalm GB. The effect of nutritional status on length of stay and clinical outcomes following liver transplantation. *J Am Diet Assoc.* 1994;94(suppl):A-38.
7. DiCecco SR, Wieners EJ, Wiesner RH, Southorn PA, Plevak DJ, Krom RAF. Assessment of nutritional status of patients with end-stage liver disease undergoing liver transplantation. *Mayo Clin Proc.* 1989;64:95-102.
8. Hasse J, Strong S, Gorman MA, Liepa G. Subjective global assessment: alternative nutrition-assessment technique for liver-transplant candidates. *Nutrition.* 1993;9:339-343.
9. Hasse JM. Adult liver transplantation. In: Hasse JM, Blue LS, eds. *Comprehensive Guide to Transplant Nutrition.* Chicago, Ill: American Dietetic Association; 2002:58-89.
10. Francisco-Ziller N, DiCecco S. Nutritional care of the pretransplant patient. *Top Clin Nutr.* 1998;13:1-14.
11. Jorgenson R, Lindor KD, Sartin J, LaRusso N, Wiesner R. Serum lipid and fat-soluble vitamin levels in primary sclerosing cholangitis. *J Clin Gastroenterol.* 1995;20:215-219.
12. Green JH, Bramley PN, Losowsky MS. Are patients with primary biliary cirrhosis hypermetabolic? A comparison before and after liver transplantation and controls. *Hepatology.* 1991;14:464-472.
13. Muller MJ, Boker KHW, Selberg O. Are patients with liver cirrhosis hypermetabolic? *Clin Nutr.* 1994;13:131-144.
14. Plevak D, DiCecco S, Wiesner R, Porayko M, Wahlstrom E, Janzow D, Hammel K, O'Keefe S. Nutritional support for liver transplantation: identifying calorie and protein requirements. *Mayo Clin Proc.* 1994;69:225-230.

15. Plauth KM, Merli M, Kondrup J, Weimann A, Ferenci P, Muller MJ. ESPEN guidelines for nutrition in liver disease and transplantation. *Nutr Clin Pract.* 1997;16:43-55.

16. Dolz C, Raurich JM, Ibaniz J, Obrador A, Marse P, Gaya J. Ascites increases the resting energy expenditure in liver cirrhosis. *Gastroenterology.* 1991;100:738-744.

17. Patton KM, Aranda-Michel J. Nutritional aspects in liver disease and liver transplantation. *Nutr Clin Pract.* 2002;17:332-340.

18. Swart GR, Zillikens MC, Vuuve JK, van den Berg JWO. Effect of a late evening meal on nitrogen balance in patients with cirrhosis of the liver. *Br Med J.* 1989;299:1202-1203.

19. Chang WK, Chao YC, Tang HS, Lang HF, Hsu CT. Effects of extra-carbohydrate supplementation in the late evening on energy expenditure and substrate oxidation in patients with liver disease. *JPEN J Parenter Enteral Nutr.* 1997;21:96-99.

20. Roberts LR, Kamath PS. Ascites and hepatorenal syndrome: pathophysiology and management. *Mayo Clin Proc.* 1996;71:874-881.

21. Azia I, Perez GO, Schiffer ER. Management of ascites in patients with chronic liver disease. *Am J Gastroenterol.* 1994;89:1949-1956.

22. Wong K, Klein BJV, Fish JA. Nutrition management of the adult with liver disease. In: Skipper A, ed. *Dietitian's Handbook of Enteral and Parenteral Nutrition.* 2nd ed. Gaithersburg, Md: ASPEN Publishers; 1998:209-238.

23. Sherlock S, Summerskill WHK, White LP, Phear EA. Portal systemic encephalopathy: neurological complications on liver disease. *Lancet.* 1954;267:453-457.

24. Menon KVN, Kamath PS. Managing the complications of cirrhosis. *Mayo Clin Proc.* 2000;75:501-509.

25. Bunout D, Aicardi V, Hirsch S, Petermann M, Kelly M, Silva G, Garay P, Ugarte G, Iturriaga H. Nutritional support in hospitalized patients with alcoholic liver disease. *Eur J Clin Nutr.* 1989;43:615-621.

26. Langnas AN. Shunt versus transplantation. *Liver Trans Surg.* 1998;4(suppl 1):S105-S107.

27. Klein S, Kinney J, Jeejeebhoy K, Alpers D, Hellerstein M, Murray M, Twomey P. Nutrition support in clinical practice: review of published data and recommendations for future research directions. *JPEN J Parenter Enteral Nutr.* 1997;21:133-156.

28. Muñoz SJ. Nutritional therapies in liver disease. *Semin Liver Dis.* 1991;11:278-291.

29. Angulo P. Nonalcoholic fatty liver disease. *N Engl J Med.* 2002;346:1221-1231.

30. Summerskill WHJ, Korman MG, Ammon HV, Baggenstoss AH. Prednisone for chronic active liver disease: dose titration, standard dose, and combination with azathioprine compared. *Gut.* 1975;16:876-883.

31. Noël PH, Pugh JA. Management of overweight and obese adults. *BMJ.* 2002;325:757-761.

32. Expert Panel on the Identification, Evaluation, and Treatment of Overweight and Obesity in Adults. Executive summary of the clinical guidelines on the identification, evaluation, and treatment of overweight and obesity in adults. *Arch Intern Med.* 1998;158:1855-1867.

33. McCaughan GW, Feller RB. Osteoporosis in chronic liver disease: pathogenesis, risk factors and management. *Dig Dis.* 1994;12:223-231.

34. Hay JE. Bone disease in cholestatic liver disease. *Gastroenterology.* 1995;108:276-283.

35. Carey E, Balan V. Metabolic bone disease in patients with liver disease. *Curr Gastroenterol Rep.* 2003;5:71-77.

36. McClain CJ, Marsano L, Burk RF, Bacon B. Trace metals in liver disease. *Semin Liver Dis.* 1991;11:321-339.

37. Riordan SM, Williams R. Treatment of hepatic encephalopathy. *N Engl J Med.* 1997;337:473-479.

38. McCullough AJ. Malnutrition in cirrhosis. In: Bacon BR, DiBisceglie AM, eds. *Liver Diseases: Diagnosis and Management.* Philadelphia, Pa: Churchill Livingstone; 2002:269-281.

39. de Ledinghen V, Beau P, Mannant PR, Borderie C, Ripault MP, Silvain C, Beauchant M. Early feeding or enteral nutrition in patients with cirrhosis after bleeding from esophageal varices? A randomized controlled study. *Dig Dis Sci.* 1997;42:536-541.

40. Pikul J, Sharpe MD, Lowndes R, Chent CN. Degree of preoperative malnutrition is predictive of postoperative morbidity and mortality in liver transplant recipients. *Transplantation.* 1994;57:469-472.

41. Hasse JM, Gonwa TA, Jennings LW. Malnutrition affects liver transplant outcomes (abstract). *Transplantation.* 1998;66(suppl):S53.

42. Zetterman RK, Belle SH, Hoofnagle JH, Lawlor S, Wei Y, Everhart J, Wiesner RH, Lake J. Age and liver transplantation. *Transplantation.* 1998;66:500-506.

43. Hebert MF, Davis CL, Limaye AP, Kowdley KV, Carither RL. Liver transplantation: long-term post-transplant management. In: Bacon BR, DiBisceglie AM, eds. *Liver Diseases: Diagnosis and Management.* Philadelphia, Pa: Churchill Livingstone; 2002:392-404.

44. Wiesner RH. Current indications, contraindications, and timing for liver transplantation. In: Busuttil RW, Klintmalm GB, eds. *Transplantation of the Liver.* Philadelphia Pa: WB Saunders Co; 1995:71-84.

CHAPTER

8 Renal Disease

The end-stage renal disease (ESRD) population is aging, and approximately 50% of patients receiving renal replacement therapy are older than 65 years (1). Transplantation is also an option for elderly dialysis patients. In 2003, 1,683 kidney transplants were performed in individuals older than 65 (2). This trend is likely to continue as the general population ages and as survival on dialysis improves.

The leading causes of chronic kidney disease (CKD) are hypertension and diabetes mellitus (1). Older adults are more likely to experience vascular disease and hypertension than is the general population (3). As expected, these clients have multiple comorbid conditions and an increased mortality rate. The incidence of malnutrition among older adults is well documented (4). Therefore, communication between the dialysis facility and the long-term-care facility is essential, to prevent development of nutritional deficiencies through early intervention and close monitoring of nutritional status.

As CKD progresses, medical nutrition therapy (MNT) becomes a challenge for dietetics professionals. The evaluation and treatment of older adults with CKD requires understanding the stages of CKD, as developed by the National Kidney Foundation Kidney Disease Outcomes Quality Initiative (NKF-K/DOQI) and illustrated in Table 8.1 (5). Creatinine clearance (CrCl) is a rough estimation of glomerular filtration rate (GFR) and can be calculated from a 24-hour timed urine collection. The most widely used method for estimating GFR is the Cockcroft-Gault formula (6):

$$\text{Men: } \frac{(140 - \text{Age}) \times \text{Wt}}{\text{Serum Creat} \times 72}$$

$$\text{Women: } \frac{(140 - \text{Age}) \times \text{Wt} \times 0.85}{\text{Serum Creat} \times 72}$$

Where: Serum Creat = serum creatinine (mg/dL); Wt = weight (kg); Age is measured in years.

As renal failure approaches stage 5 or "end-stage," some form of renal replacement therapy (RRT), such as dialysis or transplantation, may be initiated as a life-sustaining measure. Unfortunately, "renal replacement" is a misnomer, because there are several aspects of normal renal function that are not entirely corrected, and careful medical management combined with MNT is required. Nutrition recommendations for clients at all stages of kidney disease must be individualized. The guidelines presented in Table 8.2 are a starting point for nutrition care of older adults with kidney disease (7-9).

NUTRITIONAL RISKS IN KIDNEY DISEASE

The primary nutritional risks that must be addressed in CKD include protein energy malnutrition (PEM), hypertension, renal osteodystrophy, and anemia. These risks may be present in older adults at any stage of CKD (5). A brief summary of each of these risks follows.

PROTEIN ENERGY MALNUTRITION

PEM is a known risk factor for mortality and morbidity in chronic dialysis clients (10). A multitude of factors contribute to malnutrition in this population (see Box 8.1). Nutrition strategies to correct malnutrition may include liberalization of the diet, use of enteral supplements or nutrition support, renal multivitamins, gastrointestinal medications, and assistance with meals (eg, home-delivered meals, home-care services), to name a few. Dietetics professionals must ensure that protein and energy needs are met. Close monitoring of these

TABLE 8.1. Stages of Chronic Kidney Disease

Stage	Description	GFR (mL/min/1.73 m^2)	Action
	At increased risk	> 90 with CKD risk factors	Screening CKD risk reduction
1	Kidney damage with normal or increased GFR	> 90	Diagnosis and treatment, slow progression
2	Mild decreased GFR	60-89	Estimating progression
3	Moderate decreased GFR	30-59	Evaluating and treating complications
4	Severe decreased GFR	15-29	Preparation for kidney replacement therapy
5	Kidney failure	< 15 or dialysis	Replacement, if uremia present

Abbreviations: CKD, chronic kidney disease; GFR, glomerular filtration rate.

Source: National Kidney Foundation. Kidney Disease Outcomes Quality Initiative clinical practice guidelines for chronic kidney disease: evaluation, classification, and stratification. Available at: http://www.kidney.org/professionals/doqi/kdoqi/toc.htm. Accessed May 11, 2004.

clients by the use of calorie counts, weight records, assessment of laboratory values, and early medical nutrition intervention will result in better outcomes.

HYPERTENSION

Hypertension is common among older adults with CKD. Those on hemodialysis should limit sodium intake to 2 to 3 g daily. Those on peritoneal dialysis may liberalize sodium restriction to approximately 4 g per day (7,8).

RENAL OSTEODYSTROPHY

Clients with kidney disease at all stages are at risk for renal osteodystrophy, or weak, brittle bones, as well as secondary hyperparathyroidism (11). In healthy individuals, the kidneys play a role in calcium and phosphorus balance, by initially activating vitamin D in the kidneys. Vitamin D, in turn, aids in calcium absorption. As kidney function deteriorates, the body loses its ability to activate vitamin D, and serum calcium levels decrease. This drop in serum

calcium triggers the release of parathyroid hormone (PTH). PTH then triggers a response that allows calcium to be drawn from the bones to supply serum calcium. Prevention of renal osteodystrophy is most important, because once the condition occurs, correction is nearly impossible (12).

It is important that clients with CKD have normal serum levels of corrected total calcium. Hypocalcemia may cause secondary hyperparathyroidism and adverse effects on bone mineralization. Because calcium is bound to protein, calcium levels may appear falsely low if the patient has hypoalbuminemia. Ideally, an ionized calcium should be drawn to determine a more accurate calcium level (12). In the clinical setting, another way to assess the calcium level is to calculate a "corrected calcium." Although not as accurate as an ionized calcium, it is a good indicator of the approximate calcium level. The formula to determine "corrected calcium" follows (6). Only the serum albumin and the actual calcium levels are required to calculate the estimated or corrected calcium level.

TABLE 8.2. Daily Nutrient Recommendations for Chronic Kidney Disease

Nutrient	Condition				
	Chronic Kidney Disease	Hemodialysis	Peritoneal Dialysis	Posttransplant, Postoperative	Posttransplant, Chronic
Protein (g/kg)	*K/DOQI:* GFR < 25 mL/min: 0.6-0.75 ≥59% HBV	*K/DOQI:* ≥ 1.2 ≥ 50% HBV protein	*K/DOQI:* ≥ 1.2-1.3 ≥ 50% HBV protein	1.3-2.0	0.8-1.0
Energy (kcal/kg)	*K/DOQI:* ≥ 60 y of age: 30-35 < 60 y of age: 35	*K/DOQI:* ≥ 60 y of age: 30-35 < 60 y of age: 35	*K/DOQI:* ≥ 60 y of age: 30-35 < 60 y of age: 35 Include dialysate kcal	30-35	30-35
Fluid (mL)	No restriction	Output plus 1,000 mL	Maintain balance	Unrestricted	Unrestricted
Sodium (g)	Varies from 1-3 to NAS	1-3	2-4 Monitor fluid balance	2-4	2-4
Potassium (g)	Usually unrestricted unless individual's serum levels are high	2-3 Adjust to serum levels	3-4 Adjust to serum levels	2-4	2-4
Phosphorus	10-12 mg/g protein or 10 mg/kg	10-12 mg/g protein < 900 mg, adjust for protein	10-12 mg/g protein < 900 mg, adjust for protein	RDA; supplement as needed	RDA
Calcium (g)	< 2-2.5 including binder load	< 2-2.5 including binder load	< 2-2.5 including binder load	0.8-1.5	0.8-1.5
Other minerals and vitamins	RDA: Complex and vitamin C; individualize vitamin D, iron, zinc	C: 60-100 mg B-6: 2 mg Folate: 1 mg B-12: 3 µg RDA: others vitamin E: 15 IU Zinc: 15 mg Individualize iron, vitamin D	Same as hemodialysis, but may need 1.5-2 mg of vitamin B-1 because of dialysis loss	RDA, may need additional vitamin D	RDA, may need additional vitamin D

Abbreviations: GFR, glomerular filtration rate; HBV, high biological value; K/DOQI, Kidney Disease Outcomes Quality Initiative; NAS, no added salt; RDA, recommended dietary allowance.

Source: Data are from references 7-9.

Box 8.1   Risk Factors for Malnutrition

- Dietary restrictions
- Catabolic illness
- Loss of nutrients
- Blood loss
- Poor appetite
- Malabsorption/abnormal metabolism
- Social, physical, or psychological factors
- Knowledge deficit

Corrected serum calcium = [(4 – Albumin level) × 0.8] + Calcium level

Where: Calcium and albumin levels are measured in mg/dL.

Example: If a client has a calcium level of 8.8 mg/dL and an albumin level of 3.1 mg/dL, the calculations could be:

$$4 - 3.1 = 0.9$$
$$0.9 \times 0.8 = 0.72$$
$$0.72 + 8.8 = \text{Corrected calcium of } 9.52 \text{ mg/dL}$$

Recent reports suggest that abnormalities in serum phosphorus, which is the product of multiplying the serum calcium level by the serum phosphorus level (Ca x P), and PTH levels cause soft-tissue calcification and increase the risk of cardiovascular death in the end-stage renal disease (ESRD) population (13). Hyperphosphatemia is a common occurrence in CKD and another risk factor for renal osteodystrophy and bone disease. A low-phosphorus diet should be initiated, to maintain the serum phosphorus in a range of 3.5 to 5.5 mg/dL. Dietary phosphate should be restricted to 800 to 1,000 mg/day (12). This limits foods that can be consumed, such as milk products, whole grains, nuts and legumes, cola, and chocolate. The serum calcium-phosphorus product should be maintained at less than 55 mg²/mL², to minimize calcium phosphate crystals from being deposited into soft tissues (12,13).

Diet alone does not usually lower the serum phosphorus level; therefore, "phosphate binders" are often prescribed. These medications bind phosphorus from food in the gastrointestinal tract, which causes some of it to be excreted. To be most effective, phosphate binders should be taken with meals and snacks and should not be taken at the same time as iron supplements (12). Some common phosphate binders include PhosLo (calcium acetate), Tums (calcium carbonate), and Renagel (sevelamer hydrochloride). If calcium-based phosphate binders are prescribed, the total elemental calcium should not exceed 1,500 mg/day. Some clients with serum phosphorus levels greater than 7.0 mg/dL may use Amphogel (aluminum hydroxide) for short-term therapy. Aluminum binders should be used with caution, because high levels can be toxic (12).

Parathyroid hormone levels may be assessed, to determine whether the older adult is in an active stage of renal osteodystrophy. Controlling PTH levels prevents calcium from being withdrawn from the bones. Therapy with an active vitamin D sterol, such as Calcijex (calcitriol), Zemplar (paricalcitol), or Hectorol (doxercalciferol), will be prescribed if the plasma levels of intact PTH are greater than 300 pg/mL (12).

ANEMIA OF CKD

Older adults are also at risk for anemia of CKD. Anemia plays a significant role in the incidence of cardiovascular disease, the leading cause of death among those on dialysis (14). The primary cause for the anemia seen in CKD is the decreased production of the hormone erythropoietin (EPO), which is normally produced by the healthy kidney. This hormone signals the body to make red blood cells. As the kidney loses its ability to make this hormone, hemoglobin and hematocrit levels start to drop, and anemia develops (14).

Hemoglobin is the preferred test to assess anemia. The NKF-K/DOQI recommends a target hemoglobin of 11 to 12 g/dL and a hematocrit of 33% to 36% (14). In addition to measuring Hct and Hgb, iron studies will also be assessed. Adequate iron stores are necessary for EPO to work effectively. Iron studies include ferritin, iron, iron-binding capacity, and transferrin saturation. Adequate iron status is defined as follows (14):

- Transferrin > 20%
- Serum ferritin > 100 ng/mL
- Serum iron > 80 µg

If the client is iron deficient, the administration of EPO must be delayed until iron stores are repleted. Most persons requiring dialysis need iron supplementation, because iron stores quickly become depleted during erythropoiesis. Iron can be provided in either oral or intravenous preparations. Most people receive intravenous iron preparations, such as Infed (iron dextran), Venofer (iron sucrose), and Ferrlecit (iron gluconate), which is administered through the dialysis machine. Effective treatment of anemia in CKD improves survival, decreases morbidity, and improves quality of life (14).

NUTRITION CONSIDERATIONS FOR PREDIALYSIS PATIENTS

In the initial stages of kidney disease, blood chemistries become altered as the blood urea nitrogen (BUN) and creatinine levels start to rise. As the disease progresses and as waste products accumulate in the blood stream, symptoms of uremia develop. These symptoms include altered taste, poor appetite, nausea, vomiting, and weight loss (7,8).

The Modification of Diet in Renal Disease (MDRD) project, funded by the National Institutes of Health, was conducted to determine whether MNT would be beneficial in slowing the progression of kidney disease (15). The investigators concluded that blood pressure control, protein restriction, and phosphorus restriction can delay kidney disease progression. Although there may be some evidence that protein restriction may delay the progression of renal failure, the risks of such therapy in already protein-depleted older adults may outweigh any short-term benefits. Preserving lean body mass and preventing malnutrition is the main objective when prescribing protein restrictions in predialysis patients (see Table 8.2 for recommendations) (4).

As the GFR approaches 10 mL/min and as symptoms of uremia become uncontrollable with diet and medication, RRT must be initiated. The renal diet is generally more restrictive for those on hemodialysis than for those receiving peritoneal dialysis. This is primarily because of the fact that those on hemodialysis average treatment times of 3 to 4 hours, 3 days a week, for a total therapy time of 9 to 12 hours per week. Those on peritoneal dialysis average 10 to 12 hours of therapy daily, for a total treatment time of 70 to 84 hours per week. Adequate dialysis is a major factor in nutritional status, because poor dialysis leads to uremia (7). Dialysis centers routinely assess adequacy of dialysis.

HEMODIALYSIS

It is well documented that up to 50% of those requiring hemodialysis are malnourished (10). Inadequate dialysis and dialysis access problems may affect oral intake, because poor dialysis results in uremic symptoms. Although protein requirements may be slightly reduced in older adult clients, the combination of amino acid lost during dialysis, catabolic events of dialysis, and acidosis increases the protein requirement for those on dialysis (10).

Those on hemodialysis are at risk for developing hyperkalemia (potassium levels > 6.0 mg/dL), but hypokalemia (potassium levels < 3.5 mg/dL) can also be dangerous and can lead to cardiac arrest. High-potassium foods must be restricted in the diet, to control serum potassium levels. Most dialysis clients can tolerate one or two high-potassium foods a day (7,8). Examples of high-potassium foods include bananas, oranges, melons, potatoes, and tomatoes.

A sodium restriction of approximately 2 to 3 g per day is recommended for those on hemodialysis. The most difficult restriction for most on dialysis is the fluid restriction. Large interdialytic weight gains of more than 2.5 kg cannot be ultrafiltrated in a 3- to 4-hour dialysis session. Excessive fluid gains result in pulmonary edema, peripheral edema, congestive heart failure, and symptoms of cramping and low blood pressure while on the dialysis machine. Fluid restrictions typically range from 1,000 to 1,500 mL, depending on urine output (7,8).

PERITONEAL DIALYSIS

Clients with peritoneal dialysis (PD) are also at risk for malnutrition. The diet is usually less restrictive, with the diet order based on blood chemistries. Clients with PD do not require potassium or fluid restriction. They do, however, require a higher protein intake, because of the excessive loss of amino acids in the dialysate. Often these clients are unable to achieve an albumin level > 3.5 mg/dL and require modular protein powders or enteral supplements (7,8).

PD clients who have diabetes may require an adjustment in their energy requirement or an adjustment in their insulin, because of the higher concentration of glucose in the dialysate solution. A typical client with PD can absorb 300 to 600 kcal/day from the dialysate (7,8).

Another nutrition concern of PD clients is hyperlipidemia, especially elevated triglycerides. This is also related to the glucose load from the dialysate. A dietary restriction limiting fats and simple sugars may be beneficial for these clients. A lipid-lowering agent may also be prescribed (16).

PD clients are also at risk for malnutrition, renal osteodystrophy, and anemia, as previously discussed. Treatment may need to be implemented for each of these conditions. See Table 8.2 for recommendations.

NUTRITION CONSIDERATIONS FOR TRANSPLANT CLIENTS

When an older adult receives a successful kidney transplant, dietary modifications are still necessary. Transplant candidates with diabetes need to monitor sodium intake, avoid excessive weight gain, monitor fat intake, and control carbohydrate intake (17). Table 8.2 provides nutrient recommendations for the transplant population.

SUMMARY

Whether an older adult has early kidney disease or requires HD or PD, special nutrition problems can be evident. Typically, the diet needs to be liberalized because of poor appetite and weight loss. Use of polypharmacy and drug-nutrient interactions can also be factors leading to malnutrition in an older adult. Medications should be reviewed frequently for drug-nutrient interactions. It is essential that dietetics professionals have at least monthly communication with the dialysis center regarding laboratory values, oral intake, client progress on the diet, medications, and weight changes, to ensure optimal care for the older adult with kidney disease.

REFERENCES

1. US Renal Data System. *USRDS 2003 Annual Data Report.* Bethesda, Md: National Institutes of Health, National Institute of Diabetes and Digestive and Kidney Diseases; 2003.
2. 2003 Annual Report of the US Scientific Registry of Transplant Recipients and the Organ Procurement and Transplantation Network: transplant data, 1989-2003. Available at: http://www.optn.org/latestData/step2.asp?. Accessed May 11, 2004.
3. Krishnan M, Lok C, Sarbit J. Epidemiology and demographic aspects of treated end-stage renal disease in the elderly. *Semin Dial.* 2002;15:79-83.
4. Wolfson M. Nutrition in elderly dialysis patients. *Semin Dial.* 2002;15:113-115.
5. National Kidney Foundation. Kidney Disease Outcomes Quality Initiative clinical practice guidelines for chronic kidney disease: evaluation, classification, and stratification. Available at: http://www.kidney.org/professionals/doqi/kdoqi/toc.htm. Accessed May 11, 2004.
6. Walser M. Assessing renal function from creatinine measurements in adults with chronic renal failure. *Am J Kidney Dis.* 1998;32:23-31.
7. Kopple JD, Massry SG, eds. *Nutritional Management of Renal Disease.* 2nd ed. Philadelphia, Pa: Lippincott, Williams and Wilkins; 2003.
8. Mitch WE, Klahr S, eds. *Handbook of Nutrition and the Kidney.* 4th ed. Philadelphia, Pa: Lippincott, Williams and Wilkins; 2002.
9. National Kidney Foundation. Kidney Disease Outcomes Quality Initiative clinical practice guidelines for nutrition in chronic renal failure. Available at: http://www.kidney.org/professionals/kdoqi/guidelines_updates/doqi_nut.html. Accessed May 11, 2004.
10. Ikizler TA, Hakim RM. Nutrition in end-stage renal disease. *Kidney Int.* 1996;50:343-357.
11. Sprague SM, Lerrna E, McCormmick D, Abraham M, Batlie D. Suppression of parathyroid hormone secretion in hemodialysis patients: comparison of paricalcitol with calcitriol. *Am J Kidney Dis.* 2001;38:551-556.
12. National Kidney Foundation. Kidney Disease Outcomes Quality Initiative clinical practice guidelines for bone metabolism and disease in chronic kidney disease. Available at: http://www.kidney.org/professionals/kdoqi/guidelines_bone/index.htm. Accessed May 11, 2004.
13. Block G, Port G. Re-evaluation of risks associated with hyperphosphatemia and hyperparathyroidism in dialysis patients: recommendations for a change in management. *Am J Kidney Dis.* 2000;35:1226-1237.
14. Treatment of anemia of chronic renal failure. Available at: http://www.kidney.org/professionals/doqi/kdoqi/toc.htm. Accessed May 11, 2004.
15. The MDRD Study Group. Reduction of dietary protein and phosphorus in the Modification of Diet in Renal Disease Feasibility Study. *J Am Diet Assoc.* 1994;94:986-990.
16. National Kidney Foundation. Kidney Disease Outcomes Quality Initiative clinical practice guidelines for managing dyslipidemias in chronic kidney disease. Available at: http://www.kidney.org/professionals/kdoqi/guidelines_lipids/index.htm. Accessed May 11, 2004.
17. Blue LS. Adult kidney transplantation. In: Hasse JM, Blue LS, eds. *Comprehensive Guide to Transplant Nutrition.* Chicago, Ill: American Dietetic Association; 2002:44-57.

CHAPTER 9

Gastrointestinal Problems

With advancing age, persons increasingly suffer from a variety of gastrointestinal (GI) symptoms and disorders that may significantly compromise quality of life. Yet the extent to which the aging process contributes to GI maladies is unclear, in part because knowledge about the effect of age on the human GI tract is still evolving. Sufficient evidence exists, however, to support the idea that, like most other tissues, the GI tract loses some structural and functional integrity with age. Age-related changes appear to be gradual, and the GI tract normally has considerable functional reserve. Secretory, digestive, and absorptive capacities in humans normally exceed those needed to meet nutritional requirements, so long as adequate foods and nutrients are ingested. The high incidence of GI symptoms probably results more from a number of associated pathogenic problems that occur more often as the years and decades pass than from the aging process itself (1-3).

COMMON GI SYMPTOMS IN AGING

With advancing age, upper GI symptoms, such as decreased taste acuity, decreased olfactory sensation, periodontal disease and tooth loss, difficulty swallowing, heartburn, early satiety, and dyspepsia, occur with increasing frequency (see Box 9.1).

Lower GI symptoms, including bloating, abdominal cramping or gas, diarrhea, constipation, and fecal incontinence, also increase with advancing age. Most of these symptoms are more prevalent in institutionalized than in free-living older adults (4,5). The consequences of increased GI problems may include decreased variety and overall quality of foods consumed, change in textures or consistency of food, inadequate intake of micro- and macronutrients, decreased enjoyment of foods, and considerable decrease in overall quality of life (6-8).

Box 9.1 Common GI Symptoms in Older Adults

- Changes in taste and smell
- Anorexia, early satiety
- Difficulty chewing, swallowing, coughing; choking
- Heartburn, regurgitation, noncardiac chest pain
- Belching, nausea
- Dyspepsia/abdominal pain
- Gas, bloating, lower abdominal cramping/pain
- GI bleeding
- Diarrhea
- Constipation/impaction
- Incontinence

EFFECT OF AGE ON THE STRUCTURE AND FUNCTION OF THE GI TRACT

Several changes appear to occur in GI function and structure with increased age. However, in healthy older adults the changes appear to be subtle and do not, in themselves, greatly compromise the ability to digest and absorb sufficient amounts of macronutrients to maintain reasonable nutrition. It appears that age-related changes are less of a factor in the increased prevalence of GI problems than the cumulative effects of disease, infections, medications, and various toxins (1-3). But it is not clear to what extent each factor contributes to GI dysfunction or when. It is also not clear to what degree GI problems are reversible when therapies are available. The age-related effects of growing older (eg, on cell function and number) are not as well studied in the GI tract as in other organs or tissues. The normal roles of the many related hormones and neurotransmitters affecting or secreted by the GI tract and its enteric nervous system, for example, are still being unraveled. The degree to which they are altered with age is just being studied. As a result, it is likely that unraveling the age-related changes will take many years of study. A few examples of age-related changes being reported are mentioned below.

Altered Perceptions of Appetite and Satiety

Altered taste perception, diminished taste discrimination, decreased olfactory response, and decreased appetite and thirst responses occur with advancing age. The perception changes with age, however, are normally minor and are highly variable among older adults. More changes appear to occur in the olfactory function than in taste; yet the ability to smell plays an important role in the "taste" of foods (9,10). The reduced food intake commonly associated with aging may be related more to symptoms of acute and chronic disease, medications, smoking, and depression than to age-related changes in appetite (11,12).

Imbalance of Mediators Affecting Feeding and Satiety

Evidence suggests that, in older adults, several signals that normally drive hunger and accommodate feeding are reduced, and factors that tend to terminate or limit intake are increased (13-15). The net result favors early satiety and reduced food intake. For example, the neuropeptides/neurotransmitters ghrelin, nitric oxide, opioids, and neuropeptide-Y tend to induce feeding. All have been shown to be reduced with aging. Cholecystokinin (CCK) and leptin tend to signal satiety. With advancing age, leptin tends to increase in males, and CCK increases in both sexes. A number of other signaling agents for feeding and satiety may be altered with age (13-15).

Changes in Oropharyngeal, Esophageal, and Gastric Motility

Changes that have been noted in the upper alimentary tract include slower oropharyngeal transfer of food, decreased protection of the airway, increased frequency of unproductive esophageal peristalsis, and both reduced resting pressures and delayed relaxation of the upper esophageal sphincter (1,2,13,16). Although the changes with age generally are not considered major, they may contribute to the increased frequency of symptoms, such as coughing and choking spells, dysphagia, and esophagitis.

In the stomach, age-related decline in adaptive relaxation of the fundus, an increased rate of antral filling, and decreased postprandial gastric contractile force may play a role in early satiety and decreased intake (1,17,18). Other changes in gastric function include reduced gastric secretory response and compromised mucosal defense mechanisms. Studies dealing with the effect of age on rate of gastric emptying are not consistent. Although some investigators have reported delayed emptying in older adults, Tougas et al showed an increased emptying rate, at least with a low-fat meal (7,19-21). Delayed gastric emptying can clearly result from endocrine disease, neuromuscular disease, and many other degenerative diseases that may develop with advancing age. The aging process itself may make some additional contribution (7,20,21).

Intestinal and Anorectal Changes

With advancing age, cell loss, collagen accumulation, and other "normal" changes occur in the GI tract. However, the age-related functional losses in the small and large intestine do not appear to be sufficient to explain the increased prevalence of constipation, impaction, and fecal incontinence seen in older adults. One exception to relatively normal function of the aging intestine may be the anorectal segment (1,6). Anorectal changes include decreased rectal compliance, diminished ability to "sense" rectal fullness, decreased muscle strength, and decreased anal pressure. The combined result may contribute to constipation, fecal impaction, decreased call to stool, and, consequently, increased risk of fecal incontinence around the mass. The much higher incidence of constipation, impaction, and fecal incontinence in disabled individuals and in those in nursing facilities supports the likelihood that immobility and sedentary activity is a major factor (1,6). Again, prevalence of increasing organic disease, poor dietary habits, medications, and other factors likely contribute to the frequency and severity of these problems.

Changes in Immunologic Features of the GI Tract With Aging

The GI tract makes up the largest single immunologic organ. It produces large amounts of secretory immunoglobulin A (IgA), is lined with several types of lymphocytes collectively known as gut-associated lymphoid tissue (GALT), and serves as a physical barrier to entry of microorganism. The GI tract is the first line of defense against ingested and colonic microbes,

Box 9.2   Functional Age-Related Changes in the GI Tract

Altered sensory response/perception

- Appetite, minor changes in taste, smell, satiety, thirst
- Decreased sensation of sigmoid/rectal filling

Altered GI motility

- Oropharynx, esophagus
- Stomach
- Small intestine? Colon?
- Anorectal

Decreased muscle mass/strength/altered pressures

- Esophagus
- Stomach?
- Sigmoid, Anorectal

Decreased secretion/digestion?

- Salivary, gastric bicarb, biliary
- Pancreatic enzyme

- Decreased gastric acid, pepsin?
- Lactase deficiency

Decreased absorption

- Vitamin B-12?
- Calcium
- Vitamin D
- Iron

Immune function

- IgA responsiveness
- Lymphocyte subtypes
- Immune response to antigen
- Inflammatory response

General changes

- Collagen deposition
- Amyloid deposits
- Cell loss
- Diminished compliance

"?" indicates a possible altered sensory response or perception.

but the incidence of bacterial overgrowth and GI infections increases in older adults. Schmucker et al (22) stated that some immune defects appear to be seen in aged animals and humans. The compromise may be related to abnormal transport, to processing and response to antigens, and perhaps to abnormal distribution of lymphocyte types. In some studies, basal nonspecific antibody (IgA) numbers appeared to be increased in older adults, but production of additional IgA and specific subpopulations of lymphocytes in response to challenge (a better indicator of immune function) was decreased (22). Box 9.2 lists examples of functional age-related changes in the GI tract.

NUTRITIONAL IMPLICATIONS OF COMMON MALADIES IN OLDER ADULTS

GI problems are probably more closely related to specific disease processes and their treatment than to age. For example, diabetes, vascular disease, neuromuscular disorders, inflammatory disease, malignancies, infectious disease, and surgical procedures likely take their toll on the GI tract.

The new onset of most GI disorders (eg, irritable bowel syndrome [IBS] and inflammatory bowel disease [IBD]) tends to be less frequent, but the complications of existing diseases and perhaps the results of their treatment may surface with age. Some disorders with GI pathology do appear to occur more often with age (see Box 9.3), including diabetes, diverticular disease, malignancies, gall bladder disease, and atrophic gastritis (2,4,6). The incidence of IBD declines after the second decade of life but then increases after the sixth decade. Approximately 15% of new cases of IBD occur after age 65 (23). Medications taken for acute or chronic disease (eg, arthritis or infection), or exposure to irradiation or toxins, may add to the overall effect on GI dysfunction (1,20).

Nutrition plays a role in the onset and prevention of many GI maladies commonly seen in advancing age. Nutrition may also play a significant role in treatment of GI disorders. A lifetime of eating a poor-quality diet, inactivity, and other lifestyle habits (excess alcohol consumption, use of tobacco) contribute to dysfunction of the GI tract. The

Box 9.3   Potential Contributors to
Gastrointestinal Symptoms and
Maladies With Advancing Age

- Medications (eg, antibiotics, analgesics, laxatives agents, antidepressants, anticholinergics, calcium antagonists, over-the-counter and alternative supplements, cyclooxygenase inhibitors, amylase/lipase inhibitors)
- Neuromuscular disease (eg, amyotrophic lateral sclerosis, multiple sclerosis, myasthenia gravis, achalasia, stroke)
- Exposure to irradiation, toxins
- Periodontal disease, tooth decay, tooth loss
- Esophageal reflux, hiatal hernia, achalasia
- Renal failure
- Diabetes, hypothyroidism
- Diverticulosis, diverticulitis
- Poor dietary habits, malnutrition (macro and micro), inadequate hydration
- Inactivity, immobility
- Use of laxatives
- Vascular disease/stroke
- Inflammatory, autoimmune gastrointestinal disorders (eg, celiac disease, inflammatory bowel disease)
- H pylori/atrophic gastritis
- Surgical resections
- Alcoholism, tobacco use, depression

combination of age-related effects on the GI tract, consequences of disease, poor nutrition, and lifestyle factors can significantly affect quality of life. Compromised GI function and the symptoms they bring have the potential to

- increase malnutrition (14,24,25)
- increase use of medications, health care resources, and health care costs
- increase pain and discomfort and loss of sleep
- decrease overall diet quality and enjoyment of food
- decrease freedom to participate freely in activities
- decrease productivity

COMMON GI-RELATED MALADIES IN OLDER ADULTS AND THE ROLE OF DIET

Loss of Appetite, Reduced Hunger, and Early Satiety

A functional or physiologic basis for anorexia and decreased food intake may be related to several changes that occur with age, but disease and other factors are more likely to make clinically significant differences in appetite and food intake. Reduced or altered taste and smell are more common in Parkinson's disease, Alzheimer's disease, head trauma, multiple sclerosis, diabetes, hypothyroidism, renal failure, liver disease, nutrient deficiencies, malignancies, HIV, tobacco use, poor oral hygiene, dentures, sinus infection, and allergic rhinitis. Radiation therapy to the head and neck, surgical interventions, and many medications also affect taste and smell (9,11,26).

With any acute or chronic disease, several anorexic cytokines are produced in the inflammatory response that can affect appetite. Acute-phase proteins and cytokines serve as markers of the inflammatory response, and increased levels occur with arthritis, infections, cancers, and other wasting disorders. Appetite is also affected by medications, dental problems, real or perceived dietary intolerances, inactivity, and depression (1,14,18,27).

Treatment involves treating the underlying disorders to the extent possible; using appetite-enhancing medications; correcting micronutrient deficiencies; enhancing flavors of foods (25,28); increasing the visual and emotional appeal of foods; enhancing the environment in which foods are consumed; and making foods readily available, easy to prepare, and easy to consume. Dietary techniques and modifications used to improve intake are well known to dietetics professionals and may include adjusting the macro- and micronutrient density of foods, adjusting food textures, using flavor enhancers and sauces, finding foods that are familiar, and appropriately using food supplements.

Dysphagia

Swallowing disorders occur in 16% to 22% of persons older than 50 years and in 60% of persons in nursing facilities (1). Dysphagia is associated with increased risk of choking, aspiration, pneumonia, decreased intake of macro- and micronutrients, dehydration, and death. Mild degrees of oropharyngeal dysphagia may be a result of the aging process, but more significant forms of dysphagia occur with neuromuscular diseases such as Parkinson's disease, multiple sclerosis, myasthenia gravis, stroke, oramyotrophic lateral sclerosis. Oropharyngeal disorders usually involve disordered neuromuscular control of the tongue, pharynx, and upper esophageal sphincter. Symptoms include difficulty initiating swallowing, coughing, nasal regurgitation and aspiration, and poor tolerance of thin liquids and some solid foods (see Chapter 11).

Esophageal dysphagia may result from structural abnormalities (eg, rings, webs or strictures, malignancies, or achalasia). The symptoms tend to occur more with food getting caught in the upper chest or with onset of sternal pain.

Clients with oropharyngeal dysphagia generally tolerate thickened liquids and pureed foods. Nutritional concerns include ensuring sufficient energy and nutrient intake, ensuring adequate fiber and fluid intake, and maintaining good oral hygiene. Providing the right texture and viscosity are important to avoid risk of aspiration, but providing sufficient variety, appeal, and flavor are equally important to assure interest, enjoyment, and adequate amounts of food. As a general rule, when clients are not able to advance to thin liquids and solids, the likelihood for at least supplemental enteral or parenteral nutrition is increased (29,30).

Evaluation of the nature of the dysphagia and the client's ability to ingest different textures and types of food is typically the task of a multidisciplinary team, which includes physician specialists, speech pathologists, nurses, and dietetics professionals. Each team member offers a unique contribution to the overall care and evaluation of the client. Subsequent nutrition assessment and monitoring are also important functions of dietetics professionals, but other team members contribute as well.

Gastroesophageal Reflux Disease

The prevalence of heartburn and gastroesophageal reflux disease (GERD) depends on how the symptoms are described. It ranges from 20% to 40% of the older population, and, in some subsets (eg, persons with diabetes), it may even be higher (4,16,31). In addition to the potential morbidity and mortality, the reduction in quality of life associated with GERD is probably underappreciated. The symptoms can range from infrequent bouts of heartburn and regurgitation to significant daily life-altering distress. Burning sensations in the mid-chest may or may not be perceived. With long-standing reflux disease, the complications become more prevalent and significant. Complications can include frequent belching,

coughing, chest pain, esophagitis, perforation, altered motility, rings, webs and strictures, and dysphagia. Hiatal hernia may exist without GERD, but coexistence of hiatal hernia increases the likelihood of GERD symptoms and retards the clearance of gastric contents from the esophagus after reflux (32).

Typically, more GERD symptoms are experienced at night, but daytime symptoms may be worsened by position changes. Some persons may experience symptoms at all times (32).

Approximately 6% to 12% of individuals with GERD develop Barrett's esophagus, a condition resulting from severe injury of the esophageal mucosa. Barrett's esophagus describes characteristic intestinal metaplasia, the growth of intestinal columnar epithelium that is considered a potential premalignant condition. The percentage of those with Barrett's esophagus who go on to develop adenocarcinoma is not clear but may range from 10% to more than 25% (33).

Typical treatment for mild, intermittent cases of GERD include dietary measures and antacids as needed. More significant cases of GERD are usually treated with H2 receptor blockers or proton pump inhibitors. Strictures may require endoscopic procedures to dilate the occluded segment; in more severe, unrelenting cases, surgical procedures, such as fundoplication, have been used to reduce reflux with reasonable success (32).

Dietary recommendations to prevent symptoms and complications of GERD are based on a small number of studies with specific food types, and the evidence is not complete. Those recommendations that have been frequently cited in Web sites and textbooks are based on existing studies plus what may be extrapolated from the general studies on the normal effects of foods on GI secretions, motility, and gastric emptying. Most recommendations are aimed at preventing symptoms, but some may be aimed at preventing long-term complications. Duration or frequency of reflux may be reduced by (a) consuming small meals, (b) consuming meals several hours before reclining or retiring, (c) consuming low-fat meals, especially before retiring, (d) avoiding alcoholic beverages, (e) raising the head of the bed—usually by placing 4 to 6 inches of blocks under the headboard, (f) encouraging weight loss in those who are obese, and (g) wearing clothing that does not restrict the abdomen. Limiting "acid" foods may not affect the symptoms of heartburn or reflux, but those with preexisting reflux may experience burning with their consumption. Foods that have a pH less than 3 or 4 include many soft drinks, lime, lemon, orange, and tomato. Clients may complain of symptoms with "spicy" foods. When using standard dietary quantities in mixed meals, the results are rarely related to perceived symptoms. Responses may be related more to exacerbation of preexisting inflammation than to esophageal inflammation. Foods considered spicy are often high in fat and energy, are often consumed in large volumes, or are consumed with other foods (fiber, alcohol, caffeine, sugars) that may be at least partially related to the symptoms. Long-term alcohol consumption increases the risk of esophagitis and esophageal cancer (32).

Another component of diet therapy that may need attention is the possibility of stricture. In the case of partial restriction of the esophagus or disordered motility, more liquid foods may be needed, or particle size of foods may need to be reduced by chopping, dicing, or pureeing (32).

Diarrhea

Diarrhea occurs more commonly in older adults than in younger persons. Decreased immune function, altered GI motility, malnutrition, and increased use of a number of medications may increase the risk of infectious and nosocomial diarrheas in older adults (34-36). Opportunity for infection increases significantly with increased exposure to potentially infectious agents in extended hospital and nursing home stays, especially when antibiotics are used. Long-standing disease, GI surgeries, and neoplastic disease and its treatment may increase the risk of diarrhea (34-36).

Diarrhea can be episodic or continuous and unrelenting, and the consequences can be minimal or life threatening. Because the term *diarrhea* may relate to situations ranging from minor client or caretaker inconvenience to severe, life-threatening fluid and electrolyte imbalance, the descriptors for diarrhea should include the volume, frequency, and duration of the problem. Consequences include burning pain, irritation, and breakdown of the skin surrounding the anus; dehydration and electrolyte disturbances; and death. Poor dietary intake (amount and quality) may result from fear of diarrhea or incontinence. Several dietary factors may cause or contribute to diarrhea. Excessive intake of sugars, notably lactose, alcohol sugars, and fructose, may contribute to osmotic diarrhea. Osmotic diarrhea is especially likely after use of broad-spectrum antibiotics, in the presence of bacterial overgrowth, or after surgical resections of the stomach and small intestine (37).

Medical treatment of diarrhea includes eradication of the cause when possible. This may include the use of antidiarrheal medications, antimicrobials, rehydration fluids, and diet.

Dietary management includes restoration and maintenance of nutritional requirements, limitation of specific sugars (38), and adequate dietary fiber intake. Total fluid needs should be based on fecal and urinary output plus the insensible loss from respiration and evaporation. Depending on the severity and duration of diarrhea, normal fluid and electrolyte needs can be supplied by oral rehydration fluids, IV fluids, or normal diet. In healthy individuals, tolerance to lactose is about 6 to 12 g per serving (even in lactose malabsorbers) (32). Concrete threshold levels for sugar intolerance have not been established for specific diarrheal disorders, but it makes sense to limit sugars to the lowest tolerance levels in normal situations (32). Caffeine, which increases both GI secretions and motility, may also be limited. Use of foods containing adequate amounts of dietary fiber appears to help firm stools, to normalize stool weight, and to alter intestinal microflora when clients are fed orally and enterally (39,40).

Dietary fiber and oligosaccharides may serve as prebiotic material to favor the growth of "friendly" bacteria (41-45). Selected probiotic cultures have shown promise in attenuation of some forms of diarrhea, especially antibiotic-associated diarrhea (44-46). For best results, it appears that the right probiotic product must be selected for the application, the product must be the appropriate dose and concentration, and the product must be viable (46-48).

Irritable Bowel Syndrome

IBS is a common, functional bowel disorder that involves abdominal pain, abnormal bowel perceptions, and abnormal defecation patterns. IBS affects 10% to 20% of the US population, and women make up approximately 70% of those reported (49). The prevalence does not appear to increase with advancing age, and Talley et al (5) found that the prevalence of IBS-like symptoms was closer to 11% in a survey of Minnesota residents ranging from 65 to 93 years of age. The disorder does not result in increased mortality or morbidity, but it can affect quality of life, productivity, number of physician visits, absenteeism from work, and participation in social events or travel.

The cause is not completely understood, but persons with IBS tend to have abnormal GI motility and abnormal enteric neurotransmitter and neuropeptide responses to various types of emotional, GI, and dietary stimuli. Recent studies have found that at least some cases of IBS may be improved with antibiotic therapy. This finding implies that there may be an infectious etiology for some cases or for the microflora in some clients that may affect the syndrome (37).

IBS is diagnosed by screening for the possibility of organic disease that could be responsible for the symptoms and then applying the Rome II criteria for IBS. The Rome II criteria state that the patient has had at least 12 weeks of continuous or recurrent symptoms of abdominal pain or discomfort that is relieved by defecation; and/or, onset is associated with a change in frequency of stool; and/or, onset is associated with a change in form or appearance of stool. The screen includes indicators such as family history of GI cancer, IBD, celiac disease, blood in the stool, fever, nocturnal GI distress, and lab work to rule out organic disease. In addition to the basic Rome II criteria, three predominant patterns are usually described: diarrhea, alternating constipation and diarrhea, or constipation (50,51).

Medical management typically includes education and reassurance, diet, medications, and psychological or behavioral counseling for stress and anxiety reduction. No single medication is effective for all types of IBS, and treatment is aimed at the predominant form of IBS pattern. Anticholinergics, prokinetics, antispasmodics, opioid receptor agonists, stool softeners, laxatives, and antidepressants may be used for the appropriate symptoms. Recently, tagaserod, a selective 5-HT4 antagonist, has been used for the constipation-predominant pattern; and alosetron, a 5-HT3 receptor antagonist, has been used in the diarrhea-predominant pattern. Other medications that affect GI secretions and motility or that alter psychological profiles are being investigated (51,52).

Persons with IBS typically have many concerns about diet and tend to report many more food intolerances than other individuals of the same age and gender. The intolerances may or may not be related to altered physiologic GI responses to their ingestion. Some food intolerances may be associated with adverse experiences with foods—eg, when foods were consumed while stress-induced symptoms or other provoking stimuli were experienced. Some intolerances may be predictable, in that they may occur in everyone in given amounts, but perhaps the threshold for food-related symptoms may be lower for people with IBS. Lactose intolerance and intolerance to sweets, fatty foods, or caffeine are commonly mentioned. However, food allergies have not been evaluated thoroughly in IBS.

As with medical management, dietary approaches include education and reassurance. Diet therapy is also tailored to the predominant symp-toms. Those with diarrhea-predominant IBS and alternating constipation and diarrhea should be cautioned to limit lactose, fructose and sorbitol, caffeine, and alcoholic beverages. Consumption of adequate amounts of foods containing fiber is also indicated. For those with constipation-predominant symptoms, adequate fiber-containing food, exercise, and fluids (see section on constipation) should be encouraged. Use of large quantities of bran and bran cereals are no longer touted for IBS, but consumption of adequate amounts of fibrous foods throughout the day is recommended (37).

Fiber intake helps to normalize bowel function in all types of IBS, and fiber may play several roles in affecting GI microflora and GI transit, and in immune and neuroendocrine activity. Dietary fiber intake of adults in the United States averages only about 14 to 15 g per day. In older adults, fiber intake is typically closer to 10 or 11 g. The recent recommendation is to increase fiber to 25 to 38 g/day (41,42), preferably in the form of fibrous foods, as opposed to powdered supplements, because fiber from food carries the added benefit of contributing to the nutritional intake of the individual. Plant foods contribute macro- and micronutrients and electrolytes, and they add numerous protective phytochemicals and prebiotic materials. Fibrous foods can also be incorporated as purees or finely chopped and mixed into dishes or foods that are traditionally low in fiber. If the individual is unable or unwilling to take sufficient amounts of fibrous foods, liquid supplements containing fiber or powdered supplements can be used or added to foods. Like oral medications, powdered/flaked fiber supplements are not part of a normal diet and patients have the right to refuse them. Also, caution should be exercised to ensure that powdered supplements are interspersed with food or liquid or that they be taken in small amounts, rather than in a single large dose. When taken as dry powders, some products may clump or congeal in the GI tract, and use of powdered fiber supplements taken at a single time have been reported to cause obstruction and GI discomfort. Whether the diet is increased by foods or by supplements, it is probably wise to increase the diet in 5- to 10-g increments for several weeks, until the desired level is reached.

Explaining the dominant role of stress and anxiety in the disorder will help older adults understand why foods might or might not be tolerated at different times. For some individuals, variety and quantity of foods are significantly limited, and the anxiety about what to eat may itself be an additional source of stress. Clients should be advised in times of stress to be cautious about the specific foods likely to worsen symptoms, to select from foods not likely to create problems, and to consume smaller meals more frequently. When appropriate, vitamin-mineral supplements should be included. Because of the possible relationship of the host microflora and IBS symptoms, pre- and probiotics are being evaluated to treat IBS. Some probiotics may be helpful in certain situations, but additional study is warranted (53,54).

Inflammatory Bowel Disease

The first onset of IBD normally occurs before the age of 30 years, but about 10% to 15% of new cases occur after the age of 65 (2,23). The two major categories of IBD include ulcerative colitis and Crohn's disease. The etiology of both diseases is not certain, but, according to Podolsky, IBD is "thought to result from inappropriate and ongoing activation of the mucosal immune system, driven by the presence of normal luminal flora. This aberrant response is most likely facilitated by defects in both the barrier function of the intestinal epithelium and the mucosal immune system" (55). Ulcerative colitis involves continuous, fine, superficial ulceration, involving only the colon, whereas Crohn's disease typically involves the colon and ileum and may affect any segment of the alimentary canal. With Crohn's disease, mucosal involvement is typically deeper than with ulcerative colitis, and the disease may "skip" segments of bowel and continue further along the intestines (see Box 9.4). Both disorders increase the risk of GI malignancy with advancing age, and, especially in the case of the older adult with ulcerative colitis, colonic resection was likely considered if the client had been diagnosed early in life. Adequate nutrition, in terms of micro- and macronutrient intake, may be difficult in either disease. Because Crohn's disease may result in strictures, fistulas, resection of digestive and absorptive surfaces, and malabsorption, malnutrition is usually more common (37).

Medical management of IBD typically includes use of antibiotics and anti-inflammatory, immunosuppressive, and immunoregulatory agents. For Crohn's disease, monoclonal anti-TNF-alpha has been used to suppress the inflammatory effects of this pivotal cytokine. Several other medications are being evaluated. Surgical management in Crohn's disease involves repair of strictures, fistulas, and resections, when the disease is unresponsive to other therapies (37).

The long-term clinical consequences of Crohn's disease probably have greater potential to affect

---

Box 9.4   Features of Ulcerative Colitis and Crohn's Disease

Ulcerative Colitis

- Superficial mucosal involvement
- Involves only the colon
- Continuous involvement
- Fissures, strictures (fistulas rare)

Crohn's Disease

- Deep submucosal ulcerations
- Typically ileum/colon but may involve esophagus, stomach jejunum
- May skip healthy segments and continue
- Fistulas, strictures (fissures more common)

In both forms of irritable bowel disease, diarrhea, weight loss, malnutrition, malaise, and a long list of extra-intestinal manifestations (eg, arthritic, dermatologic) may occur.

---

morbidity, mortality, and quality of life than those of ulcerative colitis. If clients with ulcerative colitis have a colonic resection, the disease is resolved. Dealing with an ileostomy, a surgically created ileal reservoir, or an ileorectal pouch may be life altering, but most clients say their quality of life improves compared with the consequences of ulcerative colitis. Older adults who have had long-standing Crohn's disease are likely to be seen with the consequences of multiple intestinal surgeries, side effects of medications, malabsorption, dietary intolerances, obstructions, short bowel syndrome, and increased risk of malnutrition (37). Nutrition management is based on the status of the disease and the host (56). During maintenance/remission, the aims of nutrition management are to (a) attain a good-quality diet and meet nutritional needs; (b) allow enjoyment of as wide a variety of foods as possible; (c) alter diet to prevent GI symptoms, such as abdominal cramping, diarrhea, and obstruction; and (d) prolong remission.

Individuals with IBD need a nutritious diet even more than healthy individuals do. Fruits, vegetables, and whole-grain products can provide micronutrients and protective phytochemicals, but these foods are often lacking in the diet of persons with IBD. When older adults have strictures or narrowed segments of intestine, fibrous foods or fiber supplements may have to be provided in particulate form or in liquid dietary supplements. Boluses of fiber may clump and form a viscous mass if taken at once, and fiber supplements have been reported periodically to cause obstruction. Vitamin, mineral, and trace-element supplements should be used when malabsorption, drug-nutrient interactions, or dietary restrictions are evident (37).

Symptoms (eg, diarrhea, abdominal cramping, and malabsorption) may be lessened by (1) limiting poorly absorbed sugars, (2) limiting significant amounts of caffeine, (3) adding extra fluid and salts based on urinary and stool output (see diarrhea section), and (4) using MCT oil when lipid malabsorption is present. Evidence for dietary measures to prolong remission is still somewhat incomplete, but use of a high-quality nutritionally complete diet, improving the n-3 to n-6 ratio of dietary lipids, use of dietary fiber and prebiotics, and use of probiotics are all measures that hold much promise (56,57). Older clients with Crohn's disease who have had significant resections of the small intestine, especially of the ileum and the ileocecal valve, may require enteral or parenteral nutrition for at least supplemental hydration and nutrition support.

Nutrition may certainly play at least a complementary role in therapy for IBD. Primary or complementary nutrition treatments of IBD have included use of enteral and parenteral nutrition, n-3 fatty acids, short-chain fatty acids (especially for ulcerative colitis), and antioxidants. Because abnormal microflora or altered response to normal host flora seems to be a primary candidate for the onset or exacerbation of IBD, a promising new area of nutrition therapy includes the use of prebiotics and specific probiotics, to alter the host flora. Several animal models and small clinical trials have shown some success at changing host flora, preventing different experimental forms of colitis, and inducing or prolonging remission in persons with either ulcerative colitis or Crohn's disease. Additional work is under way to identify specific strains of probiotics, doses, concentrations, and conditions under which the products may be successful (58,59).

Constipation

Constipation may be defined by a stool frequency of two or fewer bowel movements per week, a feeling of incomplete evacuation, passing hard stools, frequent use of laxatives, and/or straining at defecation. Although the criteria for describing or defining constipation vary greatly among studies, it appears that studies showing increasing incidence of straining, hard stools, and frequent use of laxatives are consistent. When incidence of constipation is defined by stool frequency, however, the difference between free-living middle-age adults and older adults becomes less clear (60). In a survey of 1,375 persons in the United States aged 65 or older, 40% reported constipation using symptom-based criteria (61). A nationwide survey showed that use of laxatives and self-reporting of constipation increased with age, but the proportion of persons with fewer than two bowel movements per week was not greater until after the seventh decade (62). In virtually all reports, the prevalence of constipation was greater in females and was considerably greater in institutionalized older adults (60).

The causes of constipation include functional disorders, dysmotility, malignancies, neurogenic disease, medications, inactivity, inadequate hydration, and dietary patterns. Although many subtle changes occur in the aging colon, those changes, independent of comorbidities, have not been shown conclusively to be associated with increased incidence of constipation (37).

Primary lifestyle activities that affect stool weight, frequency, and consistency include diet, activity, and adequate hydration. Increasing hydration beyond the amount sufficient to meet evaporative and normal physiologic needs (about 2 L daily) does not seem to improve constipation, but constipation is more likely when adequate fluids are not provided (37). Sufficient consumption of dietary fiber (28 to 35 g/day) is essential to avoid or improve constipation. Individuals should follow recommendations for dietary fiber outlined in the section on IBS (above).

Diverticular Disease

The incidence of diverticulosis in Western countries increases progressively with age, from approximately 5% in the fifth decade to more than 50% in the ninth decade (2,63). The etiology of this disease is not completely understood, but lifelong consumption of a low-fiber diet is a primary contributor. It has been theorized that repeated attempts to transport small-caliber, firm fecal material results in creation of compartments or haustral segments around the feces, with increased intracolonic pressure. The increased pressure that results from circular and longitudinal contractions may result in herniations at weak areas of the colon (where blood vessels pass through the wall). Other contributors to the development of diverticula may include inactivity, neuromuscular dysfunction, structural abnormalities, and/or genetic factors (64,65).

Diverticular disease may be asymptomatic or associated with varying degrees of inflammation and discomfort. Diverticulitis may result in abdominal pain, bleeding, abscess, fistula, perforation, and obstruction. If medical management is not effective at resolving acute or chronic inflammation, then surgical resection, typically limited to the sigmoid, may be indicated (37).

Diet for prevention and treatment of diverticular disease involves adequate intake of dietary fiber (25 to 38 g per day), preferably coming from fruits, vegetables, legumes, and whole grains. (See section on IBS [above] for additional recommendations on dietary fiber.) Adequate hydration and activity may also help to enhance laxation.

The role of skins, seeds, nuts, and other high-fiber foods in the exacerbation of symptoms, inflammation, or obstruction in diverticular disease is the subject of much speculation and has not been studied objectively. Eating skins, hulls, and small seeds that are a part of a normal diet (eg, grapes, corn, tomatoes) has not been shown to cause obstructions or inflammation in diverticular disease. However, individuals who are suspected to have diverticular disease should avoid unusually harsh husks and hulls from foods such as peanuts shells or sunflower and pumpkin seeds (37).

REFERENCES

1. Firth M, Prather CM. Gastrointestinal motility problems in the elderly patient. *Gastroenterology*. 2002;122:1688-1700.
2. Shamburek FD, Farrar JT. Disorders of the digestive system in the elderly. *N Engl J Med*. 1990;322:438-442.
3. Muller-Lissner S. General geriatrics and gastroenterology: constipation and fecal incontinence. *Best Pract Res Clin Gastroenterol*. 2002;16:115-133.
4. Frank L, Kleinman L, Ganoczy D, McQuaid K, Sloan S, Eggleston A, Tougas G, Farup C. Upper gastrointestinal symptoms in North America. *Dig Dis Sci*. 2000;45:809-818.
5. Talley NJ, O'Keefe EA, Zinsmeister AR, Melton LJ 3rd. Prevalence of gastrointestinal symptoms in the elderly: a population-based study. *Gastroenterology*. 1992;102:895-901.
6. Siddiqui MA, Castell DO. Gastrointestinal disorders in the elderly. *Comp Ther*. 1997;23:349-359.
7. Drenowski A, Shultz JM. Impact of aging on eating behaviors, food choices, nutrition and health status. *J Nutr Health Aging*. 2001;5:75-79.
8. Jensen GL, McGee M, Binkley J. Nutrition in the elderly. *Gastroenterol Clin North Am*. 2001;30:313-333.
9. Schiffman SS. Taste and smell losses in normal aging and disease. *JAMA*. 1997;278:1357-1362.
10. Mattes RD. The chemical senses and nutrition in aging: challenging old assumptions. *J Am Diet Assoc*. 2002;120:192-196.
11. Schiffman SS, Zervakis J. Taste and smell perception in the elderly: effect of medications and disease. *Adv Food Nutr Res*. 2002;44:247-346.
12. Mowe M, Bohmer T. Reduced appetite. A predictor for undernutrition in aged people. *J Nutr Health Aging*. 2002;6:81-83.
13. Morley JE. Decreased food intake with aging. *J Gerontol A Biol Sci Med Sci*. 2001;2:81-88.
14. Chapman IM, MacIntosh CG, Morley JE, Horowitz M. The anorexia of ageing. *Biogerontology*. 2002;3:67-71.
15. Rigamonti AE, Pincelli AI, Corra B, Viarengo R, Bonomo SM, Galimberti D, Scacchi M, Scarpini E, Cavagnini F, Muller EE. Plasma ghrelin concentrations in elderly subjects: comparison with anorexic and obese patients. *J Endocrinol*. 2002;175:R1-R5.
16. Tack J, Vantrappen G. The aging oesophagus. *Gut*. 1997;41:422-424.
17. Shimamoto C, Hirata I, Hiraike Y, Takeuchi N, Nomura T, Katsu K. Evaluation of gastric motor activity in the elderly by electrogastrography and the (13) C-acetate breath test. *Gerontology*. 2002;48:381-386.
18. Morley JE. Anorexia, sarcopenia, and aging. *Nutrition*. 2001;17:660-663.
19. Tougas G, Eaker EY, Abell TL, Abrahamsson H, Boivin M, Chen J, Hocking MP, Quigley EM, Koch KL, Tokayer AZ, Stanghellini V, Chen Y, Huizinga JD, Ryden J, Bourgeois I, McCallum RW. Assessment of gastric emptying using a low-fat meal: establishment of international control values. *Am J Gastroenterol*. 2000;95:1456-1462.
20. O'Mahony D, O'Leary O, Quigley EM. Aging and intestinal motility: a review of factors that affect intestinal motility in the aged. *Drugs Aging*. 2002;19:515-527.
21. Wade PR. Aging and neural control of the GI tract: age-related changes in the enteric nervous system. *Am J Physiol Gastrointest Liver Physiol*. 2002;283:G489-G495.
22. Schmucker DL, Heyworth MF, Owen RL, Daniels CK. Impact of aging on gastrointestinal mucosal immunity. *Dig Dis Sci*. 1996;41:1183-1193.
23. Robertson DJ, Grimm IS. Inflammatory bowel disease in the elderly. *Gastroenterol Clin North Am*. 2001;30:409-426.
24. Pirlich M, Lochs H. Nutrition in the elderly. *Best Pract Res Clin Gastroenterol*. 2001;15:869-884.
25. Saltzman JR, Russel RM. The aging gut: nutrition issues. *Gastroenterol Clin North Am*. 1998;27:309-324.
26. Chauhan J, Hawrysh ZJ, Gee M, Donald EA, Basu TK. Age-related olfactory and taste changes and interrelationships between taste and nutrition. *J Am Diet Assoc*. 1987;87:1543-1550.
27. Tisdale MJ. Cancer anorexia and cachexia. *Nutrition*. 2001;17:438-442.
28. Mathey MF, Siebelink E, de Graaf C, Van Staveren WA. Flavor enhancement of food improves dietary intake and nutritional status of elderly nursing home residents. *J Gerontol A Biol Sci Med Sci*. 2001;56:M200-M205.
29. Finestone HM, Foley NC, Woodbury MG, Greene-Finestone L. Quantifying fluid intake in dysphagic stroke patients: a preliminary comparison of oral and non-oral strategies. *Arch Phys Med Rehabil*. 2001;82:1744-1746.

30. Wilkinson TJ, Thomas K, MacGregor S, Tillard G, Wyles C, Sainsbury R. Tolerance of early diet textures as indicators of recovery from dysphagia after stroke. *Dysphagia*. 2002;17:227-232.

31. Ramirez FC. Diagnosis and treatment of gastroesophageal reflux disease in the elderly. *Cleve Clin J Med*. 2002;67:755-765.

32. Beyer P. Medical nutrition therapy for upper gastrointestinal tract disorders. In: Mahan LK, Escott-Stump S, eds. *Krause's Food, Nutrition, and Diet Therapy*. 11th ed. Philadelphia, Pa: Saunders; 2004:686-704.

33. Falk GW. Barrett's esophagus. *Gastroenterology*. 2002;122:1569-1591.

34. Slotwiner-Nie PK, Brant LJ. Infectious diarrhea in the elderly. *Gastroenterol Clin North Am*. 2001;30:625-635.

35. Holt PR. Diarrhea and malabsorption in the elderly. *Gastroenterol Clin North Am*. 2001;30:427-444.

36. Hoffmann JC, Zeitz M. Small bowel disease in the elderly: diarrhoea and malabsorption. *Best Pract Res Clin Gastroenterol*. 2002;16:17-36.

37. Beyer P. Medical nutrition therapy for lower gastrointestinal tract disorders. In: Mahan LK, Escott-Stump S, eds. *Krause's Food, Nutrition, and Diet Therapy*. 11th ed. Philadelphia, Pa: Saunders; 2004:705-737.

38. Rumessen JJ, Gudmand-Hoyer E. Functional bowel disease: malabsorption and abdominal distress after ingestion of fructose, sorbitol, and fructose-sorbitol mixtures. *Gastroenterology*. 1988;95:694-700.

39. Frankenfield DC, Beyer PL. Dietary fiber and bowel function in tube fed patients. *J Am Diet Assoc*. 1991;91:590-596.

40. Marlett JA, McBurney MI, Slavin JL. Position of the American Dietetic Association: health implications of dietary fiber. *J Am Diet Assoc*. 2002;102:993-1000.

41. Institute of Medicine. *Dietary Reference Intakes for Energy, Carbohydrate, Fiber, Fat, Fatty Acids, Cholesterol, Protein, and Amino Acids*. Washington, DC: National Academy Press; 2002.

42. Nakao M, Ogura Y, Satake S, Ito I, Iguchi A, Takagi K, Nabeshima T. Usefulness of soluble dietary fiber for the treatment of diarrhea during enteral nutrition in elderly patients. *Nutrition*. 2002;18:35-39.

43. Scheppach W, Luehrs H, Menzel T. Beneficial health effects of low-digestible carbohydrate consumption. *Br J Nutr*. 2001;85(suppl 1):23-30.

44. Van Loo J, Cummings J, Delzenne N, Englyst H, Franck A, Hopkins M, Kok N, Macfarlane G, Newton D, Quigley M, Roberfroid M, van Vliet T, van den Heuvel E. Functional food properties of nondigestible oligosaccharides: a consensus report from the ENDO project. *Br J Nutr*. 1999;81:121-132.

45. Emery EA, Ahmad S, Koethe JD, Skipper A, Perlmutter S, Paskin DL. Banana flakes control diarrhea in enterally fed patients. *Nutr Clin Pract*. 1997;12:72-75.

46. D'Souza AL, Rajkumar C, Cooke J, Bulpitt CJ. Probiotics in prevention of antibiotic associated diarrhea: a meta analysis. *BMJ*. 2002;324:1361.

47. Fooks LJ, Gibson GR. Probiotics as modulators of the gut flora. *Br J Nutr*. 2002;88(suppl 1):S39-S49.

48. Cremonini F, Di Caro S, Santarelli L, Gabrielli M, Candelli M, Nista EC, Lupascu A, Gasbarrini G, Gasbarrini A. Probiotics in antibiotic-associated diarrhea. *Dig Liver Dis*. 2002;34(suppl 2):S78-S80.

49. Irritable Bowel Syndrome (IBS) Self Help and Support Group Web site. Available at: http://www.ibsgroup.org. Accessed May 10, 2004.

50. Ringel Y, Drossman DA. Irritable bowel syndrome: classification and conceptualization. *J Clin Gastroenterol*. 2002;35(suppl 1):S7-S10.

51. Thompson WG. The treatment of irritable bowel syndrome. *Aliment Pharmacol Ther*. 2002;16:1395-1406.

52. Callahan MJ. Irritable bowel syndrome neuropharmacology. A review of approved and investigational compounds. *J Clin Gastroenterol*. 2002;35(suppl 1):S58-S67.

53. Bazzocchi G, Gionchetti P, Almerigi PF, Amadini C, Campieri M. Intestinal microflora and oral bacteriotherapy in irritable bowel syndrome. *Dig Liver Dis*. 2002;34(suppl 2):48-53.

54. Floch MH, Narayan R. Diet in the irritable bowel syndrome. *J Clin Gastroenterol*. 2002;35(suppl 1):S45-S52.

55. Podolsky DK. Inflammatory bowel disease. *N Engl J Med*. 2002;347:417-428.

56. Beyer PL. Nutrient considerations in inflammatory bowel disease. In: Coulston AM, Rock CL, Monsen ER. eds. *Nutrition in the Prevention and Treatment of Disease*. San Diego, Calif: Academic Press; 2001.

57. Graham TO, Kandil HM. Nutritional factors in inflammatory bowel disease. *Gastroenterol Clin North Am*. 2002;31:203-218.

58. Kanauchi O, Mitsuyama K, Araki Y, Andoh A. Modification of intestinal flora in the treatment of inflammatory bowel disease. *Curr Pharm Des*. 2003;9:333-346.

59. Hart AL, Stragg AJ, Kamm MA. Use of probiotics in the treatment of inflammatory bowel disease. *J Clin Gastroenterol*. 2003;36:111-119.

60. De Lillo AR, Rose S. Functional bowel disorders in the geriatric patient: constipation, fecal impaction and fecal incontinence. *Am J Gastroenterol*. 2000;95:901-906.

61. Talley NJ, Fleming KC, Evans JM, O'Keefe EA, Weaver AL, Zinsmeister AR, Melton LJ 3rd. Constipation in an elderly community: a study of prevalence and potential risk factors. *Am J Gastroenterol*. 1996;91:19-25.

62. Harari D, Gurwitz JH, Avorn J, Bohn R, Minaker KL. Bowel habit in relation to age and gender. Findings from the National Health Interview Survey and clinical implications. *Arch Intern Med*. 1996;156:315-320.

63. Stollman NH, Raskin JB. Diverticular disease of the colon. *J Clin Gastroenterol*. 1999;29:241-252.

64. Simpson J, Scholefield JH, Spiller RC. Pathogenesis of colonic diverticula. *Br J Surg*. 2002;89:546-554.

65. Camilleri M, Lee JS, Viramontes B, Bharucha AE, Tangalos EG. Insights into the and mechanisms of constipation, irritable bowel syndrome and diverticulosis in older people. *J Am Geriatric Soc*. 2000;48:1142-1150.

CHAPTER 10

Nutritional Anemias

Anemia is symptomatic of a disease and is seen in as many as one third of all hospitalized older adults. It is characterized by a decrease in circulating red blood cells (RBCs), a reduction in the amount of hemoglobin, a reduction in packed red cells, or any combination of these. Anemia is classified on the basis of the pathophysiologic cause (1-3).

There is a decrease in iron in RBCs with aging. The mechanism is not known, although iron seems to be absorbed from the intestine (4). Many older adults have undiagnosed nutritional anemias. Anemia is a significant clinical finding, and efforts should be made to determine its etiology (1-3).

Anemia is defined generally as a deficiency in erythrocyte mass and hemoglobin contents. A low hemoglobin or hematocrit value needs to be evaluated further by a complete blood cell count, which includes hemoglobin concentration, hematocrit value, RBC mass, and mean corpuscular volume (MCV) (5,6). Normal ranges for these laboratory tests are listed in Table 10.1 (7). Norms assume adequate hydration. If the client is dehydrated, the values will be falsely high; overhydration produces falsely low values (5).

With aging, there is a gradual drop in RBC indexes. There is a trend toward lower hemoglobin levels after age 60 in both men and women. This is accompanied by a decrease in RBCs (8,9). Abrams et al (4) reported a mild normochromic anemia with hemoglobin levels between 11 and 12 g/dL in adults older than 70 years, with no identified underlying pathology. The significance of this drop in hemoglobin is not known.

CLASSIFICATION OF ANEMIAS

Anemias are classified using various systems. One method organizes anemias by underlying cause. The causes include blood loss, deficient erythropoiesis, and excessive hemolysis (6).

TABLE 10.1. Normal Values for Laboratory Tests for Anemia

Laboratory Test	Normal Values	
	Males	Females
Hemoglobin (g/dL)	14-18	12-16
Hematocrit (%)	42-52	37-47
Mean corpuscular volume (μm³)	80-95	80-95
Serum iron (μg/dL)	80-180	60-190
Total iron-binding capacity (μg/dL)	250-420	250-420
Ferritin (ng/mL)	12-300	10-150
Serum B-12 (pg/mL)	160-950	160-950
Folate (μg/mL)	5-25	5-25
Homocysteine (μmol/L)	4-14	4-14
Methylmalonic acid (ng/mL)	17-76	17-76

Source: Data are from reference 7.

Blood loss anemias can result from acute or chronic blood loss. Identification of the cause of the blood loss and resolution of the loss will most likely resolve the anemia. The lost erythrocyte mass and hemoglobin content will be replaced via transfusion or erythropoiesis (6). Often therapeutic supplementation of iron is ordered for 3 months. The iron levels need to be reevaluated to determine whether supplementation goals are being met (9).

Deficient erythropoiesis anemias include microcytic anemias, normochromic-normocytic anemias, and macrocytic anemias. All are characterized by low hemoglobin and hematocrit values (5,7). The distinction is made by examining the MCV (10). This test provides the average size of the client's RBCs. In microcytic anemias, the heme or globin synthesis is deficient or defective, resulting in a lower-than-normal MCV. In normocytic anemia, the bone marrow failure prevents the erythroid mass from expanding as needed, but the volume is normal, so the MCV is normal. Megaloblastic erythropoiesis results when DNA or RNA synthesis is impaired; MCV then exceeds normal values (6).

Excessive hemolysis anemias are caused by the destruction of RBCs. These are much less common and rarely associated with blood loss or bone marrow failure. These anemias are caused by defects that are either extrinsic (eg, autoimmune hemolysis) or intrinsic (eg, sickle cell disease) to the RBCs (6,7).

NUTRITIONAL ANEMIAS

There are four types of nutritional anemias: iron-deficiency anemia, anemia of chronic disease, megaloblastic anemia, and pernicious anemia. Early onset of all is evidenced by lack of energy, malaise, and decreased interest in activities of daily living and lifelong interests. However, each presents a different pattern of laboratory results from a variety of blood tests. Because the nutritional anemias present similar symptoms and may appear to be the same, it is important to look at more than one laboratory value before recommending a plan for medical nutrition therapy.

Anemias are categorized using RBC indexes about the size, weight, and hemoglobin concentration (5,7). Each of the four types is discussed below.

Iron-Deficiency Anemia

Iron-deficiency anemia may be the result of a chronic blood loss, an acute blood loss, a deficient diet, medications, malabsorption of iron, or increased need for iron. It may occur concurrently with anemia of chronic disease (11). Clinical signs and symptoms include inflammation of the tongue, lips, or mucous membranes of the mouth, and spooned nails. In its advanced state, it is described as a microcytic hypochromic anemia.

Laboratory tests used to diagnose iron-deficiency anemia include low hemoglobin concentration, low hematocrit value, low MCV, low serum iron level, elevated total iron-binding capacity

---

Box 10.1 Laboratory Test Results for Iron-Deficiency Anemia

↓ Hgb
↓ Hct
↓ MCV
↓ Serum Fe
↑ TIBC
↓ Ferritin

Key: elevated, ↑; low, ↓.

Abbreviations: Fe, iron; Hct, hematocrit; Hgb, hemoglobin; MCV, mean corpuscular volume; TIBC, total iron-binding capacity.

Box 10.2 Medications Associated With Iron Loss

- Amoxicillin
- Amoxicillin potassium
- Aspirin
- Bumetanide
- Ceftriaxone
- Clonidine
- Diflunisal
- Levodopa
- Naproxen
- Nifedipine
- Nitrofurantoin
- Piroxicam
- Procainamide
- Propylthiouracil
- Sulfamethoxazole
- Sulfasalazine
- Trimethoprim

(TIBC), and low ferritin level. In a geriatric population, all of these tests may not be available, because of cost restraint. The MCV is the key test to examine, once low hemoglobin and low hematocrit values are identified (7,11-15). Box 10.1 illustrates the pattern of laboratory values typically seen in iron-deficiency anemia. Box 10.2 lists medications associated with iron losses in the body.

Once underlying causes of iron-deficiency anemia are identified and addressed, oral iron therapy is preferred; however, a multivitamin may be better tolerated. Absorption is best on an empty stomach but may cause gastric upset. The goal of pharmacologic intervention is to increase the deficient body components while avoiding a negative impact on the total dietary intake of the older adult.

Anemia of Chronic Disease

Anemia of chronic disease manifests similarly to iron-deficiency anemia. It is often associated with a chronic infection or inflammation, congestive heart failure, and other chronic diseases. The anemia may develop after 4 to 6 weeks of illness due to a chronic infection or inflammation. The anemia is caused by a decrease in erythropoietin, which decreases RBC production and impairs iron delivery from the reticulothelium system to the bone marrow (4).

Although the physical signs and symptoms are the same, anemia of chronic disease is a normochromic-normocytic anemia seen in older adults and in those with AIDS and Crohn's disease. The following laboratory values are below normal ranges: hemoglobin, hematocrit, serum iron, and TIBC. However, the MCV and ferritin level are normal (5).

Box 10.3 illustrates the pattern of laboratory values typically seen in anemia of chronic disease. This pattern of test results suggests that the body is unable to absorb and use iron from food and mineral supplements.

A multivitamin supplement with iron or oral iron therapy may be ordered but should be carefully monitored for expected outcomes. In cases of true anemia of chronic disease, the body will not be able to absorb these additional nutrients and significantly improve the anemia. Anemia of chronic disease associated with end-stage renal disease and congestive heart failure may be treated effectively using endogenous erythropoietin (1).

Megaloblastic Anemia

Macrocytic anemias include megaloblastic anemia (folate deficiency) and pernicious anemia (vitamin B-12 deficiency). Both are normochromic and commonly seen in older adults.

Megaloblastic anemia is a folate deficiency most commonly seen in older adults. It has been associated with an increased risk for heart disease and end-stage renal disease, because of the association with elevated homocysteine levels (16-18). Megaloblastic anemia occurs after approximately 5 months of folate depletion. It may be due to increased needs, a deficient diet, malabsorption of folate, or a vitamin B-12 deficiency.

In addition, some medications are folate antagonists and interfere with nucleic acid synthesis. Box 10.4 lists the most common folate antagonists. Decreased folate levels are associated with megaloblastic anemia, hemolytic anemia, malnutrition,

---

Box 10.3 Laboratory Test Results for Anemia of Chronic Disease

↓ Hgb

↓ Hct

⇔ MCV

↓ Serum Fe

↓ TIBC

⇔ Ferritin

Key: low, ↓; normal ⇔.

Abbreviations: Fe, iron; Hct, hematocrit; Hgb, hemoglobin; MCV, mean corpuscular volume; TIBC, total iron-binding capacity.

Box 10.4 Medications That Are Folate Antagonists

- Allopurinol
- Aspirin
- Colchicine
- Hydrocortisone
- Phenobarbital
- Phenytoin
- Sulfasalazine
- Sulfamethoxazole
- Triamterene
- Trimethoprim

---

malabsorption syndromes, liver disease, and celiac disease. A vitamin B-12 deficiency will eventually cause a folate deficiency, because folate cannot be converted into an active form without vitamin B-12 (19-27).

Megaloblastic anemia is categorized as a macrocytic normochromic anemia. The initial clinical signs and symptoms of megaloblastic anemia are low levels of hemoglobin, hematocrit, and serum folate. However, elevated values are seen in serum iron, mean corpuscular volume, ferritin, and homocysteine (5,7). Box 10.5 illustrates the pattern of laboratory values typically seen in megaloblastic anemia.

The megaloblastic erythropoiesis is usually caused by impaired DNA, RNA, and/or protein synthesis. The result is abnormal cellular development and maturation. The RBCs have shortened life spans and reduced capacity to carry hemoglobin. Iron is absorbed by the body and stored as serum iron or ferritin rather than in hemoglobin. Once the folate deficiency is addressed through pharmacologic intervention, the iron stores from the serum iron and ferritin will shift back to the RBCs, and the hemoglobin and hematocrit will return to normal levels. Homocysteine levels may or may not return to normal levels with folate supplementation.

Pernicious Anemia

Pernicious anemia is a vitamin B-12 deficiency most commonly seen in older adults. It is associated with numbness of the hands and feet and with significant cognitive changes. Permanent nerve lining damage results from a B-12 deficiency.

A lack of dietary B-12 or an underuse of B-12 usually causes pernicious anemia. The most common etiology is due to a gastric mucosa defect, resulting in inadequate secretion of intrinsic factor (IF). When B-12 is ingested, it combines with IF and is absorbed in the distal part of the ileum. Without IF, B-12 cannot be absorbed, body stores are depleted, and the body produces enlarged, immature RBCs. It is categorized as a macrocytic normochromic anemia; however, about 40% of the cases are normocytic (10,28-30).

The laboratory values for pernicious anemia are very similar to megaloblastic anemia. Lower than normal values are seen for hemoglobin, hematocrit, and serum B-12. However, elevated levels are seen in serum iron, serum folate, ferritin, and homocysteine. MCV may be elevated or normal. The only definitive laboratory test is methyl malonic acid, which is elevated in B-12 deficiency and normal in megaloblastic anemia. Because the methyl malonic acid test is available in only a few laboratories in the United States, diagnosis is typically done without it (31,32).

Box 10.6 illustrates the pattern of laboratory values typically seen in pernicious anemia. Some medications are associated with lower than normal B-12 levels. These medications are listed on Box 10.7.

Treatment for pernicious anemia is based on the etiology of the anemia. Oral B-12 supplements are effective if the body can produce adequate levels of intrinsic factor. However, if the body is unable to produce intrinsic factor, then monthly injections of B-12 are recommended.

Box 10.5 Laboratory Test Results for Megaloblastic Anemia

↓ Hgb
↓ Hct
↑ MCV
↑ Serum Fe
↑ Ferritin
↓ or ⇔ Serum B-12
↓ Folate
↑ Hcy
⇔ MMA

Key: elevated, ↑; low, ↓; normal ⇔.

Abbreviations: Fe, iron; Hct, hematocrit; Hcy, homocysteine; Hgb, hemoglobin; MCV, mean corpuscular volume; MMA, methylmalonic acid.

Box 10.6 Laboratory Test Results for Pernicious Anemia

↓ Hgb
↓ Hct
↑ or ⇔ MCV
↑ Serum Fe
↑ Ferritin
↓ Serum B-12
↑ Folate
↑ Hcy
⇔ MMA

Key: elevated, ↑; low, ↓; normal ⇔.

Abbreviations: Fe, iron; Hct, hematocrit; Hcy, homocysteine; Hgb, hemoglobin; MCV, mean corpuscular volume; MMA, methylmalonic acid.

IMPLICATIONS FOR PRACTICE

Anemias are commonly seen in older adults. However, no anemic state is too trivial to investigate. It is important to identify the underlying cause before effective therapy can be administered. Because symptoms are common to different kinds of anemias,

Box 10.7 Medications Associated With Low B-12 Levels

- Allopurinol
- Cimetidine
- Phenobarbital
- Phenytoin
- Primidone

laboratory assessment is essential. Reevaluation of intervention strategies is important to determine whether the plan is working or whether the anemia is an early symptom of another disease process.

REFERENCES

1. Andrews NC. Disorders of iron metabolism. *N Engl J Med.* 1999;341:38-46.
2. Looker AC, Dallman PR, Carroll MD, Gunter EW, Johnson CL. Prevalence of iron deficiency in the United States. *JAMA.* 1997;277:973-976.
3. Rockey DC. Occult gastrointestinal bleeding. *N Engl J Med.* 1999;341:38-46.
4. Abrams WB, Beers MH, Berkow R, eds. *The Merck Manual of Geriatrics.* 3rd ed. Whitehouse Station, NJ: Merck Research Laboratories; 1995.
5. Litchford MD. *Practical Applications in Laboratory Assessment of Nutritional Status.* Greensboro, NC: CASE Software; 2002.
6. Blackwell S, Hendrix P. Common anemias: what lies beneath. *Clinician Rev.* 2001;11:53-62.
7. Pagana KD, Pagana TJ. *Mosby's Diagnostic and Laboratory Test Reference.* St. Louis, Mo: Mosby; 2002.
8. Fischbach F. *A Manual of Laboratory and Diagnostic Tests.* 5th ed. Philadelphia, Pa: Lippincott Co; 1996.
9. Corbett JV. *Laboratory Tests and Diagnostic Procedures With Nursing Diagnosis.* Stamford, Conn: Appleton and Lange; 2000.
10. Carmel R. Prevalence of undiagnosed pernicious anemia in the elderly. *Arch Int Med.* 1996;156:1097-1100.
11. Ahluwalia N, Lammi-Keefe CJ, Bendel RB, Morse EE, Beard JL, Haley NR. Iron-deficiency anemia of chronic disease in elderly women: a discriminant analysis approach for differentiation. *Am J Clin Nutr.* 1995;61:590-596.
12. Coulter JS. Red blood cell distribution width and mean corpuscular volume: clinical applications. *Adv Clin Care.* 1991;6(6):13.
13. Massey AC. Microcytic anemia: differential diagnosis and management of iron deficiency anemia. *Med Clin North Am.* 1992;76:549-566.
14. Provan D. Mechanism and management of iron deficiency anemia. *Br J Haematol.* 1999;105(suppl 1):19S-26S.
15. Shine JW. Microcytic anemia. *Am Fam Phys.* 1997;55:2455-2462.
16. Morrison HI, Schaubel D, Desmeules M, Wigle DT. Serum folate and risk of fatal coronary heart disease. *JAMA.* 1996;275:1893-1896.
17. Pancharuniti N, Lewis C, Sauberlich H. Plasma homocysteine, folate, and vitamin B12 concentrations and risk for early onset coronary artery disease. *Am J Clin Nutr.* 1994;59:940-948.
18. Robinson K, Gupta A, Dennis V, Arheart K, Chaudhary D, Green R, Vigo P, Mayer EL, Selhub J, Kutner M, Jacobsen DW. Hyperhomocystinemia confers an independent increased risk of atherosclerosis in end-stage renal disease and is closely linked to plasma folate and pyridoxine concentrations. *Circulation.* 1996;94:2743-2748.
19. Bostom AG, Shemin D, Lapane KL, Nadeau MR, Sutherland P, Chan J, Rozen R, Yoburn D, Jacques PF, Selhub J, Rosenberg IH. Folate status is the major determinant of fasting total plasma homocysteine levels in maintenance dialysis patients. *Atherosclerosis.* 1996;123:193-202.
20. Guttormsen AB, Schneede J, Ueland PM, Refsum H. Kinetics of total plasma homocysteine in subjects with hyperhomocystinemia due to folate or cobalamin deficiency. *Am J Clin Nutr.* 1996;63:194-202.
21. Hine RJ. What practitioners need to know about folic acid. *J Am Diet Assoc.* 1996;96:451-452.
22. Joosten E, van den Berg A, Riezler R, Naurath HJ, Lindenbaum J, Stabler SP, Allen RH. Metabolic evidence that deficiencies of vitamin B-12 (cobalamin), folate, and vitamin B-6 occur commonly in elderly people [correction in *Am J Clin Nutr.* 1994;60:147]. *Am J Clin Nutr.* 1993;58:468-476.
23. Koehler KM, Pareo-Tubbeh SL, Romero LJ, Baumgartner RN, Garry PJ. Folate nutrition and older adults: challenges and opportunities. *J Am Diet Assoc.* 1997;97:167-173.
24. Lewis CA, Pancharuniti N, Sauberlich H. Plasma folate adequacy as determined by homocysteine level. *Ann NY Acad Sci.* 1992;669:360-362.
25. Makoff R, Dwyer J, Rocco MV. Folic acid, pyridoxine, cobalamin, and homocysteine and their relationship to cardiovascular disease in end-stage renal disease. *J Ren Nutr.* 1996;6:2-11.
26. O'Keefe CA, Bailey LB, Thomas EA, Hofler SA, Davis BA, Cerda JJ, Gregory JF 3rd. Controlled dietary folate affects folate status in nonpregnant women. *J Nutr.* 1995;125:2717-2725.
27. Tucker KL, Selhub J, Wilson PW, Rosenberg IH. Dietary intake pattern relates to plasma folate and homocysteine concentrations in the Framingham Heart Study. *J Nutr.* 1996;126:3025-3031.
28. Allen RH, Stabler SP, Savage DG, Lindenbaum J. Diagnosis of cobalamin deficiency I: usefulness of serum methylmalonic acid and total homocysteine concentrations. *Am J Hematol.* 1990;34:90-98.
29. Pennypacker LC, Allen RH, Kelly JP, Matthews LM, Grigsby J, Kaye K, Lindenbaum J, Stabler SP. High prevalence of cobalamin deficiency in elderly outpatients. *J Am Geriatr Soc.* 1992;40:1197-1204.

30. Prentice AG, Evans IL. Megaloblastic anemia with normal MCV. *Lancet.* 1979;1:1606-1607.

31. Van Asselt DZ, Van den Broek WJ, Lamers CB, Corstens FH, Hoefnagels WH. Free and protein-bound cobalamin absorption in healthy middle-aged and older subjects. *J Am Geriatr Soc.* 1996;44:949-953.

32. Savage DG, Lindenbaum J, Stabler SP, Allen RH. Sensitivity of serum methylmalonic acid and total homocysteine determinations for diagnosing cobalamin and folate deficiencies. *Am J Med.* 1994;96:239-246.

ADDITIONAL RESOURCES

Izaka GJ, Westendorp RG, Knook DL. The definition of anemia in older persons. *JAMA.* 1999;281:2247-2248.

Melillo KD. Interpretation of laboratory values in older adults. *Nurse Pract.* 1993;18:59-67.

Smith DL. Anemia in the elderly. *Am Fam Phys.* 2000;62:1565-1572.

Stabler SP. Screening the older population for cobalamin (vitamin B-12) deficiency. *J Am Geriatr Soc.* 1995;43:1290-1297.

Yao Y, Yao SL. Prevalence of vitamin B12 deficiency among geriatric outpatients. *J Fam Pract.* 1992;35:524-528, 1992.

CHAPTER
11

Neurological Diseases

AMYOTROPHIC LATERAL SCLEROSIS

Amyotrophic lateral sclerosis (ALS), or Lou Gehrig's disease, is a classic motor neuron disease. It is a progressive, chronic disease, and it is fatal. It affects the nerves leading from the spinal cord, which is responsible for supplying electrical stimulation to the muscles. The average age for onset of the disease is 55 years; however, 80% of cases begin between the ages of 40 and 70 years, with men more often affected than women. Fifty percent of those with the disease die within 18 months of diagnosis (1).

Signs and symptoms of ALS include loss of motor functions, tripping, stumbling, loss of strength, difficulty with speech, difficulty swallowing and breathing, muscle twitching and cramping, and chronic fatigue. Upper-limb symptoms include shaking, muscle twitching, and stiffness. The lower limbs often have muscle weakness and atrophy (1,2).

Treatment measures in those diagnosed with motor neuron diseases are largely supportive, treating the complications, such as infections and general health. The treatment of ALS is also directed toward suppressing the immune inflammation, which is assumed to play a role in the degeneration of the nervous system in those diagnosed. Although there is no cure for ALS and no proven therapy that will prevent or reverse the disorder, riluzole (Rilutek) has been approved by the Food and Drug Administration and has been shown to prolong the survival of those with ALS (3).

As with many chronic diseases, good nutrition is not always easy to maintain in ALS patients. Many lose weight in the early stages of the disease because of the loss of muscle mass, depression, and overall inactivity (4). A multivitamin supplement can be taken but should include no more than 100% of the dietary reference intake (DRI) (4). Additional supplementation has been a focus of interest in

some recent research (5), but more studies are needed to prove any hypothesis and before recommending megadoses of any vitamin or mineral.

Urinary tract infections and constipation can affect individuals with ALS. These problems occur as the older adult becomes weak and has more difficulty eating solid foods and drinking thin liquids. Lower fiber intake and the potential for dehydration also result. Chronic dehydration can cause even further weakness, fatigue, and difficulty swallowing, due to thickening of saliva. It is important for dietetics professionals to educate caregivers and clients on the need for increased fluids and fiber, as tolerated, in the diet (5,6). The use of adaptive eating devices should be considered if weakness begins to hinder self-feeding. Lightweight glasses and deep-welled plates may lessen frustration and promote a sense of pride in maintaining independence while eating (see Chapter 23).

When dysphagia occurs, altered food and fluid consistency may be desirable. Tube feeding may be necessary as the disease progresses. A thorough discussion of the pros and cons of this method of nutrition should be reviewed with the client. All caregivers should honor the client's wishes regarding nutrition support and advance directives.

MULTIPLE SCLEROSIS

Multiple sclerosis (MS) is an autoimmune neurological disease associated with inflammation and scarring of the myelin sheaths, the insulating material surrounding nerve fibers of the central and peripheral nervous systems. The disease is generally progressive, and the cause is still unknown (7).

MS mainly affects young adults, with onset usually occurring somewhere between 20 and 40 years of age and peak incidence at age 30. The incidence in women is generally higher than in men (3:2 ratio), but men, in general, tend to experience a more debilitating form of the disease. MS occurs in whites twice as often as in blacks; it rarely occurs in Asians (8,9). Signs and symptoms include weakness, numbness, fatigue, tremor, stiffness, muscle spasms, pain, dizziness, double vision, clumsiness, and cognitive impairment. Secondary conditions may also surface and may include bowel problems, loss of sense of position resulting in decreased ambulation, and pressure ulcers. Reduced appetite and dysphagia are common but usually do not cause nutritional failure. However, they do affect nutritional status and quality of life (9,10).

Studies from as early as the 1950s have suggested that high consumption of saturated fat may be involved in the etiology and course of MS, because lipids are the main component of the myelin sheath (11). The most recent research completed by the Nurses' Health Study found no differences between intake of specific types of fat and the risk for the disease (12). Studies have instead implicated proinflammatory cytokines, pathological iron deposition, and oxidative stress in the pathogenesis of MS (13).

Because the cure for MS has not been found, those with the disease often seek alternative methods that promise alleviation of symptoms or delay of the disease's progression. This may cause them to make poor choices regarding nutrition. Presently, there is insufficient research to establish precise energy and protein requirements for those with MS. Dietetics professionals should work with MS clients to maintain a healthy weight, using a diet of approximately 55% of total energy from carbohydrates, 15% to 20% from protein sources, and 25% from fat, with most from polyunsaturated fatty acids (PUFA) (9). This diet will be easier to implement in those clients who are cared for in nursing facilities. Most residents will be provided a general diet, with texture modification as appropriate when needed. Higher-fiber options can also be incorporated, as the need to alleviate constipation occurs.

GUILLAIN-BARRÉ SYNDROME

Guillain-Barré syndrome is a disorder caused by nerve inflammation involving progressive muscle weakness or paralysis, which often follows an infectious illness, especially an acute respiratory or gastrointestinal illness. The exact cause of the syndrome is not known. The signs of the infection that had been treated are usually gone before the signs of Guillain-Barré begin. The inflammation damages portions of the nerve cells, resulting in muscle weakness or paralysis and sensory loss. The damage usually includes loss of the myelin sheath of the nerve that slows conduction of impulses through the nerve (6,14).

Signs and symptoms usually include weakness, which starts in the distal lower extremities, and ascends to arms, trunk, face, and head. In 10% to 30% of cases, there may be severe weakness, resulting in clients having paralysis, unstable blood pressure, and difficulty chewing and swallowing; some have severe dysphagia, anorexia, and weight loss (15,16).

Nutrition goals include maintaining usual body weight and preventing malnutrition. Diet texture may need to be modified, and a vitamin/mineral supplement provided if intake is poor. In some acute cases, enteral or parenteral feeding may be necessary (9).

PARKINSON'S DISEASE

Parkinson's disease (PD) is a slow, progressive chronic disease of the nervous system that affects the neurons in the substantia nigra area of the brain. The condition involves the decrease in the production of the substance dopamine, which coordinates muscle movement. Approximately 1 million people in the United States are affected by the disease; 60% of those with PD are more than 60 years of age (9,17-19).

Causes of PD are unclear. Some researchers hypothesize that environmental factors may influence development of the disease (20). Environmental factors implicated in the etiology of PD include intravenous drug use, dietary lipids, antioxidants, and geographic variation (ie, a greater incidence in industrialized countries).

PD is a very individualized disease. It manifests in a range of primary and secondary symptoms that affect people uniquely and to varying degrees (Box 11.1).

Nutrition goals include improving fiber intake and reducing constipation, maintaining hydration status, assessing for dysphagia and gastrointestinal problems, providing adequate energy to prevent weight loss or excessive gain due to lack of physical activity, adjusting/redistribution of protein to the evening meal or snack, and preventing bone thinning and vitamin D deficiency (21).

Use of Low-Protein or Adjusted-Protein Diets

In a very small percentage of the PD population, adjusting protein levels can be an effective treatment to allow for better mobility (6). This approach should not be considered unless a thorough assessment is completed and a comprehensive plan is formulated in conjunction with the client's physician (22).

The use of protein-adjusted diets may be appropriate when the client is prescribed a medication that

Box 11.1   Symptoms of Parkinson's Disease

Primary symptoms

- Bradykinesia
- Postural instability
- Rigidity
- Tremor

Secondary symptoms

- Bone thinning with vitamin D deficiency
- Constipation
- Dehydration
- Delay in gastric motility
- Dementia
- Depression
- Drooling
- Lack of facial expression
- Medication side effects
- Sleep disturbances
- Swallowing difficulty
- Weight loss

contains levodopa (ie, Sinemet, Sinemet CR, Laro-dopa, Madopar). Levodopa is absorbed in the small intestine and reaches peak plasma concentration in 30 minutes to 2 hours. Controlled-release products have extended the uptake to 60 to 150 minutes. The extent of absorption depends on the timing of gastric emptying and, to some extent, the contents of the food consumed. Levodopa medications compete with various amino acids for absorption (isoleukine, leukine, valine, phenylalanine, tryptophan, tyrosine), and, therefore, the rationale for the diet is to keep protein intake low throughout the day when more movement is desired. Levodopa has a very short plasma half-life and is absorbed in the small intestine. Delayed gastric emptying also needs to be considered. Protein should still be consumed at the suggested level of 0.8 to 1.0 g/kg for older adults (22). Timing of the medications is an important factor. Taking the drug 15 to 30 minutes before a meal is often sufficient to allow the balance between timing and absorption. If nausea occurs, a small low-protein snack can be given with the medication (21,23).

The assessment needed to institute this regimen needs to be comprehensive, with attention given to timing of meals, bowel movements, gastric symptoms, types of foods, and an explanation of the movements that the patient does or does not experience. The client must be guided in proper reporting of these data in a systematic manner. A chart-type format, where times, outcomes, and symptoms are recorded, should be provided, and data should be collected in 3- to 5-day periods. Correlation between client "on-off" movement times and factors such as bowel movements, meal times, medication times, and gastrointestinal distress may provide insight into diet content and timing adjustment, which may improve the client's quality of life (21).

Combining levodopa with carbidopa (Sinemet) represents a significant improvement in the treatment of PD. The addition of carbidopa prevents levodopa from being metabolized in the gut, liver, and other tissues and allows more of it to get to the brain. Therefore, a smaller dose of levodopa is needed to treat symptoms. In addition, the severe nausea and vomiting often associated with levodopa treatment are greatly reduced (24). The health care provider should consider whether the client is taking a carbidopa/levodopa medication.

Pyridoxine, Aspartame, and Levodopa

Pyridoxine (vitamin B-6) has been demonstrated to possibly reverse the effects of levodopa by increasing the rate of aromatic amino acid decarboxylation (6). Attention needs to be given to vitamin supplementation and to the intake of foods high in B-6. These foods include bananas, lima beans, whole-grain cereals, egg yolks, peanuts, and meat. It is not suggested that B-6 be eliminated or consumed at levels below usual recommendations but that unusually high intakes, seen often in those who self-administer vitamin supplements, be evaluated as part of the total assessment process (25). Because of the phenylalanine component of aspartame and its competition for absorptive sites with the medication, aspartame should be evaluated for limitation (26).

Other Research

Numerous studies evaluate how various nutrient intakes may be involved in the onset and the treatment of PD, but some of this research is unscientific or only preliminary (27,28). Such studies should not be the basis for promoting changes in dietary patterns that may not be appropriate for the nutritional health of the person with PD.

REFERENCES

1. ALS fact sheet. ALS Survival Guide. Available at: http://www.lougehrigsdisease.net/als_pages/als_fact_sheet.htm. Accessed March 12, 2004.

2. ALSlinks.com Internet Portal for the ALS Community. Available at: http://www.alslinks.com/alsdefined.htm. Accessed March 12, 2004.

3. Treatment for ALS, approved drugs. ALS Survival Guide. Available at: http://www.lougehrigsdisease.net/als_treatments.htm#Approved%20Drugs. Accessed March 12, 2004.

4. Lewis S. Nutrition and ALS. The ALS Association, Florida Chapter. Available at: http://www.als-florida.org/version1/Nutrition.html. Accessed March 12, 2004.

5. Treatment for ALS: nutrition. ALS Survival Guide. Available at: http://www.lougehrigsdisease.net/als_treatments.htm#Nutrition. Accessed March 12, 2004.

6. Mahar K, Escott-Stump S. *Krause's Food Nutrition and Diet Therapy*. 11th ed. San Diego, Calif: Elsevier Science; 2003.

7. National Multiple Sclerosis Society. About MS: what causes MS. Available at: http://www.nationalmssociety.org/What%20causes%20MS.asp. Accessed March 12, 2004.

8. National Multiple Sclerosis Society. Who gets MS? Available at: http://www.nationalmssociety.org/Who%20gets%20MS.asp. Accessed March 12, 2004.

9. Escott-Stump S. *Nutrition and Diagnosis Related Care*. 5th ed. Baltimore, Md: Lippincott, Williams, and Wilkins; 2002.

10. National Multiple Sclerosis Society. Symptoms. Available at: http://www.nationalmssociety.org/Symptoms.asp. Accessed March 12, 2004.

11. Zhang SM, Willlettt WC, Hernan MA, Olek MJ, Ascherio A. Dietary fat in relation to risk of multiple sclerosis among two large cohorts of women. *Am J Epidemiol*. 2000;152:1056-1064.

12. Zhang SM, Hernan MA, Chen H, Spiegelman D, Willett WC, Ascherio A. Intakes of vitamins E and C, carotenoids, vitamin supplements, and PD risk. *Neurology*. 2002;59:1161-1169.

13. Mehindate K, Sahlas DJ, Frankel D, Mawal Y, Liberman A, Corcos J, Dion S, Schipper HM. Proinflammatory cytokines promote glial heme oxygenase-1 expression and mitochondrial iron deposition: implications for multiple sclerosis. *J Neurochem*. 2001;77:1386-1395.

14. NINDS Guillain-Barre Syndrome Information Page. Available at: http://www.ninds.nih.gov/health_and_medical/disorders/gbs.htm. Accessed April 27, 2004.

15. National Chronic Care Consortium Web site. Available at: http://www.ncconline.org. Accessed April 27, 2004.

16. National Organization for Rare Disorders. Guillain Barre syndrome. Available at: http://www.rarediseases.org/search/rdbdetail_abstract.html?disname=Guillain%20Barre%20Syndrome. Accessed April 27, 2004.

17. National Organization for Rare Disorders. Parkinson's Disease. Available at: http://www.rarediseases.org/search/rdbdetail_abstract.html?disname=Parkinson%27s%20Disease. Accessed April 27, 2004.

18. Parkinson's Disease Foundation. Parkinson's disease: an overview. Available at: http://www.pdf.org/AboutPD. Accessed March 27, 2004.

19. Parkinson's Action Network. What is Parkinson's disease? Available at: http://www.parkinsonsaction.org/aboutparkinsons/whatisparkinsons.htm. Accessed April 27, 2004.

20. National Institute of Neurological Disorders and Stroke. Parkinson's disease backgrounder. Available at: http://www.ninds.nih.gov/health_and_medical/pubs/parkinson's_disease_backgrounder.htm. Accessed March 12, 2004.

21. Riley D. Diet and nutrition in Parkinson's disease (Living with Parkinson's Disease Web site). Available at: http://www.parkinsonsdisease.com/lwp/lwp.htm. Accessed April 27, 2004.

22. Karstaedt PJ, Pincus JH. Protein redistribution diet remains effective in patients with fluctuating Parkinsonism. *Arch Neurol*. 1992;49:149-151.

23. Parkinson's Organization. Summary points regarding dopaminergic therapy. Available at: http://www.parkinson.org/med20.htm. Accessed April 27, 2004.

24. Parkinson's Disease Foundation. Medications for Parkinson's. Available at: http://www.pdf.org/AboutPD/med_treatment.cfm. Accessed April 27, 2004.

25. Holden K. Parkinson's, B6, B12, and folate—what's the connection? Available at: http://www.parkinson.org/bvitamin.htm. Accessed April 27, 2004.

26. Food and Drug Administration. Available at: http://www.fda.gov/ohrms/dockets/dailys/03/Jan03/012203/02P-0317_emc-000201.txt. Accessed April 27, 2004.

27. National Institute of Neurological Disorders and Stroke. Parkinson's disease: hope through research—can diet or exercise programs help relieve symptoms? Available at: http://www.ninds.nih.gov/health_and_medical/pubs/parkinson_disease_htr.htm#diet. Accessed April 27, 2004.

28. The National Parkinson Foundation. Nutritional considerations of Parkinson's disease. Available at: http://www.parkinson.org/Nutrit.htm. Accessed April 27, 2004.

OTHER RESOURCES

ALS Survival Guide. Available at: http://www.lougehrigsdisease.net. Accessed March 12, 2004.

Bine JE, Frank EM, McDade HL. Dysphagia and dementia in subjects with Parkinson's disease. *Dysphagia*. 1995;10:160-164.

Cushing ML, Traviss KA, Calne SM. Parkinson's disease: implications for nutritional care. *Can J Diet Pract Res*. 2002;63:81-87.

Fats of Life Newsletter. Available at: http://www.pufanewsletter.com. Accessed July 13, 2003.

Guillain-Barré Syndrome Foundation International Web site. Available at: http://www.guillain-barre.com. Accessed April 30, 2004.

Holden K. *Parkinson's Disease: Guidelines for Medical Nutrition Therapy for Use by Nutrition Professionals*. Fort Collins, Colo: Five Star Living; 2002.

Holden K, Remig VM. *Parkinson's Disease: Assessing and Managing Unique Nutritional Needs.* Chicago, Ill: American Dietetic Association; 1999.

Johnson CC, Gorell JM, Rybicki BA, Sanders K, Peterson EL. Adult nutrient intake as a risk factor for Parkinson's disease. *Int J Epidemiol.* 1999;28:1102-1109.

National Multiple Sclerosis Society Web site. Available at: http://www.nmss.org. Accessed March 12, 2004.

Ross GW, Abbott RD, Petrovitch H, Morens DM, Grandinetti A, Tung KH, Tanner CM, Masaki KH, Blanchette PL, Curb JD, Popper JS, White LR. Association of coffee and caffeine intake with the risk of Parkinson disease. *JAMA.* 2000;283:2674-2679.

CHAPTER
12
Dementia

ISSUES IN DEMENTIA

Dementia may be defined as a loss of memory, cognitive reasoning, awareness of environment, judgment, abstract thinking, and the ability to perform usual tasks associated with self-care and day-to-day function. As the population ages, the prevalence of dementia will become an increasing burden on the health care system. Because life expectancy has increased to nearly twice what it was a century ago, the incidence of dementia appears to be increasing (1-3). Older adults are more likely to demonstrate loss of cognitive function as they live longer (1-3).

Dementia may be difficult to diagnose, because of the variability of symptoms at onset as well as the many possible etiologies that may lead to atypical behavior. Although there may be some consistency among usual changes in behavior with dementia, it is still challenging to determine the underlying pathology, because diagnostic tests are not as accurate or definitive as they could be. One of the challenges that many health professionals encounter is that of distinguishing among depression, delirium, and dementia. Most health professionals are not aware of how common depression is among older adults. It can be treated, but first it must be diagnosed (4).

Depressed individuals often experience memory impairment but demonstrate intact cognitive function and appropriate language skills for their age. Delirium is frequently a rapid-onset condition of short duration associated with some disorientation and variable recall of events. Dementia tends to be progressive, with disorientation, aphasia, and memory loss that may include loss of recognition of food versus nonfood items, forgetting how to use utensils, forgetting to swallow chewed foods, and so on. Depression and delirium are transient, treatable conditions and should be treated with appropriate interventions as soon as the condition is diagnosed (5-7).

Some dementias are reversible, particularly those that are nutrition related. If dementia is suspected, the first step in intervention should be a trial of replacing deficient nutrients and observing whether there is an improvement in cognitive function. This is a reasonable strategy that does not cost much and is noninvasive; response to treatment (medication or nutrient supplementation) usually occurs in a short time frame. Dementia caused by brain pathology is not reversible and responds poorly and unpredictably to medication (5,8).

Before an individual is diagnosed with dementia, a condition known as mild cognitive impairment (MCI) may be apparent (9). Individuals with MCI may complain about memory problems, but they generally score well on diagnostic tests, such as evaluation of activities of daily living (the ability to care for self) and the mini-mental state examination, a standardized test of cognition (10). Clients who demonstrate symptoms of MCI have a higher risk for developing Alzheimer's disease (9). Early diagnosis can contribute to early intervention, which may be helpful for individuals who have reversible forms of dementia.

There are many etiologies for dementia, but most contribute to the loss of intellectual function, memory impairment, loss of judgment, and personality changes. Dementia tends to be progressive and is often irreversible. However, there are dementias that can be resolved with treatment of the underlying disease process. Reversible causes of dementia include central nervous system infection; brain trauma or tumors; multi-infarct dementia related to chronic cerebrovascular disease; normal pressure hydrocephalus; Wernicke-Korsakoff syndrome; vitamin-deficiency diseases; and neurological disorders, such as multiple sclerosis, Huntington's disease, Parkinson's disease, and others (11).

Diagnosing dementia as early in its development as possible allows for aggressive intervention that may slow the progression of disease (11). The two most common and irreversible causes of dementia are vascular disease and Alzheimer's disease (12). Vascular dementia has been described as the second most common type of dementia in older adults (13). Because the two leading causes of morbidity and mortality are related to vascular disease, stroke, and ischemic heart disease, it is possible that vascular disease is also a factor in other dementias as well. Large-vessel disease in the brain is associated with multi-infarct dementia, where there is a progressive loss of tissue. Small-vessel disease usually leads to lacunar strokes (12). Cardiovascular diseases, particularly coronary artery bypass grafts (CABG) associated with the use of cardiopulmonary bypass machines, and congestive heart failure are also associated with progressive dementia. Patients with CABG may develop dementia from emboli associated with their surgery. Emboli may occur because of bubbles from nitrous oxide or anesthetic gases or because of thrombi from the vessels in the heart; emboli may also be fat or inorganic. There may be more dementia related to vascular disease than is currently being diagnosed (12).

The most common form of dementia is Alzheimer's disease. The progression of this type of dementia is variable, and symptoms may develop at different rates among individuals (14). Exploration of the physiologic etiology and processes of Alzheimer's disease is active and continues to identify characteristics, such as the presence of Lewy bodies (characteristic eosinophilic structures in neuron cytoplasm) (15), which may offer information that will result in prevention or treatment of this terrible disease. Acetyl cholinesterase inhibitors, nonsteroidal anti-inflammatory drugs, hormones, vitamins, and herbal remedies have been tried to inhibit the progression of the disease (16,17). Although some of these remedies hold promise, carefully controlled, conclusive clinical trials have not yet been reported.

Recently, a newer syndrome, called mixed dementia, has been identified. It seems to have pathologies and manifestations of both vascular dementia and Alzheimer's disease (18). Virtually all the current literature strongly asserts that additional research is essential to determine the etiology of dementia, its diagnosis, and treatment modalities that slow or stop progression of the disease, or at the very least, permit a greater quality of life for those who develop dementia in later life (17).

REASONS FOR CONCERN

Losses associated with dementia may include decreased or abnormal senses of smell and taste, which manifest as olfactory or oral hallucinations in which food smells rotten or tastes burnt. Those with dementia may lose their ability to recognize food, and nonfood items that are visually appealing (eg, flowers, plants, brightly colored paper objects) may be consumed. Individuals with dementia may lack memory of what utensils are for and how they are appropriately used; they may also exhibit abnormal or lost perceptions of other objects or hazards in the environment that may cause them injury or harm. In advanced dementia, individuals may forget that they have eaten recently, consume nonfood items, chew and forget to swallow, pocket food, spit food out, or demonstrate other unusual eating behaviors (19,20).

Those with dementia may also demonstrate significant changes in body weight. Although there have been many theories about why this happens, there are presently no clear explanations. It has been hypothesized that there is a change in metabolism associated with dementia, but no one has been able to demonstrate this in a controlled environment (21-27). Some individuals may develop pacing or wandering behaviors that contribute to an increase in energy expenditure; others may become more sedentary and not require as many calories for energy. Some medications cause loss of appetite; others cause an increase in appetite. Some drugs may have adverse gastrointestinal side effects. It is difficult to categorize changes that occur with dementias without recognizing that each individual has a unique symptomatology and must be treated accordingly.

Eating behavior may be sporadic, unpredictable, and unusual. It is best to have meals associated with a low-stress environment, where noise and visual stimulation are kept to a minimum. A quiet, well-lit room without too many people around will minimize mealtime stress and distraction. Developing a routine that can be sustained over time will be a first step to successful meals. Many dementia clients have a very short attention span; although it is time consuming and labor intensive, having one person spend the mealtime with an uninterrupted feeding schedule may contribute to an increase in food consumption in those whose attention drifts easily. Even developing a routine meal pattern with similar and familiar foods every day may serve as a cue for those with dementia to eat. Families often report that their loved one will eat when a member of the family is there to assist them; this may be associated with a sense of familiarity with the family member and the undivided attention provided in this situation (28).

When those with dementia demonstrate behaviors such as repetitive chewing, pocketing foods, or an unwillingness to allow someone to assist them, a skillful staff can overcome some of these behaviors. Speech pathologists who are experts in swallowing disorders can help teach some of the necessary skills to staff responsible for assisting clients (see Chapter 23) (7).

Some individuals with memory loss may not recall having eaten and may look for additional food between meals. When this pattern emerges, dividing meals into small portions to create six or eight smaller meals may help the client to maintain a sense of control over his environment as well as to prevent an unintended weight gain. A similar strategy of providing snacks or small meals between regularly scheduled mealtimes may also contribute to maintaining weight in agitated older adults or those who demonstrate pacing or wandering behaviors (7).

It is important for the health professional to be aware when an unusual event occurs to a dementia client. Fevers, infection, injuries, influenza, and other illnesses may increase the need for energy, protein, and fluid. Choosing higher-energy foods (eg, substituting whole milk for low-fat milk; adding cream to cooked breakfast cereals or mashed potatoes; adding butter or margarine to vegetables, soups, or casseroles) may be the simplest strategy to use in these cases. Offering between-meal frozen desserts, such as slushes or Popsicles, can be an effective way to increase fluid intake in a client with a fever. For dementia clients, immediate medical goals should take priority over long-term health concerns, such as managing blood lipid levels or other chronic conditions (except for diabetes or renal disease). A rational approach to dietary priorities is essential when caring for dementia clients.

In the advanced stages of dementia, older adults may become unaware of their surroundings and may require total care. For those who are no longer able to ingest food without risk of choking or aspiration, tube feeding may be considered if it is in accordance with advance directives. Nasogastric tubes may present a risk for these older adults, because they may pull at the tube, which can cause aspiration of formula into the lungs or injury to the esophageal, pharyngeal, laryngeal, or oral mucosa. Most decision makers opt for a gastrostomy for feeding, because it can be well anchored, offers easy access, and poses

the least risk to the client. Providing adequate energy, protein, vitamins, minerals, and fluid may be a challenge in tube-fed older adults. It is not unusual to have inadequate volumes of formula ordered, which do *not* meet the nutritional needs of an individual. Many formulations require 1,800 mL to provide 100% of the daily nutrient needs of older adults. It is important to read labels carefully and to select formulas that provide an adequate diet, including the best nutrient profile to meet the older adult's unique requirements. Tube feeding is not a benign procedure; it does require skilled nursing care to be safe and effective (29,30).

Starting an aggressive nutritional modality in a severely demented older adult does demand some thought as to the risks and benefits for the client. Tube feeding is often instituted without a plan that addresses goals for outcomes. These plans should be thoroughly discussed and formulated before tube insertion and with some consideration of the burden that may be placed on the older adult as well as the family and care providers. Serious consideration should be given to the costs, benefits, and burdens on older adults and caregivers if parenteral nutrition is raised as an option for feeding. Clear, short-term goals that are agreed on by all the decision makers (family, physician, nursing staff, dietetics professionals) are essential for successful parenteral intervention. This option is generally not recommended for terminally demented older adults (27).

SUMMARY
Providing adequate nutrition and appropriate feeding for older adults with dementia is a challenge in nursing facilities. Assessing the client's eating skills, including chewing and swallowing, interest in food, attention span, resources to support help with feeding, potential need for nutrition support, and prognosis, is essential to develop a rational care plan for maintaining or improving nutritional status.

REFERENCES

1. Berg RL, Cassells JS, eds. *The Second Fifty Years: Promoting Health and Preventing Disability,* Washington, DC: National Academy Press; 1990.
2. Volicer L. Management of severe Alzheimer's disease and end-of-life issues. *Clin Geriatr Med.* 2001;17:377-391.
3. Gonzalez-Gross M, Marcos A, Pietrzik K. Nutrition and cognitive impairment in the elderly. *Br J Nutr.* 2001;86:313-321.
4. Cegles KA. Psychosocial aspects of aging. In: Lewis CB, ed. *Aging: The Health Care Challenge.* 4th ed. Philadelphia, Pa: FA Davis; 2002:18-42.

5. Marcus DL, Freedman ML. The role of vitamin and mineral metabolism in cognition. *Clin Appl Nutr.* 1991;1:71-80.

6. Hall GR. Challenges in feeding patients with chronic dementia. *Clin Appl Nutr.* 1991;1:81-89.

7. Claggett MS. Nutritional factors relevant to Alzheimer's disease. *J Am Diet Assoc.* 1989;89:392-396.

8. Gray GE. Nutrition and dementia. *J Am Diet Assoc.* 1989;89:1795-1802.

9. Brandt J. Mild cognitive impairment [editorial]. *Am Fam Phys.* 2001;63:620-623.

10. Folstein MF, Folstein SE, McHugh PR. "Mini-mental state": a practical method for grading the cognitive state of patients for the clinician. *J Psychiatr Res.* 1975;12:196-198.

11. Santacruz KS, Swagerty D. Early diagnosis of dementia. *Am Fam Phys.* 2001;63:703-713, 717-718.

12. Dickson DW. Neuropathology of Alzheimer's disease and other dementias. *Clin Geriatr Med.* 2001;17:209-228.

13. Román GC. Vascular dementia may be the most common form of dementia in the elderly. *J Neurol Sci.* 2002;203-204:7-10.

14. Bianchetti A, Trabucch M. Clinical aspects of Alzheimer's disease. *Aging.* 2001;13:221-230.

15. Simard M, van Reekum R. Dementia with Lewy bodies in Down's syndrome. *Int J Geriatr Psychiatry.* 2001;16:311-320.

16. Schneider LS. Treatment of Alzheimer's disease with cholinesterase inhibitors. *Clin Geriatr Med.* 2001;17:337-358.

17. Grossberg GT, Desai AK. Management of Alzheimer's disease. *J Gerontol.* 2003;58A:331-353.

18. Zekry D, Hauw JJ, Gold G. Mixed dementia: epidemiology, diagnosis, and treatment. *J Am Geriatr Soc.* 2002;50:1431-1438.

19. White HK. Dementia. In Bales CW, Ritchie CS, eds. *Handbook of Clinical Nutrition and Aging.* Totowa, NJ: Humana Press; 2004:349-366.

20. Riviere S, Gillette-Guyonnet S, Andrieu S, Nourhashemi F, Lauque S, Cantet C, Salva A, Frisoni G, Vellas B. Cognitive function and caregiver burden: predictive factors for eating behaviour disorders in Alzheimer's disease. *Int J Geriatr Psychiatry.* 2002;17:950-955.

21. Poehlman ET. Regulation of energy expenditure in aging humans. *J Am Geriatr Soc.* 1993;41:552-559.

22. Niskanen L, Piirainen M, Koljonen M, Uusitupa M. Resting energy expenditure in relation to energy intake in patients with Alzheimer's disease, multiinfarct dementia and in control women. *Age Aging.* 1993;22:132-137.

23. Gillete-Guyonnet S, Nourhashemi F, Andrieu S, deGlisezinski I, Ousset PJ, Riviere D. Weight loss in Alzheimer's disease. *Am J Clin Nutr.* 2000;71(suppl):637S-647S.

24. Riviere S, Gillette-Guyonnet S, Nourhashemi F, Vellas B. Nutrition and Alzheimer's disease. *Nutr Rev.* 1999;57:363-367.

25. Poehlman ET, Dvorak RV. Energy expenditure in Alzheimer's disease. *J Nutr Health Aging.* 1998;2:115-118.

26. Spindler AA, Renvall MJ, Nichols JF, Ransdell JW. Nutritional status of patients with Alzheimer's disease: a 1-year study. *J Am Diet Assoc.* 1996;96:1013-1018.

27. Wolf-Klein GP, Silverstone FA, Lansey SC, Tesi D, Ciampaglia C, O'Donnell M, Galkowski J, Jaeger A, Wallenstein S, Leleiko NS. Energy requirements in Alzheimer's disease patients. *Nutrition.* 1995;11:264-268.

28. Young KW, Binns MA, Greenwood CE. Meal delivery practices do not meet needs of Alzheimer patients with increased cognitive and behavioral difficulties in a long term care facility. *J Gerontol.* 2001;56:M656-M661.

29. Chernoff R. Nutritional support for the elderly. In Chernoff R, ed. *Geriatric Nutrition: The Health Professional's Handbook.* Gaithersburg, Md: Aspen Publishers; 1999:416-434.

30. Finucane TE, Christmas C, Travis K. Tube feeding in patients with advanced dementia. *JAMA.* 1999;282:1365-1370.

CHAPTER

13

Taste and Smell

With the global improvement of health and medical services, life expectancy has increased dramatically. By 2050, the world population is projected to reach 9.37 billion, with one in 10 individuals older than 65 years (1). A large proportion of this older population will have age-related taste and smell losses that can impair their overall health, self-sufficiency, and quality of life (2).

Impairment of the chemical senses of taste and smell can have a profound impact on nutritional status, because it reduces the motivation to eat, alters food choices and nutrient intake, and diminishes the ability to detect spoiled food. Current data indicate that approximately 14 million older adults in the United States suffer from olfactory losses (3). In a population-based, cross-sectional study of 2,491 residents of Beaver Dam, Wisconsin, aged 53 to 97 years, Murphy and associates found that the prevalence of impaired olfaction was 24.5% for the group as a whole, and it increased with age to 62.5% for individuals 80 to 97 years of age (3). For persons 70 to 79 years, the prevalence was 29.2%; and for persons 60 to 69 years, the prevalence was 17.3% (3). In 2000, the US census counted approximately 60 million Americans older than 55 years (4). Therefore, if one extrapolates from Murphy's findings (3), 14 million older adults currently may have an impaired ability to detect odor signals.

These numbers will continue to increase. By 2015, 77 million American adults are projected to be 55 years and older (5), and approximately 18 million will have olfactory disorders. Worldwide, the number of older adults projected to have olfactory impairments by 2050 is at least 230 million, based on United Nations projections of global population growth as well as prevalence data from Murphy et al (3). The prevalence of taste disorders, unlike smell disorders, is not known.

FUNCTIONS OF TASTE AND SMELL

The senses of taste and smell play important roles in nutritional status for many reasons (2,6). First, chemosensory stimuli prepare the body to process and digest food by triggering salivary, gastric, pancreatic, and intestinal secretions, called cephalic phase responses (7). Second, taste and smell sensations modulate food choices and meal size. This occurs because there is a learned association between a food's taste and smell and its postingestive effects that helps us select foods that meet our biological needs. Third, chemosensory sensations enhance feelings of enjoyment and satiety from a meal and are primary reinforcers of eating. Sensory stimulation derived from food is especially important in older adults, for whom other sources of gratification and happiness may be less frequent. Fourth, taste and smell sensations warn of potential dangers of spoiled food. Given these important functions that are served by the chemical senses, it is not surprising that taste and smell impairment have been shown experimentally to interfere with appetite, appropriate food choices, and nutrient intake in older adults (8-10).

LOSSES OF TASTE PERCEPTION IN OLDER ADULTS

Taste impairments are classified as follows: ageusia (absence of taste), hypogeusia (diminished sensitivity of taste), and dysgeusia (distortion of normal taste). Dysgeusia is not necessarily associated with loss of sensitivity but can occur in the presence or absence of a tastant. In hypogeusia, there can be impairment at both threshold and suprathreshold concentrations. Taste detection thresholds (lowest concentration that can be detected) and taste recognition thresholds (lowest concentration that is correctly identified) tend to be elevated in healthy older individuals for prototypical tastes, such as sweet, sour, salty, and bitter. The prevalence of threshold impairments, however, is much higher for older adults who have chronic medical conditions (especially Alzheimer's disease) or who take multiple medications than for those who have no diseases and who take no medications (2). Studies of suprathreshold taste perception suggest that older adults tend to perceive a broad range of tastes as less intense than young persons; the ability to discriminate intensity differences between various concentrations of a tastant is also impaired (11). Marked losses in regional taste sensitivity also occur over different areas of the tongue in older adults (12,13).

The anatomic and physiologic causes of these impairments of taste perception in older adults are not well understood. Taste sensations occur when chemicals in foods and beverages come in contact with cells clustered into taste buds that are scattered on the dorsal surface of the tongue, soft palate, pharynx, larynx, epiglottis, uvula, and first third of the esophagus (11). Three cranial nerves transmit taste signals from the taste buds to the medulla in the brain stem, and ultimately the information is transmitted to the brain. Data regarding anatomic losses at the level of the taste buds or neural projections to the brain in older adults have been equivocal (14). Some studies have found reduced numbers of taste buds in older adults, but other studies have not. One possible cause of the discrepancy in the anatomic findings may be the level of malnutrition experienced by older adults. Malnutrition (eg, lack of protein) can impair the reproduction of taste cells, which are normally replaced every 10 to 10.5 days (2).

Medications and medical conditions definitely play a role in taste losses and taste distortions in both healthy and wasting older adults (2,6,11,15). Clinical reports suggest that more than 250 drugs alter taste sensations, including psychotropic, cardiovascular, antirheumatic, antimicrobial, and antineoplastic medications. Drugs can impact taste at several levels, including peripheral receptor cells, chemosensory neural pathways, and/or the brain. Drugs can also be secreted into the saliva, producing a taste of their own. Anticholinergic medications cause symptoms of dry mouth that often accompany taste complaints (16). Many medical conditions, including cancer, impair taste perception (2,6). Dentures are another factor that can affect taste perception when they occlude and cover taste receptors in the soft palate.

LOSSES OF SMELL PERCEPTION IN OLDER ADULTS

Olfactory impairments are usually classified as follows: anosmia (absence of smell), hyposmia (diminished sensitivity of smell), and dysosmia (distortion of normal smell). Dysosmia, like dysgeusia, does not necessarily involve loss of sensitivity and can occur in the presence or absence of a stimulus. The term *parosmia* refers to the situation in which distortion of odor perception occurs when an odor is present. *Phantosmia* refers to cases in which odor sensations occur in the absence of an odor stimulus, such as a hallucination. Hyposmia, in which there is impairment at threshold and/or suprathreshold concentrations, tends to become noticeable at around 60 years of age and becomes progressively greater with advancing years. Olfactory losses become more severe in persons older than 70 years (2,17).

Olfactory impairment occurs during the normal course of the aging process and is the result of degenerative processes in olfactory sensory neurons, the olfactory bulb, and central neural processing centers (18). Odorants interact with olfactory sensory neurons that are located in the olfactory epithelium at the upper portion of the nasal cavity. The number of proliferating basal cells and of immature neurons in the olfactory epithelium decreases with age (19), and individual olfactory sensory neurons from older adults are less selective in their responses to odorants (20). Axons of olfactory sensory cells traverse through small holes in the cribriform plate of the ethmoid bone to the olfactory bulb to synapse in intricate neural masses called glomeruli. The olfactory tract projects from the olfactory bulb to the anterior olfactory nucleus, the olfactory tubercle, the prepyriform cortex, and the amygdala. During the aging process, there is atrophy in the olfactory bulb (21,22) and along the olfactory tract (23,24). Anatomic studies have found that all the central nervous system (CNS) targets of the olfactory pathways undergo structural and anatomic degeneration, including the temporal lobe, entorhinal cortex, hippocampus, and amygdala (18). Event-related brain potentials (ERPs) show reduced amplitude and longer latency to olfactory stimulation in the elderly (25).

There are many causes of smell losses, including normal aging, medical conditions, medication side effects, medical treatments such as radiation, and environmental exposures (2,3,6,17,26,27). Common triggers of smell loss include upper respiratory infections, head injuries, polyps in the nasal cavities, hormonal disturbances, and exposure to insecticides and solvents. Many medical conditions, such as diabetes, hypertension, malnutrition, Parkinson's disease, Alzheimer's disease, multiple sclerosis, and Korsakoff's psychosis, are accompanied (or even signaled clinically) by smell disorders. Malnutrition can impair smell sensitivity by affecting the turnover of olfactory sensory neurons. Olfactory sensory neurons continually replace themselves with a turnover approximately every 30 days (2). Some older adults may recover their ability to smell when an illness causing their olfactory problem resolves; however, most smell losses in older adults are permanent.

IMPACT OF CHEMOSENSORY LOSSES ON NUTRITION, HEALTH, AND DISEASE

Taste and smell losses in older adults can have a negative impact on food selection, nutritional status, morbidity, and mortality (2). Research studies have shown conclusively that chemosensory losses interfere with appetite, food choices, and nutrient intake in the older adult (8-10). Diminished appetite is of special concern, because reduced motivation to eat can lead to inadequate intake of macro- and micronutrients. Inadequate protein-energy intake may be as high as 12% in community-dwelling older adults (28), and many ingest an inadequate amount of certain nutrients (29-32). Inadequate intake is usually not caused by the lack of availability of food but rather by loss of appetite resulting in part from smell and taste losses (2). Undernutrition subsequent to taste and smell losses is a major cause of progressive involuntary weight loss (wasting), increased disease susceptibility, and decreased immunocompetence in frail elderly persons (33). Weight loss not only increases the risk for morbidity and mortality in older adults but also contributes to decreased functional independence and poor quality of life (34).

DETECTION OF SPOILED OR CONTAMINATED FOOD

One of the most serious problems associated with chemosensory losses is the inability to recognize spoiled food. Food spoilage is produced by microbial growth, chemical reactions, and/or enzymatic processes, and it is generally associated with changes in the odor and taste of the food (35). Odorous volatile compounds (called odorants), produced by many types of microorganisms, alert us to food spoilage (36-38). Older adults are at elevated risk for foodborne illness from pathogens because of their reduced ability to detect off-odors from spoiled food. The annual incidence of food poisoning in the United States is approximately 76 million cases, with 325,000 hospitalizations and 5,000 deaths each year (39). Deaths from food poisoning are more likely to occur in vulnerable populations that are known to have compromised olfactory functioning, such as older adults and severely debilitated persons (40,41). Furthermore, although the most common clinical conditions associated with foodborne disease are acute (diarrhea, vomiting, or other gastrointestinal manifestations), a number of chronic sequelae may result, including arthropathies, renal disease, cardiac and neurological disorders, and nutritional and other malabsorptive disorders (42-44). Sequelae such as arthropathies can have a disproportionate impact on older adults who already suffer from joint disease.

Food spoilage (and its associated odors) can be produced by chemical and enzymatic processes as well as by pathogenic microorganisms. A subtle but severe problem of food spoilage that can have profound effects on the nutritional status and health of older adults is chemical oxidation. At room temperature, oxygen reacts with unsaturated fatty acids to form peroxides, along with a variety of other compounds with objectionable odors. Young persons with a good sense of smell can detect this development of rancidity in the early stages, whereas older adults with an impaired sense of smell cannot. Consumption of partially oxidized lipids appears to play a role in chronic conditions caused by oxidative stress, such as cardiovascular disease (45). Ursini and Sevanian (46) reported that consumption of oxidized lipids at a meal increases the plasma level of lipid hydroperoxides and increases the susceptibility to oxidation of low-density lipids. Consumption of highly oxidized corn oil by human subjects increased 4.7-fold the concentrations of conjugated dienes in the chylomicron fraction of their postprandial serum, compared with a meal of nonoxidized corn oil (47). The level of conjugated dienes is an indicator of the level of oxidized lipids.

FLAVOR ENHANCEMENT OF FOOD

At present, there are no pharmacological methods to treat age-associated decrements to taste and smell, and the prognosis for recovery of chemosensory functioning is poor. However, amplification of foods with simulated food flavors has been helpful in treating clients with hyposmia who have reduced ability to detect odors but can perceive more intense aromas (48). Simulated food flavors can be added to meats, vegetables, and other nutritious foods to amplify the odor intensity. Some food flavors, such as butter, cheese, and bacon flavors, are commercially available at grocery stores. Simulated flavors are mixtures of odorous molecules that are extracted from natural products or synthesized after chromatographic analysis of the target food. Food flavors have an advantage over spices in that they add sensory appeal without irritating the stomach like spices. Flavor enhancement has been shown to improve appetite, increase total number of lymphocytes (including T cells and B cells), increase the secretion rate of salivary IgA, and improve functional status in older adults (33,48-50).

SUMMARY

Losses in taste and smell are pervasive in all segments of the elderly population, but the magnitude of the losses are largest in those with a variety of diseases (especially Alzheimer's disease) and those taking multiple medications. Taste and smell losses in older adults have a negative impact on food selection, nutritional status, morbidity, and mortality. Amplification of flavor levels of food can compensate in part for these losses.

REFERENCES

1. United Nations Population Division. *World Population Prospects 1950-2050 (The 1996 Revision)* [diskette]. New York: United Nations; 1996.
2. Schiffman SS. Taste and smell losses in normal aging and disease. *JAMA.* 1997;278:1357-1362.
3. Murphy C, Schubert CR, Cruickshanks KJ, Klein BEK, Klein R, Nondahl DM. Prevalence of olfactory impairment in older adults. *JAMA.* 2002;288:2307-2312.
4. US Census Bureau. Statistical Abstract of the United States, 2001. Section 1. Population Table No. 11. Resident Population by Sex and Age Group: 1990 and 2000. Available at: http://www.census.gov/prod/2002pubs/01statab/stat-ab01.html. Accessed January 8, 2003.
5. US Census Bureau. United States Census 2000. Summary File 1 (SF 1) Table QT-01. Profile of General Demographic Characteristics for the United States: 2000. Available at: http://www.census.gov/main/www/cen2000.html. Accessed March 12, 2004.
6. Schiffman SS. Taste and smell in disease. *N Engl J Med.* 1983;308:1275-1279,1337-1343.
7. Giduck SA, Threatte RM, Kare MR. Cephalic reflexes: their role in digestion and possible roles in absorption and metabolism. *J Nutr.* 1987;117:1191-1196.
8. de Jong N, Mulder I, de Graaf C, van Staveren WA. Impaired sensory functioning in elders: the relation with its potential determinants and nutritional intake. *J Gerontol A Biol Sci Med Sci.* 1999;54:B324-B331.

9. Griep MI, Verleye G, Franck AH, Collys K, Mets TF, Massart DL. Variation in nutrient intake with dental status, age, and odour perception. *Eur J Clin Nutr.* 1996;50:816-825.
10. Duffy VB, Backstrand JR, Ferris AM. Olfactory dysfunction and related nutritional risk in free-living, elderly women. *J Am Diet Assoc.* 1995; 95:879-884.
11. Schiffman SS, Zervakis J. Taste and smell perception in the elderly: effect of medications and disease. *Adv Food Nutr Res.* 2002;44:247-346.
12. Matsuda T, Doty RL. Regional taste sensitivity to NaCl: relationship to subject age, tongue locus and area of stimulation. *Chem Senses.* 1995;20:283-290.
13. Bartoshuk LM, Rifkin B, Marks LE, Bars P. Taste and aging. *J Gerontol.* 1986;41:51-57.
14. Mistretta CM. Aging effects on anatomy and neurophysiology of taste and smell. *Gerodontology.* 1984;3:131-136.
15. Lewis IK, Hanlon JT, Hobbins MJ, Beck JD. Use of medications with potential oral adverse drug reactions in community-dwelling elderly. *Spec Care Dent.* 1993;13:171-176.
16. Smith RG, Burtner AP. Oral side-effects of the most frequently prescribed drugs. *Spec Care Dent.* 1994;14:96-102.
17. Doty RL, Shaman P, Applebaum SL, Giberson R, Siksorski L, Rosenberg L. Smell identification ability: changes with age. *Science.* 1984;226:1441-1443.
18. Schiffman S, Orlandi M, Erickson RP. Changes in taste and smell with age: biological aspects. In: Ordy JM, Brizzee K, eds. *Sensory Systems and Communication in the Elderly.* New York, NY: Raven Press; 1979:247-268.
19. Loo AT, Youngentob SL, Kent PF, Schwob JE. The aging olfactory epithelium: neurogenesis, response to damage, and odorant-induced activity. *Int J Dev Neurosci.* 1996;14:881-900.
20. Rawson NE, Gomez G, Cowart B, Restrepo D. The use of olfactory receptor neurons (ORNs) from biopsies to study changes in aging and neurodegenerative diseases. *Ann NY Acad Sci.* 1998;855:701-707.
21. Smith CG. Incidence of atrophy of the olfactory nerves in man. *Arch Otolaryngol.* 1941;34:533-539.
22. Meisami E, Mikhail L, Baim D, Bhatnagar KP. Human olfactory bulb: aging of glomeruli and mitral cells and a search for the accessory olfactory bulb. *Ann NY Acad Sci.* 1998;855:708-715.
23. Bhatnagar KP, Kennedy RC, Baron G, Greenberg RA. Number of mitral cells and the bulb volume in the aging human olfactory bulb: a quantitative morphological study. *Anat Rec.* 1987;218:73-87.
24. Jones N, Rog D. Olfaction: a review. *J Laryngol Otol.* 1998;112:11-24.
25. Murphy C, Morgan CD, Geisler MW, Wetter S, Covington JW, Madowitz MD, Nordin S, Polich JM. Olfactory event-related potentials and aging: normative data. *Int J Psychophysiol.* 2000;36:133-145.
26. National Institute on Deafness and Other Communication Disorders. Smell and smell disorders. Available at: http://www.nidcd.nih.gov/health/pubs_st/smell.htm#diagnosed. Accessed May 27, 2002.

27. Murphy C. Nutrition and chemosensory perception in the elderly. *Crit Rev Food Sci Nutr.* 1993;33:3-15.

28. Thomas DR. Causes of protein-energy malnutrition. *Z Gerontol Geriatr.* 1999;32:S38-S44.

29. Salva A, Pera G. Screening for malnutrition in dwelling elderly. *Public Health Nutr.* 2001;4:1375-1378.

30. Morley JE, Thomas DR. Anorexia and aging: pathophysiology. *Nutrition.* 1999;15:499-503.

31. Chapman KM, Nelson RA. Loss of appetite: managing unwanted weight loss in the older patient. *Geriatrics.* 1994;49:54-59.

32. Blumberg J. Nutritional needs of seniors. *J Am Coll Nutr.* 1997;16:517-523.

33. Schiffman SS, Wedral E. Contribution of taste and smell losses to the wasting syndrome. *Age Nutr.* 1996;7:106-120.

34. Toth MJ, Poehlman ET. Energetic adaptation to chronic disease in the elderly. *Nutr Rev.* 2000;58:61-66.

35. Schuler G, Hurst W, Reynolds E, Christian J; revised by Tybor PT. Food Spoilage and You. The University of Georgia College of Agricultural & Environmental Sciences Cooperative Extension Service. Bulletin 906 (reprinted July 1992). Available at: http://www.ces.uga.edu/pubcd/b906-w.html. Accessed January 17, 2003.

36. Nakai S, Wang ZH, Dou J, Nakamura S, Ogawa M, Nakai E, Vanderstoep J. Gas chromatography/principal component similarity system for detection of *E. coli* and *S. aureus* contaminating salmon and hamburger. *J Agric Food Chem.* 1999;47:576-583.

37. Pittard BT, Freeman LR, Later DW, Lee ML. Identification of volatile organic compounds produced by fluorescent pseudomonads on chicken breast muscle. *Appl Environ Microbiol.* 1982;43:1504-1506.

38. Macfie HJ, Gutteridge CS, Norris JR. Use of canonical variates analysis in differentiation of bacteria by pyrolysis gas-liquid chromatography. *J Gen Microbiol.* 1978;104:67-74.

39. Mead PS, Slutsker L, Dietz V, McCaig LF, Bresee JS, Shapiro C, Griffin PM, Tauxe RV. Food-related illness and death in the United States. *Emerg Infect Dis.* 1999;5:607-625.

40. Food Safety and Inspection Service, United States Department of Agriculture. Backgrounders: Campylobacter. November 1997. Available at: http://www.fsis.usda.gov/OA/background/campy_qa.htm. Accessed March 12, 2004.

41. Hingley A. Focus on food safety: initiative calls on government, industry, consumers to stop food-related illness [originally published in *FDA Consumer.* September-October 1997; revised May 1998]. Available at: http://www.fda.gov/fdac/features/1997/697_safe.html. Accessed March 12, 2004.

42. Bunning VK. Immunopathogenic aspects of foodborne microbial disease. *Food Microbiol.* 1994;11:89-95.

43. Bunning VK, Lindsay JA, Archer DL. Chronic health effects of foodborne microbial disease. *World Health Stat Quart.* 1997;50:51-56.

44. Lindsay JA. Chronic sequelae of foodborne diseases. *Emerg Infect Dis.* 1997;3:443-452. Available at: http://www.cdc.gov/ncidod/EID/vol3no4/lindsay.htm. Accessed March 12, 2004.

45. Parthasarathy S, Khan-Merchant N, Penumetcha M, Santanam N. Oxidative stress in cardiovascular disease. *J Nucl Cardiol.* 2001;8:379-389.

46. Ursini F, Sevanian A. Wine polyphenols and optimal nutrition. *Ann NY Acad Sci.* 2002;957:200-209.

47. Staprans I, Rapp JH, Pan X-M, Kim KY, Feingold KR. Oxidized lipids in the diet are a source of oxidized lipid in chylomicrons of human serum. *Arterioscler Thromb.* 1994;14:1900-1905.

48. Schiffman SS, Graham BG. Taste and smell perception affect appetite and immunity in the elderly. *Eur J Clin Nutr.* 2000;54(suppl):S54-S63.

49. Schiffman SS, Miletic ID. Effect of taste and smell on secretion rate of salivary IgA in elderly and young persons. *J Nutr Health Aging.* 1999;3:158-164.

50. Schiffman SS, Warwick ZS. Effect of flavor enhancement of foods for the elderly on nutritional status: food intake, biochemical indices and anthropometric measures. *Physiol Behav.* 1993;53:395-402.

ADDITIONAL RESOURCES

Nakamoto T. Odor handling and delivery systems. In: Pearce TC, Schiffman SS, Nagle HT, Gardner JW, eds. *Handbook of Machine Olfaction: Electronic Nose Technology.* Weinheim, Germany: Wiley VCH; 2003:chap 3.

US Census Bureau. (NP-T3-D) Projections of the Total Resident Population by 5-Year Age Groups, and Sex with Special Age Categories: Middle Series, 2011 to 2015. Population Projections Program, Population Division, US Census Bureau. Available at: http://www.census.gov/population/projections/nation/summary/np-t3-d.txt. Accessed January 8, 2003.

CHAPTER 14

Oral Health

"Nutrition is an integral component of oral health" (1,2). This position of the American Dietetic Association is particularly important with respect to older adults. Local oral factors, such as tooth loss (edentulism), ill-fitting dentures, and soft-tissue disorders, as well as systemic disease and medications, can impact the integrity of the oral cavity and subsequent function and sensory perception. All these factors can have a significant impact on diet quality and nutritional status. Similarly, malnutrition may impact the integrity of the oral cavity, which influences wound healing and the ability to recover from infection and surgery.

THE BIG PICTURE

Older adults frequently have one or more chronic diseases and/or other factors that can affect their oral health. Those with partial (missing some) or full (missing all) edentulism and those wearing ill-fitting dentures are at greater nutritional risk. Poor oral health has been shown to be a significant contributory factor in involuntary weight loss and compromised diet quality (2-5). New patterns of oral infectious diseases are seen in today's older adults as individuals retain their natural teeth longer and live longer. With the increasing incidence of chronic disease in older adults, oral manifestations of diseases such as diabetes may impact oral health and the integrity of the oral mucosa. Xerostomia (dry mouth), a common side effect of more than 600 medications, may occur because of the polypharmacy experienced by this population. It may also occur as a result of dehydration, autoimmune disease associated with xerostomia, or undetected damage to the salivary gland (6). The relationship between osteoporosis and tooth loss has been documented; this may have a significant impact on the oral health of older adults, par-

ticularly women (1). The negative impact of edentulism and dentures on eating habits, biting and chewing, sense of taste, and gastrointestinal disorders has been documented (6,7).

FUNCTIONAL ABILITY OF THE ORAL CAVITY

The term "oral invalids" (8) has been coined for individuals who wear dentures. Researchers have found that they have about one fifth the chewing ability of their dentate counterparts (9) and take more drugs, including laxatives and anti-reflux agents, for gastrointestinal disorders (7).

THE ROLE OF DIETETICS PROFESSIONALS

Nutritional risk evaluation, at a minimum, includes subjective statements relative to diet, oral health, and weight history, as well as objective assessment of height, weight, and the condition of the oral cavity. Nutritional risk factors are defined as "characteristics that are associated with an increased likelihood of poor nutritional status" (10). Oral health nutritional risk factors are outlined in Box 14.1 (11). Nutritional risk is based on the type and extent of risk factors present. At significant risk is the older adult who lives alone, has lost more than 10 lb in 6 months, and has difficulty chewing.

Despite clear evidence of the relationship between diet and nutritional status and oral problems faced by older adults, dietary quality can be achieved when nutrition counseling is a routine component of dental practice (9,12,13). Conversely, when planning medical nutrition therapy (MNT), qualified dietetics professionals should be encouraged to routinely consider the oral manifestations of diseases and medications or the oral problems faced by those who wear dentures and experience related

Box 14.1   Oral Nutrition Risk Factors in Older Adults

- Altered or painful taste
- Arthropathies
- Autoimmune diseases
- Cranial nerve disorders
- Dental procedures altering ability to eat a usual diet
- Extensive root or coronal caries
- Inadequate diet
- Masticatory compromise (biting/chewing/ swallowing difficulty)
- Oral infections

- Oral surgeries
- Oro-facial pain
- Osteoporosis
- Polypharmacy
- Poverty
- Substance abuse
- Type 2 diabetes
- Ulcerations/lesions in the mouth
- Unintentional weight change
- Xerostomia

Source: Reprinted from Touger-Decker R, Mobley C. American Dietetic Association Position Paper: nutrition and oral health. *J Am Diet Assoc.* 1996;96:184-189, with permission from American Dietetic Association (ADA). For updated ADA position, see: Touger-Decker R, Mobley CC; American Dietetic Association. Position of the American Dietetic Association: oral health and nutrition. *J Am Diet Assoc.* 2003;103:615-625.

problems (2,9,14). The Nutrition Screening Initiative (NSI), introduced in 1990 as a national approach to early detection of nutritional risk and its potential causes in older adults, is an example of a rapid strategy to detect combined nutritional and oral health problems (10). This initiative exemplifies multidisciplinary care by dental and dietetics professionals. The DETERMINE Your Nutritional Health Checklist and the separate Oral Health Risk Factor Checklist identify oral problems contributing to nutritional risk in the older adult population (10).

Box 14.2 lists recommended strategies for dietetics professionals to integrate the oral exam and a consultation into MNT. First and foremost, dietetics professionals should perform an oral exam on all older adult clients. This exam, which typically takes a maximum of 10 minutes, can help detect factors that impact functional and systemic diet and nutrition needs. The American Dietetic Association offers a video-based training course for dietetics professionals interested in learning these skills (15); the University of Medicine and Dentistry of New Jersey, Newark, also offers training. An alternative route of training is to ask a dental professional (dentist or registered dental hygienist) to train the dietetics professional in the performance of an oral screening exam.

The oral examination should include looking in the mouth at the integrity of the oral tissue to

Box 14.2   Approaches to Oral Nutrition Management for Dietetics Professionals

- Include oral health screening exams as part of nutrition assessment protocols (ie, cranial nerve function, integrity of the soft tissue, occlusion, edentulism, masticatory ability, swallowing, salivary adequacy).
- Recognize oral manifestations of systemic diseases, and provide patients with guidelines to maximize oral intake.
- Confer with and refer patients (via consults) to dental practitioners for management of oral diseases and/or risk factors for oral diseases.
- Consult with dental professionals in interpretation of oral-nutrition assessment findings and planning in the long-term-care setting.

determine the degree of edentulism (missing teeth) and occlusion (how teeth come together) of the remaining teeth or prosthodontics (removable dentures or fixed crowns and bridges) (1,16). Occlusion refers to the pattern of teeth and how they come together. For example, an individual may have four maxillary anterior teeth (teeth on their top jaw in

Box 14.3 Nutritional Risk Questions to Ask Patients About Oral Symptoms

1. Do you have any difficulties biting or chewing food?
   - If yes, which (biting or chewing)?
   - If yes, what foods/fluids cause difficulty and how?
2. Do you have any difficulty swallowing?

   If yes, do you have difficulty with liquids, thin or thick solids, semisolids, or all textures?

   If yes, has this difficulty been progressive in degree of difficulty and in types of foods?
3. Is swallowing painful?

   If yes, when?
4. Can you eat a meal or snack without extra liquids?

   If *no,* how many cups of liquids do you need to consume?
5. How would you describe changes in tastes that have occurred?

   What types of food or beverage taste different?

   Has your medication (prescription or over-the-counter) changed at all during this time?
6. How often during the day do you eat, including meals and snacks?

7. How many times a day do you drink sweetened coffees, teas, soda, juices, or other sweetened beverages?
8. When in the course of the day do you brush your teeth?

Questions to Ask About Osteoporosis Risk

1. How many servings of dairy products do you have on a typical day?

   (1 serving = 1 ounce of cheese or 1 cup of yogurt or milk)
2. Do you take a calcium supplement?

   If yes, what is the name and how much do you take in a day?
3. Do you get any exercise in the course of a day or week?

   If yes, how many times a week and for how long?
4. Are you peri- or postmenopausal? (Asked of women only)
5. Have you, or has a first-degree relative, broken one or more bones?

---

the front) and four mandibular (lower jaw) molars. This individual has no teeth in occlusion. Consequently, biting (which is typically done with anterior teeth) and chewing (typically done with posterior teeth) are both compromised. The older adult should be asked questions, as noted in Box 14.3, about masticatory ability. The importance of routine oral exams was highlighted in a letter to the editor in the *Journal of the American Medical Association* (17). An older adult client aspirated a four-unit bridge; a radiograph noted the bridge located in the esophagus. The authors concluded that the bridge was aspirated several weeks before the client's illness; however, no one had noted the problem, and the client was on a gastrostomy feeding. Routine oral exams could prevent such a problem.

Adequacy of saliva can be determined with simple subjective questions, noted in Box 14.3. Any indication of salivary difficulties should be referred to the dentist for further evaluation.

Cranial nerve function may have already been examined. If not, it is within the realm of dietetics practice to perform a cranial nerve examination. Cra-

nial nerve function will provide information relative to biting, chewing, swallowing, and taste. The following nerves should be evaluated for their possible contribution to oral function or dysfunction: trigeminal, facial, vagus, glossopharyngeal, and hypoglossal. Brody et al (18) developed a dysphagia screening tool for dietetics professionals that includes assessment of cranial nerve function. The trigeminal nerve affects jaw strength and movement, and the facial nerve affects taste and muscles of facial expression that can impact both biting and chewing function. The glossopharyngeal nerve affects taste, gag reflex, and swallowing function, contributing to the assessment of dysphagia, as does the vagus nerve (gag reflex and swallow), and the hypoglossal nerve (tongue range of motion and strength).

Box 14.4 (18) shows a dysphagia prescreening tool. Box 14.5 (18) shows a dysphagia screening tool used by dietitians.

A soft-tissue exam simply involves looking at the tongue, palate, and oral mucosa for any non-normal coloration, lesions, or alterations in appearance. Normally, mucosa is pink and moist, without

Box 14.4 Dysphagia Prescreening Tool Used by Registered Dietitians

Chart review

Age
Diagnosis*
Diet/feeding order†
History of dysphagia
History or diagnosis of aspiration pneumonia
Tracheostomy
Cranial nerve dysfunction (V, VII, IX, X, XII)
Altered mental status
Nutritional risk level (mild, moderate, severe)‡

Documentation by physician or nurse

Drooling
Difficulty swallowing solids, medications, or fluids
Prolonged eating time
Pocketing food or medications
Choking during or after meals

Patient is eligible for dysphagia screening by dietitian if diagnosis and/or diet order meet screening criteria AND/OR if one or more of the other prescreening criteria are present.

*Most prevalent diagnoses included cerebral vascular accident, intracerebral bleeding, transient ischemic attack, traumatic brain injury, and brain tumor.

†Eligible diet orders include puree, restriction of liquids, "dysphagia diet," and transitional feedings (enteral or parenteral feeding plus oral diet).

‡Nutritional risk was determined in accordance with the institutional policy for nutrition assessment. Predominant factors considered in nutrition assessment were diagnosis, weight status/change, albumin level, degree of metabolic stress, presence of decubitus ulcers, and need for nutrition support.

Source: Reprinted from Brody R, Touger-Decker R, O'Sullivan-Maillet J. The effectiveness of dysphagia screening by an RD on the determination of dysphagia risk. *J Am Diet Assoc.* 2000;100:1029-1037, with permission from American Dietetic Association.

Box 14.5 Dysphagia Screening Tool Used by Registered Dietitians

Observe the patient and ask if he or she has a recent history (within the past month) of any of the following:

Drooling of liquids?
Drooling of solids?
Coughing during a swallow?
Coughing after a swallow?
Facial or tongue weakness?
Difficulty managing own secretions?
Pocketing?
Change in voice quality ("wet"/hoarse)?
Poor head control or posture?
Failure to consume more than 50% of meal?
Prolonged eating time?

Conduct test of following:

Voluntary cough
Dry swallow

Source: Reprinted from Brody R, Touger-Decker R, O'Sullivan-Maillet J. The effectiveness of dysphagia screening by an RD on the determination of dysphagia risk. *J Am Diet Assoc.* 2000;100:1029-1037, with permission from American Dietetic Association.

lesions or infection. Any non-normal findings should be referred to the dentist. Oral manifestations of systemic disease may also be determined through the soft-tissue exam. Uncontrolled diabetes may be manifested by burning mouth (19) and candidiasis. A B-12 or folate deficiency may manifest itself on the tongue (20).

After the oral exam, it is incumbent on the dietetics professional to confer with and refer clients (via consults) to dental practitioners for management of oral diseases and/or risk factors for oral diseases. Consultation with dental professionals in interpretation of oral-nutrition assessment findings and planning in the long-term-care setting is also necessary in order to provide for comprehensive care.

In summary, the 10-minute oral exam includes looking at the presence and patterns of teeth (how many and do they come together), the integrity of the saliva and surrounding oral tissues and structure, and the sensory and nervous function as determined by a cranial nerve exam. Dietetics professionals can attend courses for instruction on these skills or can seek individualized instruction from a licensed dentist or registered dental hygienist. Competencies in these skills should become a routine part of dietetics practice.

DIET MANAGEMENT GUIDELINES FOR COMPROMISED ORAL HEALTH

Diet management for compromised oral health focuses primarily on modification of the typical diet to meet functional changes in the oral cavity. The more common changes experienced include xerostomia and adjustment to dentures.

Eating hints for older adults with xerostomia include the use of moist, temperate foods and the limiting of obviously salty or dry foods, such as chips, pretzels, and salted crackers. Frozen grapes and other fruits with high water content are good snacks because they moisten the oral cavity as they melt. Individuals with xerostomia should be cautioned to avoid sucking on sugared hard candies or lozenges or chewing regular chewing gum, because these foods add to their already increased risk of tooth decay. Juices, sodas, and other sugared beverages should be limited to mealtimes only. A water bottle should be the constant companion for an individual with dry mouth. Sugar-free lozenges, mints, and gums, particularly those sweetened with xylitol, are an excellent alternative. A five-carbon sugar that is not hydrolyzed by salivary amylase, xylitol does not contribute to tooth decay, and, unlike some of the other sugar alcohols, it may even have some anticariogenic benefits. Regular dental checkups should be encouraged, because individuals with xerostomia are at increased risk of dental caries by nature of the lack of saliva. In instances of severe xerostomia, when the individual's ability to consume a typical diet is altered, the dietetics professional should consult with the dental professional regarding salivary stimulants.

Denture placement does not ensure adequacy of intake. Diet issues to consider in older adults with dentures include the impact on gastric emptying time and chewing ability, which may affect food group choices and the motivation to learn how to eat with the prostheses. Guidelines for eating with dentures are listed in Box 14.6. These should be modified to meet the individual diet needs of older adults. Simply stating "resume normal diet" does not work in this instance, because individuals may have not consumed a "normal" diet for many months or years, depending on the duration and extent of their edentulism. Older adults should be encouraged to try biting at the corners of their mouth with a full denture, because it may reduce the potential of breaking the "seal" between the denture and the gingiva (gum). Nuts, rice, and seeds, as well as other foods that may disintegrate into small pieces ini-

---

Box 14.6   Guidelines for Eating With Dentures

- Let your knife and fork serve as teeth, cut food into smaller pieces.
- Try biting toward the corners of the mouth, as opposed to using the front teeth.
- Season foods to taste.
- Initially avoid soft, chewy rolls or breads, rice, nuts, and seeds.
- During the first week after denture insertion:
  - Start slowly and progress gradually.
  - Begin with soups, cereals, yogurts, eggs, canned cut fruits, and chopped cooked vegetables.
  - Advance to pastas, mashed potatoes, cut and moistened meats/poultry, and cut fruits and vegetables (soft, fresh, or canned).
- After the initial week(s), progress to whole foods, fresh fruits and vegetables, rice, and seeds.

---

tially in the mouth, should be avoided at first because they may be hard to maneuver with the new dentures. White bread and other soft chewy breads and rolls may be difficult to chew and swallow initially. It is important to note that these guidelines should be interpreted individually for each client, depending on (a) their systemic health; (b) the functional ability of their oral cavity and surrounding tissues, muscles, and nerves; and (c) whether they are receiving a mandibular (lower) or a maxillary (upper) denture, or both.

Edentulism also alters the individual's ability to eat. The guidelines in Box 14.6 can be adapted for the edentulous older adult. Interestingly, those with edentulism may report better chewing ability without dentures. Such individuals may be resistant to getting dentures or may use them only for cosmetic appearances.

SUMMARY

It has been said that "there is no shortcut to longevity; it is the work of a lifetime of habits" (author unknown). This statement is quite true regarding oral health and nutrition habits. Functional changes in the oral cavity of older adults are not typically due to a short-term problem. They are more likely the result of many years of gradual reduction in functional dentition due to oral and systemic disease.

Consequently, eating habits cannot be changed overnight. It is incumbent on the dietetics professional, however, to conduct an oral exam, and to determine through the exam, through the history, and perhaps through a consultation with the dental professional the degree of oral function of the older adult and to tailor diet modifications accordingly. Diet modification is, in fact, an iterative process, with needs changing as oral function changes. The guidelines provided for assessment and management should be tailored to meet the individual needs of the client.

REFERENCES

1. Touger-Decker R, Mobley CC; American Dietetic Association. Position of the American Dietetic Association: nutrition and oral health. *J Am Diet Assoc.* 2003;103:615-625.

2. Sahyoun N, Chien-Lung L, Krall E. Nutritional status of the older adult is associated with dentition status. *J Am Diet Assoc.* 2003;103:61-66.

3. Morais JA, Heydecke G, Pawliuk J, Lund JP, Feine JS. The effects of mandibular two-implant overdentures on nutrition in elderly edentulous individuals. *J Dent Res.* 2003;82:53-58.

4. Ritchie CS, Joshipura K, Hung HC, Douglass CW. Nutrition as a mediator in the relation between oral and systemic disease: associations between specific measures of adult oral health and nutrition outcomes. *Crit Rev Oral Biol Med.* 2002;13:291-300.

5. Mojon P, Budtz-Jørgensen E, Rapin C. Relationship between oral health and nutrition in very old people. *Age Aging.* 1999;28:463-468.

6. Budtz-Jorgensen E, Chung J, Rapin C. Nutrition and oral health. *Clin Gastroenterol.* 2001;15:885-896.

7. Brodeur JM, Laurin D, Vallee R, Lachapelle D. Nutrient intake and gastrointestinal disorders related to masticatory performance in the edentulous elderly. *J Prosthet Dent.* 1993;70:468-473.

8. Slagter AP, Olthoff LW, Bosman F, Steen WH. Masticatory ability, denture quality, and oral conditions in edentulous subjects. *J Prosthet Dent.* 1992;68:299-307.

9. Moynihan P, Bradbury J. Compromised dental function and nutrition. *Nutrition.* 2001;17:177-178.

10. *Nutrition Interventions Manual for Professionals Caring for Older Americans.* Washington, DC: Nutrition Screening Initiative; 1992.

11. Touger-Decker R, Mobley C. American Dietetic Association Position Paper: nutrition and oral health. *J Am Diet Assoc.* 1996;96:184-189.

12. Ettinger RL. Changing dietary patterns with changing dentition: how do people cope? *Spec Care Dent.* 1998;18:33-39.

13. Shinkai RSA, Hatch JP, Sakai S, Mobley CC, Saunders MJ, Rugh JD. Oral function and diet quality in a community-based sample. *J Dent Res.* 2001;80:1625-1630.

14. Allen F, McMillan A. Food selection and perceptions of chewing ability following provision of implant and conventional prostheses in complete denture wearers. *Clin Oral Implants Res.* 2002;13:320-326.

15. Dietitians in Nutrition Support. Nutrition focuses physical assessment skills for dietitians [video and study guide]. Chicago, Ill: American Dietetic Association; 2000.

16. Mobley C, Saunders MJ. Oral health screening guidelines for nondental health care providers. *J Am Diet Assoc.* 1997;97(suppl 2):S120-S122.

17. Aspiration of a dental appliance in a patient with Alzheimer's disease. *JAMA.* 2002;288:2543-2544.

18. Brody R, Touger-Decker R, O'Sullivan-Maillet J. The effectiveness of dysphagia screening by an RD on the determination of dysphagia risk. *J Am Diet Assoc.* 2000;100:1029-1037.

19. Touger-Decker R, Sirois D. Diet and dental health in diabetes. In: Powers M, ed. *Handbook of Diabetes Nutritional Management.* 2nd ed. Rockville, Md: Aspen Publishers; 1996.

20. Touger-Decker R. Oral manifestations of nutrient deficiencies. *Mt Sinai J Med.* 1998;65:355-361.

CHAPTER 15

Cancer

Although the number of deaths from cancer has declined from 1999 to 2003, the American Cancer Society reports that the total number of new cancer cases in the United States will continue to increase from 1.2 million in 1999 to more than 1.3 million (estimated) in 2004. Because the single most important risk factor for cancer is age and because the US population is both growing and aging, it is estimated that about 76% of the new cancers diagnosed in 2004 will be in people 55 years and older (1).

Many factors contribute to nutritional decline in older adults diagnosed with cancer, and any degree of malnutrition affects the immune system adversely. It is estimated that approximately 20% of older adults are malnourished, and many more are at risk for malnutrition (2). Older adults may present with malnutrition even before a diagnosis of cancer. Weight loss is one of the most common symptoms noted by older adults on physical exams.

Individuals with cancer face unique nutritional challenges, and ensuring proper nutrition is integral to cancer care. Early screening and assessment techniques will help to identify those people who would benefit most from nutrition interventions. The ultimate goals of nutrition support are to improve survival, to promote tolerance of therapy, to maintain nutritional and functional status, and to enhance quality of life.

METABOLIC COMPONENTS OF CANCER

Nutritional status can be affected by the tumor itself or by treatments aimed to cure or palliate the symptoms from the cancer. Surgery, chemotherapy, and radiation therapy each pose distinct nutritional threats to older adults. Weight loss and poor nutritional status can exacerbate the toxicities associated with cancer treatments and may interfere with the ability to respond effectively to the treatment.

Many factors can contribute to one's inability to ingest, digest, or absorb nutrients. These problems can occur as a result of the tumor location within the body or as a symptom of the treatments; they can often be corrected by medication and/or dietary modification if caught early enough. The presence of a tumor may affect biochemical and metabolic functions. The tumor, which is responsible for initiating these changes, can influence normal metabolism, thus increasing basal metabolic rate.

Several hypotheses are being explored to explain this metabolic change, including cytokine activity, circulating hormones, and neurophysiologic pathway changes. Although there are no strict criteria used to diagnose cachexia, some common clinical signs include anorexia; early satiety; and body composition changes, which include weight loss, fat depletion, and muscle atrophy. Weakness, fatigue, impaired immune function, decreased motor and mental skills, and a decline in attention span and concentration abilities generally follow (3). It should be noted that dietary modifications to increase energy and protein intake may not always be effective in significantly improving the outcomes or in reducing the catabolism.

Nutritional status can be evaluated by a variety of assessment methods. Physical assessment techniques, such as weight, height, and analyses of body fat and lean body mass, are usually combined with some laboratory studies to make an accurate assessment of the nutrition needs of older adults. Evaluating weight loss over time remains a key assessment tool and is readily available in all settings. Involuntary weight loss, of more than 5% of usual body weight in a 1-month period or of 10% in a 6-month period, has been shown to statistically increase the risk of morbidity and mortality in those with cancer (4,5).

NUTRITIONAL REQUIREMENTS

Nutrient requirements for those with cancer are dependent on many factors and cannot be generalized. Energy requirements in those with cancer vary considerably. Approximately 25% of individuals with cancer can be categorized as hypermetabolic, with increased energy needs. Hypermetabolism is often seen in those diagnosed with gastrointestinal malignancies and pulmonary diseases. Thirty percent of those diagnosed with cancer will be hypometabolic, with reduced energy needs. Hypometabolism is commonly seen in those diagnosed with nonmetastatic breast and prostate cancers. Box 15.1 provides some estimated energy requirements for older adults.

Weight loss is often accompanied by loss of lean body mass and depleted protein stores. Depleted protein stores have a negative effect on immune status and can contribute to fatigue and poor tolerance to treatments. The recommended daily allowance of protein for healthy adults is estimated at 0.8 to 1 gram per kilogram of body weight. Older adults diagnosed with cancer require 1 to 1.5 grams per kilogram of body weight to prevent catabolism, and those with severe malnutrition may require 2 grams per kilogram of body weight (6).

Box 15.1 Quick Guide to Estimating Energy Needs in Adults

These equations are useful as initial estimates of energy needs. Energy needs should be adjusted as the patient's nutritional status changes. Actual body weight is used; however, it is recommended that ideal body weight (IBW) be used in obese patients (> 120% IBW), because adjusted body weight for obesity has not been validated.

20 kcal/kg	Initial refeeding of malnourished/depleted patient
21–25 kcal/kg	Obese patients for maintenance
25–30 kcal/kg	Maintenance/standard
30–35 kcal/kg	Malnourished and/or extensive treatment/bone marrow transplant
35–45 kcal/kg	Depleted and/or hypermetabolic

Source: Reprinted from Martin C. Calorie, protein, fluid, and micronutrient requirements. In: McCallum PD, Polisena CG, eds. *The Clinical Guide to Oncology Nutrition.* Chicago, Ill: American Dietetic Association; 2000:45, with permission from American Dietetic Association.

EFFECTS OF TREATMENT MODALITIES ON NUTRITIONAL STATUS

Surgery, chemotherapy, and radiation therapy can each affect nutritional status. Nutrition care focuses on controlling the symptoms associated with the treatment modality. A proactive and interactive approach to care with all members of the health care team will offer the best outcomes possible. Side effects of cancer treatment vary among individuals and are affected by many factors. Surgical interventions to the alimentary or gastrointestinal tract have specific nutritional implications, which can range from difficulty ingesting or digesting foods to difficulties absorbing specific nutrients, such as fat. Fatigue, temporary appetite loss, and changes in bowel function are also common problems associated with surgery. Chemotherapy regimens can create a multitude of nutrition-impacting symptoms, which can interfere with the older adult's ability to obtain adequate nutrients. Many of the symptoms, such as nausea, are treatable with pharmacological agents, but dietary modifications may provide adequate symptom management for certain side effects, such as constipation, diarrhea, taste changes, and weight loss. The symptoms from radiation therapy are very site-specific; hence, the nutrition-impacting symptoms will vary, based on (*a*) the area of the body treated with radiation, (*b*) the dosage, (*c*) the type of radiation therapy given, and (*d*) the patient's tolerance of the symptoms. Nutrition-related side effects are most common in those receiving external beam radiation therapy to any part of the head or neck region, esophagus, or pelvis. The nutrition goals vary for each client, and individualization of the care plan is essential. Radiation therapy to the head and neck region can contribute to taste changes, reduced salivary function, and severe mucositis. The nutrition needs for these clients are very different from those experiencing diarrhea or malabsorption secondary to the radiation therapy of the pelvic region (7).

Many persons with cancer treat themselves with dietary supplements and herbal products, and dietetics professionals should inform themselves about the use of such treatments. The frequency of use of dietary supplements among older adults is high, compared with the general population. Results from the Third National Health and Nutrition Examination Survey indicated that between 1988 and 1994, 56% of middle-aged and older adults took at least one supplement on a daily basis, as compared with 40% in the general population (8). Scientific evidence about

TABLE 15.1.   Nutrition-Impact Signs and Symptoms

Global	Upper Aerodigestive Tract	Gastrointestinal Tract
Anorexia	Stomatitis	Nausea
Pain	Odynophagia	Vomiting
Fever	Sensory changes of taste and smell	Dyspepsia
Fatigue, muscle weakness	Loose denture, edentulous	Early satiety
Depression, anxiety	Poor oral hygiene	Delayed gastric emptying
Dementia, delirium	Xerostomia	Abdominal pain
Food aversions	Dysphagia	Cramping, bloating
Financial problems	Esophagitis	Excessive flatus
		Constipation
		Diarrhea
		Food intolerances
		Fat malabsorption

Source: Reprinted from McMahon K, Decker G, Ottery FD. Integrating proactive nutritional assessment in clinical practices to prevent complications and cost. *Semin Oncol.* 1998;25(suppl 6):23, with permission from Elsevier.

the safety and benefits of dietary supplements for older adults varies. Not all supplements are safe, and the inappropriate use of some supplements can result in adverse consequences. For example, some supplements may not interact well with prescription drugs or other treatments for cancer (9).

Because using a combination of treatment modalities is becoming more common in treating patients with cancer and because people are using more over-the-counter supplements, having an adequate screening and assessment program in place will set the stage for proactive care and may help to prevent many of the nutrition-related side effects associated with the various forms of treatment. Table 15.1 lists common nutrition-impact signs and symptoms associated with cancer and its treatments (10).

METHODS OF MEETING NUTRITIONAL REQUIREMENTS

The goals of nutrition support are to provide for adequate nutrients to minimize weight loss, to reduce or prevent any nutrition-related symptoms associated with the cancer treatments, and to prevent or correct any underlying nutritional deficiencies. Symptom control is the first step in preventing weight loss and malnutrition in those with cancer. When necessary, oral feedings should be augmented with more nutrient-dense foods and fluids, to provide adequate nutrients to meet the higher energy

needs of those with cancer. Modifications in diet consistency may be necessary for those experiencing symptoms of dysphagia or mucositis. Modifications in specific components or nutrients may be used to relieve symptoms of diarrhea, constipation, or malabsorption. Various high-energy, high-protein nutrition products are available to supplement the diet if oral intake is not adequate (11).

When oral intake is inadequate, regardless of attempts to achieve the client's goal, then enteral nutrition is warranted if in accordance with advance directives. Once enteral nutrition support is underway, nutrition needs can be easily met. If the gastrointestinal tract is unavailable, or if enteral feedings are contraindicated, then total parenteral or peripheral parenteral nutrition may be indicated. Each form of nutrition support must be evaluated not only for efficacy, cost, and possible side effects, but also with regard to patient preferences and quality of life (12).

Adding more energy and protein to the diet or modifying the diet to control symptoms is not always enough to maintain adequate nutritional status. Pharmacological interventions are sometimes useful in helping to treat the cancer-related weight loss. There are four main categories of medications for treating involuntary weight loss in those with cancer, all producing different results: (*a*) drugs to treat symptoms that interfere with adequate nutrition, (*b*) appetite stimulants, (*c*) drugs that affect metabolic or specific humeral and inflammatory responses, and (*d*) anabolic agents, used to improve body composition by maintaining or replenishing lean body mass (13).

The key to managing cancer in older adults is individualized care. Because many older adults may present at the time of diagnosis with a multitude of health, social, and nutrition problems, early intervention is paramount. By using a proactive approach to nutrition support, the older adult and the caregiver will feel empowered to take a more active role in the treatment plan.

REFERENCES

1. American Cancer Society. Facts and figures 2004. Available at: http://www.cancer.org. Accessed March 20, 2004.
2. Balducci L, Extermann M. Management of cancer in the elderly. *Home Health Care Consultant.* 1999;6(3):2-8.
3. Ottery FD. Supportive nutrition to prevent cachexia and improve quality of life. *Semin Oncol.* 1995;22 (suppl 3):98-111.
4. Dewys WD, Begg C, Lavin PT, Band PR, Bennett JM, Bertino JR, Cohen MH, Douglass HO Jr, Engstrom PF, Ezdinli EZ, Horton J, Johnson GJ, Moertel CG, Oken MM, Perlia C, Rosenbaum C, Silverstein MN, Skeel RT, Sponzo RW, Tormey DC. Prognostic effect of weight loss prior to chemotherapy in cancer patients. *Am J Med.* 1980;69:491-497.
5. Inui A. Cancer anorexia-cachexia syndrome: current issues in research and management. *CA Cancer J Clin.* 2002;52:72-91.
6. Martin C. Calorie, protein, fluid, and micronutrient requirements. In: McCallum PD, Polisena CG, eds. *The Clinical Guide to Oncology Nutrition.* Chicago, Ill: American Dietetic Association; 2000:45-52.
7. American Cancer Society. Handling side effects. Available at: http://www.cancer.org/docroot/MBC/MBC_6_1_what_to_do_about_side_effects.asp. Accessed March 20, 2004.
8. National Institutes of Health. Dietary supplement use in the elderly (conference proceedings). Available at: http://dietarysupplements.info.nih.gov/showpage.aspx?pageid=148. Accessed March 20, 2004.
9. National Center for Complementary and Alternative Medicine. Herbal supplements, consider safety too. Available at: http://nccam.nci.nih.gov/health/supplement-safety. Accessed March 20, 2004.
10. McMahon K, Decker G, Ottery FD. Integrating proactive nutritional assessment in clinical practices to prevent complications and cost. *Semin Oncol.* 1998;25(Suppl 6):S23.
11. Bloch AS. Special considerations for nutrition intervention with oncology patients. *Oncology.* 2003;17(Suppl):S17-S18.
12. Tchekmedyian NS. Pharmacoeconomics of nutritional support in cancer. *Semin Oncol.* 1998;25 (Suppl 6):S62-S69.
13. Von Roenn JH. Pharmacologic interventions for cancer-related weight loss. *Oncology Issues.* 2002;17(suppl):S18-S21.

CHAPTER 16

Nutrition Assessment

CLIENT NUTRITION SCREENING

Nutrition screening is the process of identifying characteristics known to be associated with nutrition problems. Its purpose is to pinpoint older adults who are malnourished or at nutritional risk. Assessment and intervention take place after screening occurs. A member of the health care team, such as a dietetics professional, a nurse, a physician, or another qualified health care professional, can complete the nutrition screen.

As defined in the *Journal of the American Dietetic Association,* the screening process has the following characteristics* (1):

- It may be completed in any setting (eg, via personal contact or on-site survey).
- It facilitates completion of early intervention goals.
- It includes the collection of relevant data on risk factors and the interpretation of data for intervention or treatment.
- It determines the need for nutrition assessment.
- It is cost effective.

On a nutrition screen, an older adult with a high score is identified as at risk for malnutrition. Numerous settings across the continuum of care can use the DETERMINE Your Nutritional Health

(Figure 16.1), developed by the Nutrition Screening Initiative (NSI), to determine those at nutritional risk (2). Using DETERMINE, NSI suggests that scores be placed in the following risk groups for intervention (2):

- *Scores of 0 to 2 indicate low risk of poor nutritional status.* The organization may want to distribute educational literature on nutrition and fitness.
- *Scores of 3 to 5 indicate moderate risk.* Clients may be directed to health education and wellness programs, selected health care professionals, or a case manager. It may be appropriate to direct older adults to services such as home-delivered meals/meals on wheels or to counseling services. The checklist should be re-administered in 3 months.
- *Scores of 6 and above indicate high nutritional risk.* Persons who score in this range need additional care.

Level I or II screens (Figures 16.2 and 16.3) are used for clients who need further intervention (3,4).

NUTRITION ASSESSMENT

Nutrition assessment is a comprehensive approach, completed by a dietetics professional, which defines nutritional status using medical, nutrition, and medication histories; physical examination; anthropometric measurements; and laboratory data. It "includes the organization and evaluation of information to declare a professional judgment" (5) and involves interpretation of data gathered during nutrition screening as well as data from other health professionals (such as physical or occupational therapists) (1).

*List reprinted from: Identifying patients at risk: ADA's definitions for nutrition screening and nutrition assessment. Council on Practice (COP) Quality Management Committee. *J Am Diet Assoc.* 1994;94:838-839, with permission from American Dietetic Association.

Figure 16.1

DETERMINE your Nutritional Health form. Reprinted with permission by the Nutrition Screening Initiative, a project of the American Academy of Family Physicians and the American Dietetic Association, funded in part by a grant from Ross Products Division, Abbott Laboratories Inc.

The Warning Signs of poor nutritional health are often overlooked. Use this checklist to find out if you or someone you know is at nutritional risk.

DETERMINE YOUR NUTRITIONAL HEALTH

Read the statements below. Circle the number in the yes column for those that apply to you or someone you know. For each yes answer, score the number in the box. Total your nutritional score.

	YES
I have an illness or condition that made me change the kind and/or amount of food I eat.	2
I eat fewer than 2 meals per day.	3
I eat few fruits or vegetables, or milk products.	2
I have 3 or more drinks of beer, liquor or wine almost every day.	2
I have tooth or mouth problems that make it hard for me to eat.	2
I don't always have enough money to buy the food I need.	4
I eat alone most of the time.	1
I take 3 or more different prescribed or over-the-counter drugs a day.	1
Without wanting to, I have lost or gained 10 pounds in the last 6 months.	2
I am not always physically able to shop, cook and/or feed myself.	2
	TOTAL

Total Your Nutritional Score. If it's —

0-2   **Good!** Recheck your nutritional score in 6 months.

3-5   **You are at moderate nutritional risk.** See what can be done to improve your eating habits and lifestyle. Your office on aging, senior nutrition program, senior citizens center or health department can help. Recheck your nutritional score in 3 months.

6 or more   **You are at high nutritional risk.** Bring this checklist the next time you see your doctor, dietitian or other qualified health or social service professional. Talk with them about any problems you may have. Ask for help to improve your nutritional health.

These materials developed and distributed by the Nutrition Screening Initiative, a project of:

 AMERICAN ACADEMY OF FAMILY PHYSICIANS

 THE AMERICAN DIETETIC ASSOCIATION

 NATIONAL COUNCIL ON THE AGING, INC.

Remember that warning signs suggest risk, but do not represent diagnosis of any condition. Turn the page to learn more about the Warning Signs of poor nutritional health.

Figure 16.2
Level 1 screen. Reprinted with permission by the Nutrition Screening Initiative, a project of the American Academy of Family Physicians and the American Dietetic Association, funded in part by a grant from Ross Products Division, Abbott Laboratories Inc.

Level 1 Screen

Body Weight

Measure height to the nearest inch and weight to the nearest pound. Record the values below and mark them on the Body Mass Index (BMI) scale to the right. Then use a straight edge (ruler) to connect the two points and circle the spot where this straight line crosses the center line (body mass index). Record the number below.

Healthy older adults should have a BMI between 24 and 27.

Height (in):_____
Weight (lbs):_____
Body Mass Index:_____
(number from center column)

Check any boxes that are true for the individual:

☐ Has lost or gained 10 pounds (or more) in the past 6 months.

☐ Body mass index <24

☐ Body mass index >27

For the remaining sections, please ask the individual which of the statements (if any) is true for him or her and place a check by each that applies.

NOMOGRAM FOR BODY MASS INDEX

WEIGHT
KG LB

BODY MASS INDEX
$[WT/(HT)^2]$

HEIGHT
CM IN

WOMEN — OBESE / OVERWEIGHT / *ACCEPTABLE*

MEN — OBESE / OVERWEIGHT / *ACCEPTABLE*

© George A. Bray 1978

Eating Habits

☐ Does not have enough food to eat each day

☐ Usually eats alone

☐ Does not eat anything on one or more days each month

☐ Has poor appetite

☐ Is on a special diet

☐ Eats vegetables two or fewer times daily

☐ Eats milk or milk products once or not at all daily

☐ Eats fruit or drinks fruit juice once or not at all daily

☐ Eats breads, cereals, pasta, rice, or other grains five or fewer times daily

☐ Has difficulty chewing or swallowing

☐ Has more than one alcoholic drink per day (if woman); more than two drinks per day (if man)

☐ Has pain in mouth, teeth, or gums

Living Environment

☐ Lives on an income of less than $6000 per year (per individual in the household)

☐ Lives alone

☐ Is housebound

☐ Is concerned about home security

☐ Lives in a home with inadequate heating or cooling

☐ Does not have a stove and/or refrigerator

☐ Is unable or prefers not to spend money on food (<$25-30 per person spent on food each week)

Functional Status

Usually or always needs assistance with (check each that apply):

☐ Bathing   ☐ Walking or moving about

☐ Dressing   ☐ Traveling (outside the home)

☐ Grooming   ☐ Preparing food

☐ Toileting   ☐ Shopping for food or other necessities

☐ Eating

Figure 16.3

Level 2 screen. Reprinted with permission by the Nutrition Screening Initiative, a project of the American Academy of Family Physicians and the American Dietetic Association, funded in part by a grant from Ross Products Division, Abbott Laboratories Inc.

Level II Screen

Complete the following screen by interviewing the patient directly and/or by referring to the patient chart. If you do not routinely perform all of the described tests or ask all of the listed questions, please consider including them but do not be concerned if the entire screen is not completed. Please try to conduct a minimal screen on as many older patients as possible, and please try to collect serial measurements, which are extremely valuable in monitoring nutritional status. Please refer to the manual for additional information.

Anthropometrics

Measure height to the nearest inch and weight to the nearest pound. Record the values below and mark them on the Body Mass Index (BMI) scale to the right. Then use a straight edge (paper, ruler) to connect the two points and circle the spot where this straight line crosses the center line (body mass index). Record the number below; healthy older adults should have a BMI between 24 and 27; check the appropriate box to flag an abnormally high or low value.

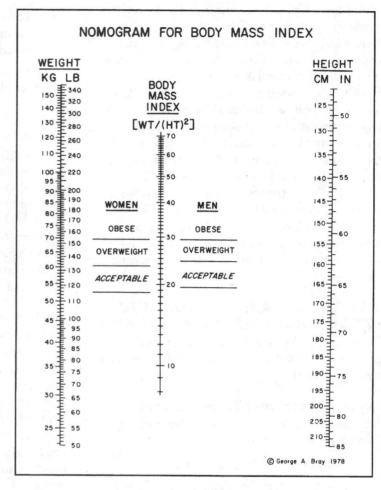

Height (in):_____
Weight (lbs):_____
Body Mass Index
(weight/height^2):_____

Please place a check by any statement regarding BMI and recent weight loss that is true for the patient.

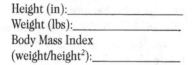

❑ Body mass index <24

❑ Body mass index >27

❑ Has lost or gained 10 pounds (or more) of body weight in the past 6 months

Record the measurement of mid-arm circumference to the nearest 0.1 centimeter and of triceps skinfold to the nearest 2 millimeters.

Mid-Arm Circumference (cm):_____
Triceps Skinfold (mm):_____
Mid-Arm Muscle Circumference (cm):_____

Refer to the table and check any abnormal values:

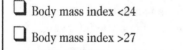

❑ Mid-arm muscle circumference <10th percentile

❑ Triceps skinfold <10th percentile

❑ Triceps skinfold >95th percentile

Note: mid-arm circumference (cm) - {0.314 x triceps skinfold (mm)}= mid-arm *muscle* circumference (cm)

For the remaining sections, please place a check by any statements that are true for the patient.

Laboratory Data

❑ Serum albumin below 3.5 g/dl

❑ Serum cholesterol below 160 mg/dl

❑ Serum cholesterol above 240 mg/dl

Drug Use

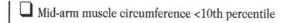

❑ Three or more prescription drugs, OTC medications, and/or vitamin/mineral supplements daily

NUTRITION RISK ASSESSMENT FORMS

The Nutrition Risk Assessment form is the result of a collaborative effort by Consultant Dietitians in Health Care Facilities (CD-HCF), the American Dietetic Association (ADA), the alliances organization that partners with ADA/CD-HCF, and the Health Care Financing Administration (now Centers for Medicare & Medicaid Services [CMS]). This form is currently in the process of being validated. Strategies and interventions are included as a guide for the health care team providing care for the resident. The form can be found in Appendix C.

The Mini Nutritional Assessment is a validated measure of nutritional risk (6). This assessment is commonly used for community-based residents before they enter a nursing facility. It has a self-assessment section but does not address biochemical measures. The form can be found in Appendix B.

RISK FACTORS AND CATEGORIES TO BE CONSIDERED DURING ASSESSMENT

The following risk factors and risk categories are guides to help the dietetics professional determine a client's risk level.

Psychological and Social Factors

This category includes history or evidence of the following risk factors* (1):

- Literacy level or language barriers
- Cultural factors that alter intake of desired nutrients, calories, or food groups
- Religious beliefs that alter intake of desired nutrients, calories, or food groups
- Emotional disturbances (eg, depression, stress), with associated feeding problems
- Caregiver or social support system
- Social isolation (motivational level for self-care)
- Eating or feeding disorders (eg, bulimia, early satiety, autism, rapid pace of eating)
- Limited resources for food preparation or limited access to transportation to obtain food
- Substance or alcohol abuse

*List reprinted from: Identifying patients at risk: ADA's definitions for nutrition screening and nutrition assessment. Council on Practice (COP) Quality Management Committee. *J Am Diet Assoc.* 1994;94:838-839, with permission from American Dietetic Association.

- Limited or low income (eg, below poverty level)
- Limited ability, use, or knowledge of normal nutrition, food preparation, food safety, and community resources
- Lack of ability to communicate needs (eg, dyspraxia)

Cultural Factors

Cultural factors that alter intake of desired nutrients, energy, or food groups can affect the nutritional status. The dietetics professional must be aware of specific groups of food that are eliminated based on cultural or religious preference.

A food preferences form, such as the one shown in Figure 16.4, can be used to gather data that help to determine food choices. This simple form is useful in any setting. Figure 16.5 outlines characteristics of selected ethnic diets (7).

ANTHROPOMETRY

Anthropometry is the measurement of body size, weight, and proportions and is used to evaluate the nutritional status of clients. Low body weight, when associated with illness or injury, increases the risk of morbidity (8). Obesity is common among nonambulatory clients whose energy expenditure is low. The dietetics professional should ensure that the methods used to weigh and measure older adults are reliable, because accurate height and weight data are imperative. Loss of height, for example, is an early indicator of osteoporosis (9). Dietetics professionals should measure and record height annually or per facility policy and procedure.

Standard Measures

Stature

To obtain height for an ambulatory client, the health professional should do the following:

- Have the person being measured wear minimum clothing, so that posture can be clearly seen.
- Instruct the person to stand tall, with bare heels as close together as possible, legs straight, arms at sides, shoulders relaxed, head erect, and eyes looking straight ahead.
- Have the person take a deep breath.
- Take measurement at the point of the person's maximum inspiration with your eyes at headboard level, to avoid errors due to parallax.

Figure 16.4
Food preferences chart. Reprinted with permission from MEP Healthcare Dietary Services, Inc., Evansville, Ind.

FOOD PREFERENCES					
MILK	YES	NO	**VEGETABLES**	YES	NO
Sweet	___	___	Asparagus	___	___
Buttermilk	___	___	Beets	___	___
Chocolate	___	___	Broccoli	___	___
			Brussels sprouts	___	___
FRUITS			Black-eyed peas	___	___
Apples	___	___	Cabbage	___	___
Applesauce	___	___	Carrots	___	___
Apricots	___	___	Cauliflower	___	___
Grapefruit	___	___	Corn	___	___
Pears	___	___	Cucumbers	___	___
Pineapple	___	___	Green beans	___	___
Plums	___	___	Lettuce	___	___
Prunes/juice	___	___	Lima beans	___	___
Peaches	___	___	Navy beans	___	___
Bananas	___	___	Onions	___	___
Fruit cocktail	___	___	Peas	___	___
Watermelon	___	___	Potatoes	___	___
Cantaloupe	___	___	Pumpkin	___	___
Oranges	___	___	Sauerkraut	___	___
Orange juice	___	___	Squash	___	___
			Spinach	___	___
BREADS/CEREAL			Tomatoes (canned)	___	___
Cornflakes	___	___	(fresh)	___	___
Branflakes	___	___	Yams/sweet potatoes	___	___
Oatmeal	___	___			
Rice	___	___	**SALAD DISHES**		
Cream of Wheat	___	___	Lettuce	___	___
Spaghetti	___	___	Coleslaw	___	___
Macaroni	___	___	Cottage cheese	___	___
Biscuits	___	___	American cheese	___	___
Cornbread	___	___	Gelatin	___	___
Pancakes/			Cranberry sauce	___	___
French Toast	___	___	Macaroni salad	___	___
			Potato chips	___	___
SOUPS			Pea salad	___	___
Chili	___	___	Mixed bean salad	___	___
Potato	___	___			
Tomato	___	___	**MEATS**		
Vegetable	___	___	Eggs, favorite style	___	___
Beef	___	___	Sausage	___	___
Bacon	___	___	Wieners	___	___
Bean	___	___	Chicken (baked)	___	___
Other	___	___	Ham	___	___
			Turkey	___	___
			Pork chop/Pork roast	___	___
			Roast beef	___	___
			Hamburger	___	___
			Meat loaf	___	___
			Fish (baked)	___	___
			(fried)	___	___
			Tuna	___	___
			Liver	___	___
			Casseroles	___	___
			Other:	___	___

NAME _____   **ROOM #** _____

Figure 16.5

Characteristics of Selected Ethnic Diets

HISPANIC AMERICANS FROM CUBA, HAITI, PUERTO RICO

Include:
- Steamed white rice; wheat breads
- Starchy vegetables (beans, cassavas, yuccas); plantains; green peppers; tomatoes; garlic
- Dried, salted fish; chicken; pork
- Lard; olive oil; sugar; jams and jellies; sweet pastries; sugared fruit juices; coffee

Exclude:
- Green, leafy vegetables
- Milk as a beverage for adults
- Fish other than dried and salted

HISPANIC AMERICANS FROM MEXICO, CENTRAL AMERICA

Include:
- Steamed rice, corn products such as tortillas
- Many varieties of beans; chili peppers; tomatoes; mangoes; prickly pear fruit; potatoes
- Meat and sausages; fish; poultry; eggs
- Lard; chocolate and coffee drinks; cakes; pastries

Exclude:
- Green, leafy vegetables; yellow vegetables
- Milk as a beverage for adults

BLACK AMERICANS FROM WEST INDIES, CENTRAL OR SOUTH AMERICA, AND RECENT AFRICAN IMMIGRANTS

Include:
- Millet, corn, wheat, rice, or barley
- Starchy roots such as cassavas, yams; plantains; bananas; coconuts; peanuts; fresh fruits; hot peppers; tomatoes; onions, okra
- Palm oil; fruit wine; tea; coffee; honey; molasses

Exclude:
- Milk and milk products (meat and fish limited use)

SOUTHERN BLACK AMERICANS FROM WEST AFRICA
(Many generations in United States)

Include:
- Rice; hominy grits; biscuits; cornmeal and cornbread
- Legumes; potatoes; onions, tomatoes; hot peppers; green leafy vegetables; okra; sweet potatoes; squashes; corn; cabbage; melons; peaches
- Smoked pork; meats and poultry; fish; thick stews
- Pecans; butter, shortening, and lard; sugar; bread puddings, pies, and sweets

Exclude:
- Milk and milk products
- Yeast breads

CHINESE AMERICANS FROM CHINA
(Diets sometimes vary with region.)

Include:
- Rice and rice gruel; wheat noodles; soy bean noodles
- Corn; cabbage-like vegetables; squashes; cucumbers; eggplant; leafy vegetables; various shoots (bamboo, mung, and soy); sweet potatoes; radishes; onions; peas and pods; mushrooms; roots; local vegetables; pickled vegetables; sea vegetables; plums; peaches; tangerines; kumquats; citrus fruits; litchis; longans; mangoes; papayas; pomegranates

continued

110

- Soybean products (tofu and soy milk); meat; fish with bones; poultry; seafood
- Soup or tea as beverage; soy sauce; sugar

Exclude:
- Milk and most milk products

JAPANESE AMERICANS FROM JAPAN

Include:
- Rice
- Vegetables (including pickled and sea); fruits; salads
- Soy (miso, tofu, bean paste); fish with bones; seafood
- Sugars as seasoning; ginseng; soy sauce

Exclude:
- Milk and milk products

KOREAN AMERICANS FROM SOUTH KOREA

Include:
- Rice; noodles
- Leafy vegetables; kimchi (hot pickled cabbage); sea vegetables; hot peppers; seasonal fruits; mushrooms
- Small fish with bones; grilled beef; chicken; squid; octopus; lobster; mussels; eggs
- Lard and vegetable fat for frying; sesame oil; nuts and seeds; ginger; sugar as seasoning

Exclude:
- Milk and milk products

VIETNAMESE AMERICANS FROM VIETNAM

Include:
- Rice; rice noodles; french bread and croissants
- Hot peppers; curries of asparagus and potatoes; salads; tropical fruits and vegetables; lemons and limes
- Small portions of poultry; eggs; fish pates; nuoc nam (a strong, fermented fish sauce)
- Sweets, candies; sweetened drinks; coffee; tea; butter

Exclude:
- Milk and milk products

NATIVE AMERICANS

Include:
- Southeast: corn; cornmeal; coontie (palmlike plant flour); fried breads; pumpkins; squashes; papayas; alligator, snake, wild hog, duck, fish, and shellfish
- Northeast: blueberries; cranberries; beans; corn; pumpkins; fish; lobster; wild game; maple syrup
- Midwest: bison; beans; corn; melons; squashes; tomatoes
- Southwest: corn (many varieties); beans; squash; pumpkins; chili peppers; melons; pinenuts; cactus
- Northwest: salmon; caviar; fish; otter; seal; elk; whale; bear; other game; wild fruits, nuts, and greens

Exclude:
- Milk and milk products

ITALIAN AMERICANS FROM ITALY

Include:
- Northern Italy: egg-based, ribbon-shaped pastas; cheese; cream; butter; meat; eggs
- Southern Italy: wheat pastas; artichokes, eggplants, peppers, and tomatoes; beans; olive oil

- Record measurement to the nearest 0.1 cm or 0.125 in; repeated measurements should agree within 1 cm or 0.5 in.

- Compare present measurement with previous stature measurement(s) and with reference tables or graphs, to determine change and to aid with interpretation of measurements.

To estimate height of nonambulatory persons, use the following method (measurement must be documented as an estimate) (10,11). For both men and women, arm span measurement is roughly equal to height at maturity (within approximately 10%). Span measurement is calculated as follows:

- With the upper extremities, including the hands, fully extended and parallel to the ground at a 90° angle to the torso, measure the distance between the tip of one middle finger and the tip of the other middle finger.

- Span measurement remains constant in spite of decreasing height and is an acceptable alternate method of establishing height.

For those clients who cannot hold arms out straight, calculate as follows (12):

- Measure from the midsternum to the tip of the middle finger.

- Double this number.

- Document as estimated height.

This method may not provide accurate measurements for Asians, African Americans, or clients with spinal deformities or contractures (12).

Weight

The ambulatory client should be weighed on the same scale each time. If the nonambulatory client can sit, a movable wheelchair balance or a wheel scale is used. The total weight minus the weight of the wheelchair equals the weight of the client. Bed scales should be used for weighing bedfast clients.

To obtain an accurate standing weight, the dietetics professional should do the following:

- Be familiar with the use of the instrument.

- Calibrate scale to zero.

- Weigh client at same time of day on the routine schedule and, if possible, by same caregiver.

- Weigh client nude or in light underclothing, without shoes.

- Position client's feet over center of platform.

- Adjust weights on balance beam, then read and accurately record measurement to nearest 0.25 lb; on a digital scale the reading should be to the nearest 0.1 kg/lb.

- Compare present measurement with previous weight measurement(s) and with reference tables or graphs, to determine change and to aid with interpretation of measurements.

Suggestions for an accurate seated or prone measurement are as follows:

- For chair scale, position subject upright in center of chair, leaning on backrest.

- Weigh client and wheelchair, then weigh the wheelchair alone and subtract that weight.

- For bed scale, position subject comfortably in center of sling.

A second measurement using either method must be taken, to verify accuracy of weight. Frequent checking and adjustment of the zero weight on the horizontal beam of the scale are necessary to ensure accuracy. The main and fractional sliding weights should be placed at their respective zero positions, and the zeroing weight should then be checked with a set of standard weights or by a dealer of weights and measures at least two or three times a year. Accurate weights are critical for the dietetics professional when evaluating the nutritional status of a client.

BODY MASS INDEX

Body mass index (BMI) is used as an indicator of body composition and health risk in clinical and epidemiological research (13). BMI is a weight-to-height ratio composed of body weight (in kilograms) divided by the square of the height in meters. BMI is highly correlated with body fat, but increased lean body mass or a large body frame can also increase BMI. It is generally agreed that a normally hydrated person with a BMI of 30 would be obese and that a person with a BMI of more than 27 would be at major risk for obesity (14). BMI categories are as follows (15):

- Healthy weight: BMI 18.5 to 24.9
- Overweight: BMI 25 to 29.9
- Obese: BMI of 30 or higher (obese persons are also overweight)

However, BMI does not consider the variable height loss with age. Thus, if height decreases while weight remains stable, an individual's BMI increases, which may not be a true indication of nutritional status.

In a study of seriously ill, hospitalized stroke patients, baseline measures of nutritional status, including BMI (< 20), were lower for those who died or remained in the hospital than for those who were discharged (16). A US multicenter study examining the relationship of BMI to subsequent mortality among seriously ill hospitalized patients reported that a low BMI (equal to the 15th percentile) was associated with an increased risk of mortality within 6 months of admission, after factors such as serum albumin and weight loss were controlled (17).

Body mass index is difficult to obtain for residents who have difficulty standing up straight. Although it is not done in most long-term-care settings, it is recommended that midarm circumference be measured. This measure is highly correlated with BMI (the Spearman rank correlation coefficient of midarm circumferences with BMI for institutionalized older adults is 0.69 for men and 0.89 for women). Low weight for height calculated as BMI may indicate poor nutritional status (18-21).

Table 16.1 shows height factors (HFs) for given heights; HFs can be used to determine BMI. Table 16.2 (22) shows BMI at specific heights and weights. The following are three formulas for calculating BMI:

$$BMI = Wt\ (kg)/Ht\ (m)^2$$
$$BMI = HF \times Wt\ (lb)$$
$$BMI = [Wt\ (lb)/Ht\ (in)^2] \times 705$$

AMPUTATION

Adjusted Weight

The percentages shown in Figure 16.6 (23) can be used as a guide when calculating an adjusted weight for an amputation.

Example:
Previous target weight range: 131 lb to 161 lb
Adjusted weight range with above-the-knee amputation (AKA)

TABLE 16.1. Body Mass Index Height Factors

Height	HF	Height	HF	Height	HF
4'7"	0.232	5'3"	0.177	5'11"	0.139
4'8"	0.224	5'4"	0.172	6'0"	0.136
4'9"	0.216	5'5"	0.166	6'1"	0.132
4'10"	0.209	5'6"	0.161	6'2"	0.128
4'11"	0.202	5'7"	0.157	6'3"	0.125
5'0"	0.195	5'8"	0.152	6'4"	0.122
5'1"	0.189	5'9"	0.148	6'5"	0.119
5'2"	0.183	5'10"	0.143	6'6"	0.116

Abbreviation: HF, height factor.

Calf and foot (5.9% of total body weight [TBW]) + $\frac{1}{2}$ thigh (5.05% of TBW) = 10.95% of TBW

131 lb × 0.1095 (10.95%) = 14.3 lb
161 lb × 0.1095 (10.95%) = 17.62 lb

Adjusted body weight: 117 lb to 144 lb

Formula for Body Mass Index (BMI) in Amputees

Using the percentages shown in Figure 16.6, Himes has provided a formula for estimating TBW, including missing limb segments, for amputees who can be weighed. The TBW estimate can then be used to calculate the individual's BMI (24).

$$Wt_E = Wt_O/(1 - P)$$

Where: Wt_E is estimated TBW; Wt_O is the observed body weight; and P is the percentage of TBW represented by the missing limb segment(s).

Example (24):
A below-the-knee amputation is 5.9% or 0.059 of TBW.

Observed weight is 70 kg.

$$Wt_E = 70\ kg \div (1 - 0.059)$$
$$= 70\ kg \div (0.941)$$
$$= 74.4\ kg$$

Studies document unique care issues for people with amputations (25), and a low BMI was a predictor of death in a 15-month period after an amputation (26).

TABLE 16.2. Body Mass Index (BMI) at Specific Heights and Weights

Height (in)	Body Weight (lb)																	
58	91	96	100	105	110	115	119	124	129	134	138	143	148	153	158	162	167	172
59	94	99	104	109	114	119	124	128	133	138	143	148	153	158	163	168	173	178
60	97	102	107	112	118	123	128	133	138	143	148	153	158	163	168	174	179	184
61	100	106	111	116	122	127	132	137	143	148	153	158	164	169	174	180	185	190
62	104	109	115	120	126	131	136	142	147	153	158	164	169	175	180	186	191	196
63	107	113	118	124	130	135	141	146	152	158	163	169	175	180	186	191	197	203
64	110	116	122	128	134	140	145	151	157	163	169	174	180	186	192	197	204	209
65	114	120	126	132	138	144	150	156	162	168	174	180	186	192	198	204	210	216
66	118	124	130	136	142	148	155	161	167	173	179	186	192	198	204	210	216	223
67	121	127	134	140	146	153	159	166	172	178	185	191	198	204	211	217	223	230
68	125	131	138	144	151	158	164	171	177	184	190	197	203	210	216	223	230	236
69	128	135	142	146	155	162	169	176	182	189	196	203	209	216	223	230	236	243
70	132	139	146	153	160	167	174	181	188	195	202	209	216	222	229	236	243	250
71	136	143	150	157	165	172	179	186	193	200	208	215	222	229	236	243	250	257
72	140	147	154	162	169	177	184	191	199	206	213	221	228	235	242	250	258	265
73	144	151	159	166	174	182	189	197	204	212	219	227	235	242	250	257	265	272
74	148	155	163	171	179	186	194	202	210	218	225	233	241	249	257	264	272	280
75	152	160	168	176	184	192	200	208	216	224	232	240	248	256	264	272	279	287
76	156	164	172	180	189	197	205	213	221	230	238	246	254	263	271	279	287	295
BMI	19	20	21	22	23	24	25	26	27	28	29	30	31	32	33	34	35	36

Height (in)	Body Weight (lb)																	
58	177	181	186	191	196	201	205	210	215	220	224	229	234	239	244	248	253	258
59	183	188	193	198	203	208	212	217	222	227	232	237	242	247	252	257	262	267
60	189	194	199	204	209	215	220	225	230	235	240	245	250	255	261	266	271	276
61	195	201	206	211	217	222	227	232	238	243	248	254	259	264	269	275	280	285
62	202	207	213	218	224	229	235	240	246	251	256	262	267	273	278	284	289	295
63	208	214	220	225	231	237	242	248	254	259	265	270	278	282	287	293	299	304
64	215	221	227	232	238	244	250	256	262	267	273	279	285	291	296	302	308	314
65	222	228	234	240	246	252	258	264	270	276	282	288	294	300	306	312	318	324
66	229	235	241	247	253	260	266	272	278	284	291	297	303	309	315	322	328	334
67	236	242	249	255	261	268	274	280	287	293	299	306	312	319	325	331	338	344
68	243	249	256	262	269	276	282	289	295	302	308	315	322	328	335	341	348	354
69	250	257	263	270	277	284	291	297	304	311	318	324	331	338	345	351	358	365
70	257	264	271	278	285	292	299	306	313	320	327	334	341	348	355	362	369	376
71	265	272	279	286	293	301	308	315	322	329	338	343	351	358	365	372	379	386
72	272	279	287	294	302	309	316	324	331	338	346	353	361	368	375	383	390	397
73	280	288	295	302	310	318	325	333	340	348	355	363	371	378	386	393	401	408
74	287	295	303	311	319	326	334	342	350	358	365	373	381	389	396	404	412	420
75	295	303	311	319	327	335	343	351	359	367	375	383	391	399	407	415	423	431
76	304	312	320	328	336	344	353	361	369	377	385	394	402	410	418	426	435	443
BMI	37	38	39	40	41	42	43	44	45	46	47	48	49	50	51	52	53	54

Figure 16.6

Percentage of total body weight contributed by individual body parts. Reprinted from Osterkamp LK. Current perspective on assessment of human body proportions of relevance to amputees. *J Am Diet Assoc.* 1995;95:215–218, with permission from American Dietetic Association.

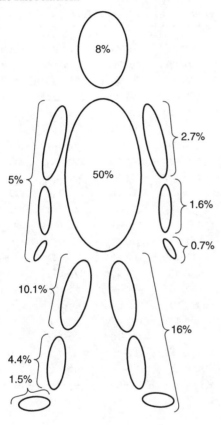

PARAPLEGICS AND QUADRIPLEGICS

In individuals with spinal cord injuries, body composition changes, such as water shifts, muscle atrophy from disease, and increased percentage of body fat, affect the interpretation of anthropometric measures. To calculate the ideal body weight (IBW) for a client who is paralyzed, first determine the IBW for a similar individual without paralysis. Next, subtract the appropriate value from that weight. The value subtracted depends on the degree of paralysis: for paraplegics, subtract 10 to 15 lb from IBW of an individual without paralysis; for quadriplegics, subtract 15 to 20 lb from IBW of an individual without paralysis (27,28).

Box 16.1   Hamwi Formula To Calculate Ideal Body Weight (IBW)*

Women: 100 lb + 5 lb for each inch of height above 5 ft

> **Example:** height 5'6"
> 100 + (6 × 5)
> 100 + 30 = 130
> IBW = 130 lb

Men: 106 lb + 6 lb for each inch of height above 5 ft

> **Example:** 5'10"
> 106 + (10 × 6)
> 106 + 60 = 166
> IBW = 166 lb

*For a large frame, add 10%. For a small frame, subtract 10%.

HEIGHT AND WEIGHT

Weight and body composition change with age. Weight tends to peak in the sixth decade, with a gradual decrease beyond the seventh decade. Shifts in body composition are noted, and the proportion of body weight that is fat increases, averaging 30% of the TBW in older adults, as compared with 20% in younger people. The Hamwi formula (Box 16.1) is frequently used to calculate desirable or IBW for older adults (29). Table 16.3 illustrates the use of the Hamwi formula and frame size.

Table 16.4 represents average weights and heights of white Americans aged 65 to 94 (30). However, some older adult clients may have a target or usual weight that does not correlate with any table. An 85-year-old woman may never reach a weight of 100 lb, and an obese client may never achieve an "ideal" weight. The important issue is achieving a stable weight for a period of 6 months or more. Usual body weight (UBW) is the preferred standard for older adults.

Weight Variances

Variances in weight have significant impact on nutritional health; degree of weight change has positive correlations with impact on health status (8).

TABLE 16.3. Ideal Body Weight (Women and Men)

Women					**Men**				
	Weight Based on Frame Size and Height (lb)			Weight Based on Height (lb)		Weight Based on Frame Size and Height (lb)			Weight Based on Height (lb)
Height	Small Frame	Medium Frame	Large Frame	General Range	Height	Small Frame	Medium Frame	Large Frame	General Range
4'6"	—	—	—	79-107	4'10"	78-88	89-99	100-110	80-97
4'7"	—	—	—	83-101	4'11"	84-94	95-105	106-116	85-104
4'8"	—	—	—	85-103	5'0"	90-100	101-111	112-122	95-117
4'9"	—	—	—	85-103	5'1"	96-106	107-117	118-128	101-123
4'10"	—	—	—	86-106	5'2"	100-111	112-123	124-135	106-130
4'11"	—	—	—	88-108	5'3"	107-117	118-129	130-141	112-136
5'0"	85-95	96-105	106-115	90-110	5'4"	110-122	123-135	136-148	117-143
5'1"	90-100	101-110	111-121	95-116	5'5"	117-127	128-141	142-155	122-150
5'2"	94-104	105-115	116-126	99-121	5'6"	121-133	134-147	148-161	128-156
5'3"	99-109	110-120	121-132	104-127	5'7"	128-138	139-153	154-168	133-163
5'4"	103-113	114-125	126-137	108-132	5'8"	134-144	145-159	160-174	139-169
5'5"	108-118	119-130	131-141	113-136	5'9"	139-149	150-165	166-181	144-176
5'6"	112-122	123-135	136-148	117-143	5'10"	144-154	155-171	172-188	149-183
5'7"	117-127	128-140	141-154	122-149	5'11"	150-160	161-177	178-194	155-189
5'8"	121-131	132-145	146-159	126-154	6'0"	155-165	166-183	184-201	160-196
5'9"	126-136	137-150	151-165	131-160	6'1"	161-171	172-189	190-207	166-202
5'10"	130-140	141-155	156-170	135-165	6'2"	166-176	177-195	196-214	171-209
5'11"	135-145	146-160	161-176	140-171	6'3"	171-181	182-201	202-221	176-216
6'0"	139-149	150-165	166-181	144-176	6'4"	177-187	188-207	208-227	182-222

Source: Used with permission from Miller's Health Systems Inc.

When evaluating weight variances, it is important to determine possible causes, such as recent surgery or treatment initiation (eg, radiation or diuretic therapy affect weight status). Weight variances can also occur when caregivers fail to use correct procedures or weigh clients at different times of the day. Procedures and protocols for addressing weight change need to be in place to ensure accurate weights. Significant weight loss should be reported to both the physician and the dietetics professional to ensure proper intervention.

Evaluating the Significance of Weight Loss

The formula to determine weight change is as follows:

Weight loss % = [(UBW – CBW)/UBW] × 100

Where: UBW = usual body weight; CBW = current body weight

Example:

[(115 – 105)/115] × 100 = 8.7% weight loss

The severity of weight loss can be categorized as follows (31,32):

- Significant weight loss:
  - 10% in 6 months
  - 7.5% in 3 months
  - 5% in 1 month
  - 2% in 1 week
- Severe weight loss:
  - > 10% in 6 months

TABLE 16.4. Average Heights and Weights of Americans Aged 65 to 94 Years

Height (in)	Ages (y)					
	65-69	70-74	75-79	80-84	85-89	90-94
Men						
61	128-156	125-153	123-151			
62	130-158	127-155	125-153	122-148		
63	131-161	129-157	127-155	122-150	120-146	
64	134-164	131-161	129-157	124-152	122-148	
65	136-166	134-164	130-160	127-155	125-153	117-143
66	139-169	137-167	133-163	130-158	128-156	120-146
67	140-172	140-170	136-166	132-162	130-160	122-150
68	143-175	142-174	139-169	135-165	133-163	126-154
69	147-179	146-178	142-174	139-169	137-167	130-158
70	150-184	148-182	146-178	143-175	140-172	134-164
71	155-189	152-186	149-183	148-180	144-176	139-169
72	159-195	156-190	154-188	153-187	148-182	
73	164-200	160-196	158-192			
Women						
58	120-146	112-138	111-135			
59	121-147	114-140	112-136	100-122	99-121	
60	122-148	116-142	113-139	106-130	102-124	
61	123-151	118-144	115-141	109-133	104-128	
62	125-153	121-147	118-144	112-136	108-132	107-131
63	127-155	123-151	121-146	115-141	112-136	107-131
64	130-158	126-154	123-151	119-145	115-141	108-132
65	132-162	130-158	126-154	122-150	120-146	112-136
66	136-166	132-162	128-157	126-154	124-152	116-142
67	140-170	136-166	131-161	130-158	128-156	
68	143-175	140-170				
69	148-180	144-176				

Source: Adapted with permission from Master AM, Laser RP, Beckman G. Tables of average weight and height of Americans aged 65 to 94 years. *JAMA.* 1960;172:658. Copyright © 1960, American Medical Association. All rights reserved.

- > 7.5% in 3 months
- > 5% in 1 month
- > 2% in 1 week

Evaluating Obesity

An adjusted IBW is often used to calculate energy and protein for the obese client (32).

Adjusted body weight =
[(Current weight – IBW) × 0.25] + IBW

Example:

145 lb = [(220 lb – 120 lb) × 0.25] + 120

ENERGY NEEDS

An estimate of energy needs must be completed for each client. To estimate kilocalories, calculate the basal energy expenditure (BEE), as specified in Tables 16.5 and 16.6, and multiply it by the activity factor and the injury factor (Box 16.2 and Box 16.3) (33). Table 16.7 shows a shortcut method for estimating adult energy needs per kilogram (34-36).

TABLE 16.5. Basal Energy Expenditure (BEE): Males*

Weight

lb	kg	kcal	lb	kg	kcal
88.0	40	616	187.0	85	1235
90.2	41	630	189.2	86	1249
92.4	42	644	191.4	87	1263
94.6	43	658	193.6	88	1276
96.8	44	671	195.8	89	1290
99.0	45	685	198.0	90	1304
101.2	46	699	200.2	91	1318
103.4	47	713	202.4	92	1331
105.6	48	726	204.6	93	1345
107.8	49	740	206.8	94	1359
110.0	50	754	209.0	95	1373
112.2	51	768	211.2	96	1386
114.4	52	781	213.4	97	1400
116.6	53	795	215.6	98	1414
118.8	54	809	217.8	99	1428
121.0	55	823	220.0	100	1441
123.2	56	836	222.2	101	1455
125.4	57	850	224.4	102	1469
127.6	58	864	226.6	103	1483
129.8	59	878	228.8	104	1496
132.0	60	891	231.0	105	1510
134.2	61	905	233.2	106	1524
136.4	62	919	235.4	107	1538
138.6	63	933	237.6	108	1551
140.8	64	946	239.8	109	1565
143.0	65	960	242.0	110	1579
145.2	66	974	244.2	111	1593
147.4	67	988	246.4	112	1606
149.6	68	1001	248.6	113	1620
151.8	69	1015	250.8	114	1634
154.0	70	1029	253.0	115	1648
156.2	71	1043	255.2	116	1661
158.4	72	1066	257.4	117	1675
160.6	73	1070	259.6	118	1689
162.8	74	1084	261.8	119	1703
165.0	75	1098	264.0	120	1716
167.2	76	1111	266.2	121	1730
169.4	77	1125	268.4	122	1744
171.6	78	1139	270.6	123	1758
173.8	79	1153	272.8	124	1771
176.0	80	1166			
178.2	81	1180			
180.4	82	1194			
182.6	83	1208			
184.8	84	1221			

Height

ft in	in	cm	kcal
4' 7"	55	139.7	699
8	56	142.2	711
9	57	144.8	724
10	58	147.3	737
11	59	149.9	749
5' 0"	60	152.4	762
1	61	154.9	776
2	62	157.5	787
3	63	160.0	800
4	64	162.6	813
5' 5"	65	165.1	825
6	66	167.6	838
7	67	170.2	851
8	68	172.7	864
9	69	175.3	876
5' 10"	70	177.8	889
11	71	180.3	902
6' 0"	72	182.9	914
1	73	185.4	927
2	74	188.0	940
6' 3"	75	190.5	953
4	76	193.0	965
5	77	195.6	978
6	78	198.1	991
7	79	200.7	1003
6' 8"	80	203.2	1016
9	81	205.7	1029
10	82	208.3	1041
11	83	210.8	1054
7' 0	84	213.4	1067

Age

y	kcal	y	kcal	y	kcal
18	122	48	324	78	527
19	128	49	331	79	534
20	135	50	331	80	541
21	142	51	345	81	548
22	149	52	352	82	554
23	155	53	358	83	561
24	162	54	365	84	568
25	169	55	379	85	575
26	176	56	379	86	581
27	183	57	385	87	588
28	189	58	392	88	595
29	196	59	399	89	602
30	203	60	406	90	608
31	210	61	412	91	615
32	216	62	419	92	622
33	223	63	426	93	629
34	230	64	433	94	635
35	237	65	439	95	642
36	243	66	446	96	649
37	250	67	453	97	656
38	257	68	460		
39	264	69	466		
40	270	70	473		
41	277	71	480		
42	284	72	487		
43	291	73	493		
44	297	74	500		
45	304	75	507		
46	311	76	514		
47	318	77	521		

*Based on the Harris-Benedict equation: BEE = 655.19 + (13.75 × weight in kg) + (5.0 × height in cm) − (6.76 × age in years).

Source: Harris J, Benedict F. *A Biometric Study of Basal Metabolism in Man.* Washington, DC: Carnegie Institute; 1919:40-44. Publication 279.

How to use this table:

Step 1: Obtain weight, height, and age of male subject.

Step 2: BEE = weight kcal + height kcal − age kcal

Example: 70-kg, 178-cm, 45-year-old male

BEE = 1029 + 889 − 304

BEE = 1614

Source: Adapted with permission from Guidelines for Nutritional Care, ©1994, reprinted with permission by Nutrition Education Center.

TABLE 16.6. Basal Energy Expenditure (BEE): Females*

Weight

lb	kg	kcal	lb	kg	kcal
77.0	35	990	171.6	78	1401
79.2	36	999	173.8	79	1410
81.4	37	1009	176.0	80	1420
83.6	38	1018	178.2	81	1429
85.8	39	1028	180.4	82	1439
88.0	40	1038	182.6	83	1449
90.2	41	1047	184.8	84	1458
92.4	42	1057	187.0	85	1468
94.6	43	1066	189.2	86	1477
96.8	44	1076	191.4	87	1487
99.0	45	1085	193.6	88	1496
101.2	46	1095	195.8	89	1506
103.4	47	1104	198.0	90	1516
105.6	48	1114	200.2	91	1526
107.8	49	1124	202.4	92	1535
110.0	50	1133	204.6	93	1544
112.2	51	1143	206.8	94	1554
114.4	52	1152	209.0	95	1563
116.6	53	1162	211.2	96	1573
118.8	54	1171	213.4	97	1582
121.0	55	1181	215.6	98	1592
123.2	56	1190	217.8	99	1602
125.4	57	1200	220.0	100	1611
127.6	58	1210	222.2	101	1621
129.8	59	1219	224.4	102	1630
132.0	60	1229	226.6	103	1640
134.2	61	1238	228.8	104	1649
136.4	62	1248	231.0	105	1659
138.6	63	1257	233.2	106	1668
140.8	64	1267	235.4	107	1678
143.0	65	1277	237.6	108	1688
145.2	66	1286	239.8	109	1697
147.4	67	1296	242.0	110	1707
149.6	68	1305	244.2	111	1716
151.8	69	1315	246.4	112	1726
154.0	70	1324	248.6	113	1735
156.2	71	1334	250.8	114	1745
158.4	72	1343	253.0	115	1755
160.6	73	1353	255.2	116	1764
162.8	74	1363	257.4	117	1774
165.0	75	1372	259.6	118	1783
167.2	76	1382	261.8	119	1793
169.4	77	1391			

Height

ft in	in	cm	kcal
4' 0"	48	121.9	226
1	49	124.5	230
2	50	127.0	235
3	51	129.5	240
4	52	132.1	244
4' 5"	53	134.6	249
6	54	137.2	254
4' 7"	55	139.7	258
8	56	142.2	263
9	57	144.8	268
4' 10	58	147.3	273
11	59	149.9	277
5' 0"	60	152.4	282
1	61	154.9	287
2	62	157.5	291
5' 3"	63	160.0	296
4	64	162.6	301
5	65	165.1	305
6	66	167.6	310
7	67	170.2	315
5' 8"	68	172.7	320
9	69	175.3	324
10	70	177.8	329
11	71	180.3	334
6' 0"	72	182.9	338

Age

y	kcal	y	kcal	y	kcal
18	84	48	225	78	365
19	89	49	229	79	370
20	94	50	234	80	374
21	98	51	239	81	379
22	103	52	243	82	384
23	108	53	248	83	388
24	112	54	253	84	393
25	117	55	257	85	398
26	122	56	262	86	402
27	126	57	267	87	407
28	131	58	271	88	412
29	136	59	276	89	417
30	140	60	281	90	421
31	145	61	285	91	426
32	150	62	290	92	431
33	154	63	295	93	435
34	159	64	300	94	440
35	164	65	304	95	445
36	168	66	309	96	449
37	173	67	314	97	454
38	178	68	318	98	459
39	183	69	323	99	463
40	187	70	328	101	468
41	192	71	332	102	477
42	197	72	337		
43	201	73	342		
44	206	74	346		
45	211	75	351		
46	215	76	356		
47	220	77	360		

*Based on the Harris-Benedict equation: BEE = 66.47 + (9.56 × weight in kg) + (1.85 × height in cm) − (4.68 × age in years).

Source: Harris J, Benedict F. *A Biometric Study of Basal Metabolism in Man.* Washington, DC: Carnegie Institute; 1919:40-44. Publication 279.

How to use this table:

Step 1: Obtain weight, height, and age of female subject.

Step 2: BEE = weight kcal + height kcal − age kcal

Example: 55-kg, 163-cm, 45-year-old female

BEE = 1189 + 302 − 211

BEE = 1271

Source: Adapted with permission from Guidelines for Nutritional Care, ©1994, reprinted with permission by Nutrition Education Center.

Box 16.2 Activity Factors

1.2	for clients confined to bed
1.3	for ambulatory clients
1.5-1.75	for most normally active persons
2.0	for extremely active persons

Source: Reprinted with permission from Consultant Dietitians in Health Care Facilities. *CD-HCF Pocket Resource for Nutrition Assessment, 2001 Revision.* Chicago, Ill: Consultant Dietitians in Health Care Facilities; 2001:39.

TABLE 16.7. Shortcut Method for Estimating Adult Energy Needs

Condition	Daily Energy Requirement (kcal/kg body weight)
Nonobese	25-35
Obese, Critically Ill	21
Paraplegic*	28
Quadriplegic*	23

*Because immobilized patients lose muscle, estimated energy needs for paraplegic and quadriplegic individuals are adjusted by reducing calculated desirable body weights.

Source: Data are from references 34-36.

Box 16.3 Injury Factors

1.00-1.05	Postoperative (no complication)
1.05-1.25	Peritonitis
1.10-1.45	Cancer
1.15-1.30	Long bone fracture
1.20-1.60	Wound healing
1.25-1.50	Blunt trauma
1.30-1.55	Severe infection/multiple trauma
1.50-1.70	Multiple trauma with client on ventilator
1.60-1.70	Trauma with steroids
1.75-1.85	Sepsis

Burns (% total body surface)

1.00-1.50	0%-20%
1.50-1.85	20%-40%
1.85-2.05	40%-100%

Source: Reprinted with permission from Consultant Dietitians in Health Care Facilities. *CD-HCF Pocket Resource for Nutrition Assessment, 2001 Revision.* Chicago, Ill: Consultant Dietitians in Health Care Facilities; 2001:39-40.

PROTEIN REQUIREMENTS

The protein content of the body changes with age, as muscle diminishes and body fat increases. Older adults can expect a 2% to 3% loss of lean body mass per decade (37). Munro and Young (38) recommend that 12% to 14% of the total energy consumed by older adults be in the form of protein if energy intakes are decreased. This may necessitate increased protein intake. The exact protein intake for older adults has not been established, but the range is probably 1 to 1.25 g/kg/day for severe protein depletion (albumin level < 2.1) (39). UBW is used in calculating the dietary protein requirements for an underweight person. See Box 16.4 (33).

FLUID REQUIREMENTS

Baseline fluid requirements are determined by various methods. In older adults, water accounts for approximately 50% of the person's weight, 10% less than in a young adult. The decrease is associated with a corresponding decrease in lean body mass (37). Older adults tend to have a decreased thirst sensation; even healthy adults have reduced thirst after extended water deprivation. Meeting fluid needs is critical.

Special consideration for fluid replacement should be given to older adults with severe vomiting or diarrhea or elevated temperature, because dehydration is a concern. When calculating needs, select the method most appropriate for the client (see Box 16.5 [40] and Box 16.6 [33]).

ORAL NUTRITION INTAKE: FOOD AND FLUIDS

Although not required by federal regulations, documentation of the client's intake of foods and fluids is an essential part of the assessment process.

Box 16.4 Protein Needs for Adults

Condition	Albumin Level (g/dL)	Protein Requirements (g/kg/d)
Normal nutrition (healthy adults)	3.5	0.8
Normal nutrition (elderly adults)	> 3.5	0.8-1.0
Mild depletion	2.8-3.5	1.0-1.2
Moderate depletion	2.1-2.7	1.2-1.5
Severe depletion	2.1	1.5-2.0

COPD 100-125 g protein/day total

Exceptions:	Protein requirement (g/kg/d)
Renal failure	
Nondialyzed	0.5-0.6
Hemodialyzed	1.0-1.2
Peritoneal-dialyzed	1.2-1.5
Hepatic failure	0.25-0.5

Another method of calculating protein needs is as a ratio of grams nitrogen to nonprotein kilocalories (6.25 g protein = 1 g N).

Patient Conditions	Ratio of Nonprotein kcal:1 g N
Adult medical	125-150:1
Minor catabolic	125-180:1
Severe catabolic	150-250:1
Hepatic or renal failure	250-400:1

Source: Reprinted with permission from Consultant Dietitians in Health Care Facilities. *CD-HCF Pocket Resource for Nutrition Assessment, 2001 Revision.* Chicago, Ill: Consultant Dietitians in Health Care Facilities; 2001:42-43.

Box 16.5 Fluid Status

- Congestive heart failure/edema = 25 mL/kg of body weight
- Normal fluid status = 25-30 mL/kg of body weight
- 1 mL/kcal
- 100 mL/kg for first 10 kg body weight + 50 mL/kg for second 10 kg body weight + 15 mL/kg for remaining kg body weight.

OR shortcut to this method
[Body Wt (kg) – 20] × 15 + 1,500 mL

Source: Adapted from Chidester JC, Spangler AA. Fluid intake in the institutionalized elderly. *J Am Diet Assoc.* 1997;97:23-28, with permission from American Dietetic Association.

A food intake record (Figure 16.7) reports the percentage of food eaten at the meal and records fluid intake in ounces. This type of record is useful to document replacements that are offered. Food replacements should be offered to older adults at risk for malnutrition, such as those eating less than 50% to 75% of the meal. It is important to document percentage of snacks that are offered. Accurate food intake records are a challenge in nursing facilities, because they represent only one aspect of care performed by caregivers who have multiple tasks to perform during the day. Intake records should be completed immediately after the meal.

MEDICATIONS

Chronic use of medication, either self-administered or prescribed, has the potential to significantly affect nutritional status. Many people mix prescribed drugs

Box 16.6   Factors That May Alter Fluid Requirements

The following may INCREASE fluid needs:

- Anabolism
- Burns
- Constipation
- Dehydration
- Diarrhea
- Emesis
- Fever*
- Fistulas/drains
- Hemorrhage
- Hot or dry environments
- Hyperventilation
- Hypotension
- Medications
- Nasogastric suctioning
- Polyuria[†]

The following may DECREASE fluid needs:

- Cardiac disease (especially congestive heart failure)
- Edema
- Fluid overload
- Hepatic failure with ascites
- Medications
- Renal failure
- Syndrome of inappropriate secretion of antidiuretic hormone (SIADH)
- Significant hypertension
- "Third spacing" of fluids

*Fluid needs increase 7% for each degree Fahrenheit above normal; 13% for each degree Celsius.

[†]Poor glucose control; excess alcohol, caffeine; osmotic diuresis

Source: Reprinted with permission from Consultant Dietitians in Health Care Facilities. *CD-HCF Pocket Resource for Nutrition Assessment, 2001 Revision.* Chicago, Ill: Consultant Dietitians in Health Care Facilities; 2001:45.

with over-the-counter medication. The dietetics professional should review the medical record and interview the older adult to determine all the medications and supplements taken. Anorexia, nausea, altered bowel functions, taste alterations, and drug-nutrient interactions are just a few examples of potential side effects. Lewis et al (41) reported an average of two potential drug-nutrient interactions for each older adult in a nursing facility (see Chapter 18).

Many of the drugs used to treat cognitive disorders, such as antidepressants, antipsychotics, antianxiety agents, and anticholinergics, have the potential to cause significant side effects. Increased or decreased appetite, nausea, dry mouth, dehydration, changes in bowel status, drowsiness, and anorexia are potential complications (42).

RISK FACTORS THAT AFFECT NUTRITION

Many physical conditions and diseases/disorders can negatively affect nutritional status (see Table 16.8).

Chewing and Swallowing

Any problems encountered while chewing or swallowing foods, beverages, or medication are risk factors and should be noted on the assessment. The dietetics professional should examine the mouth for broken or missing teeth or swollen or bleeding gums, which may indicate a vitamin C deficiency. A dry mouth with reduced saliva production may be a sign of dehydration or a result of medications (eg, bronchodilator, psychotropics, etc). Lesions in the mouth and sore or bleeding gums affect oral intake.

Dental problems, such as loose-fitting dentures, may require the assistance of the social service director to contact the dentist and correct the problem. Carefully observe the older adult who is edentulous, has poor teeth, or has ill-fitting dentures before recommending a consistency alteration. Oral status includes evaluation of texture modification. An older adult who has difficulty swallowing may also require texture modification. The dietetics professional, speech language pathologist, and occupational therapist should work as a team in evaluating the need for thickened liquids, texture modifications, and self-help feeding devices.

Figure 16.7
Food Intake Record

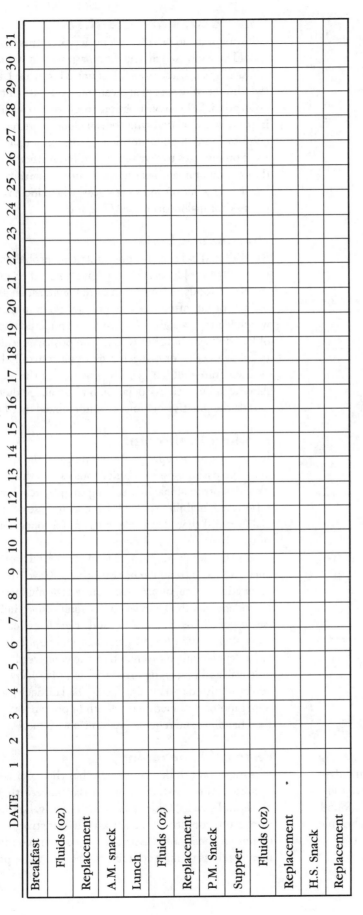

DATE	1	2	3	4	5	6	7	8	9	10	11	12	13	14	15	16	17	18	19	20	21	22	23	24	25	26	27	28	29	30	31
Breakfast																															
Fluids (oz)																															
Replacement																															
A.M. snack																															
Lunch																															
Fluids (oz)																															
Replacement																															
P.M. Snack																															
Supper																															
Fluids (oz)																															
Replacement																															
H.S. Snack																															
Replacement																															

Replacement noted for insulin, calorie-controlled diabetics, and consumption of 50% or less

Guidelines for Determining Meal Percentages Follow schedule outlined below:

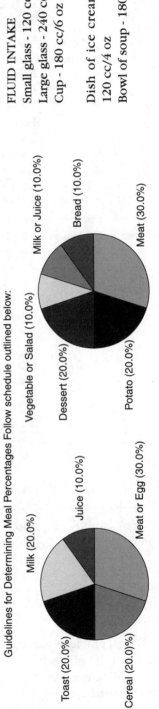

Milk (20.0%)
Vegetable or Salad (10.0%)
Dessert (20.0%)
Milk or Juice (10.0%)
Bread (10.0%)
Meat (30.0%)
Potato (20.0%)
Meat or Egg (30.0%)
Juice (10.0%)
Toast (20.0%)
Cereal (20.0%)

An item is eaten less than 1/4 of amount served - no credit shall be given.

FLUID INTAKE
Small glass - 120 cc/4 oz
Large glass - 240 cc/8 oz
Cup - 180 cc/6 oz

Dish of ice cream or Jello - 120 cc/4 oz
Bowl of soup - 180 cc/6 oz

TABLE 16.8. Risk Factors That May Lead to Undernutrition

Type of Risk	Examples
Social issues	Lack of socialization No help with meals Poverty
Mechanical barriers	Diminished/altered taste Eats slowly Ethnic preferences not available Poor eyesight Poor health Poor hygiene Poor motor coordination Requires culturally accepted food
Medical conditions	Interference with eating due to: • Cholelithiasis • Congestive heart failure • Diabetic gastroparesis • Malabsorption syndromes Increased energy needs due to: • Burns • Cancer • Chronic obstructive pulmonary disease • Fractures • Infections • Wounds
Psychological conditions	Anorexia Dementia Depression Late-life paranoia

Dental problems may contribute to mild dysgeusia or a chronic taste in the mouth. One study of 6,832 Minimum Data Set (MDS) records found that poor intake, eating dependency, and chewing problems were associated with weight loss (43) (see Chapter 14).

Constipation and Diarrhea

Constipation and diarrhea are both risk factors that should be addressed in a nutrition assessment. Older adults frequently use over-the-counter laxatives. Laxative abuse is widespread and can induce a state of malabsorption. When constipation progresses to fecal impaction, associated symptoms include anorexia, confusion, and fecal incontinence, and thus impaction itself predisposes to dehydration and to further diminution of nutritional status. Chronic diarrhea can lead to dehydration and weight loss, which increases the risk for malnutrition (see Chapter 9).

Therapeutic Diets

Restricted diets can also pose nutrition problems, especially for older adults who have enjoyed eating a variety of foods. A limitation of nutrients, such as sodium or fat, often leads to a reduction in intake, which leads to weight loss. Studies conducted with older adults with diabetes found no positive results to following a caloric-specific diet vs a controlled carbohydrate diet (44,45). The position of the American Dietetic Association on liberalized diets details the positive benefits of a liberalized diet (46).

Feeding Limitations

Review of the occupational therapist and the speech language pathologist's consultations assists the dietetics professional in assessing the physical limitations (eg, inability to drink from a cup, use of special utensils) that play a role in the nutritional status of the client.

Is the older adult alert, able to voice food preferences, and able to remember mealtimes? Have the older adult's thought processes altered the ability to eat independently? Does the older adult display indications of paranoia related to food or meal service? An older adult may be forgetful but may still be able to eat independently if prompted by the caregivers. Sidenvall and Ek (47) reported that 16 of 18 older adults admitted to a nursing facility had difficulty with upper motor dysfunction or mouth or pharyngeal food handling and required assistance with meals.

Physical Functioning

It is important to determine whether the older adult requires limited, extensive, or no assistance with meals and snacks. Older adults with physical limitations from conditions such as arthritis or strokes commonly need some assistance in opening condiment packets or milk containers, because these procedures involve hand-eye coordination. Physical concerns that affect eating are paralysis, lack of hand dexterity, or contracture to hands, which affect the ability to handle feeding utensils. Paralysis can result in chewing or swallowing problems, which require modifying the texture of the food. Some older adults have the stamina to feed themselves breakfast and lunch but tire before dinner.

Sensory Impairment

Visual impairments can contribute to decreased food intake at meals. Interviewers should alert caregivers to give verbal cues for meal placement using the clock method. Decreased peripheral vision requires moving the food into the line of sight. Ask the older adult (not family or friends) how much help is needed. For example: Should meat be cut? Should bread be buttered? Should the location of the food on the plate be described? Many persons who have lost their sight have worked out solutions to locating their food and do not like being treated as if they cannot help themselves. Smoking may alter taste and smell, and this change may impair oral intake and decrease meal satisfaction (48).

Individuals who experience difficulties with aspects of taste perception may have similar problems with perception of smell. The ability to identify common food odors and to discriminate among foods may be impaired. Some studies indicate that there is a decline in olfactory function during the lifespan (49). Older adults who smoke are less sensitive to smell than nonsmokers. A positive association between olfactory impairment and BMI has been reported (50). There may be a variety of diseases and drugs that alter taste. See Table 16.9 (51) and Chapter 13.

Other Potential Risk Factors

Depression is a common psychosocial problem that can often go undetected. Disinterest in cooking, shopping, and preparing food is observed in the depressed person, which contributes to functional decline. The decline is perpetuated by unfamiliar settings as the individual is transferred across the continuum of care from the least restrictive home care environment to extended-care facilities. Depression was reported as a major factor in nursing home residents with failure to thrive (52).

The prevalence of cognitive impairment, clinical depression, depressive symptoms, dementia, other psychiatric disorders, and psychological disturbances, along with their potential impact on nutritional status, are considerable in older adults (53). Dementia has been associated with B-12 deficiency (54), and malnutrition is often associated with dementias and depression caused by metabolic disorders, drug toxicity, hypothyroidism, and confusion (54).

Infections, acute and chronic, can result in weight loss (55). *Clostridium difficile* bacteria causes diarrhea, which results in weight loss for approximately one fourth of residents (56). Poor nutrient absorption in older adults is a consequence of *Helicobacter pylori* bacteria (57).

Laboratory Values

Laboratory values should be specific to the age and gender of the client. In the spirit of cost effectiveness, payers of health care, including managed care organizations (MCOs) and Medicare, limit the type and number of laboratory tests. The registered dietitian should request only those tests essential and diagnostically related to assessing and determining intervention (58). Physical assessment, along with anthropometric measurements and observation at mealtime, indicates those at risk for poor nutritional status. Laboratory values often support the interventions recommended by registered dietitians (see Chapter 17).

Skin Conditions

The older adult's skin condition should be observed for signs of dehydration, edema, and ascites. These signs may be indicative of protein deficiency, renal disease, or hepatic disease. All have potential nutritional significance. Loose skin may be evidence of weight loss, and the interviewer should question the older adult about his or her usual weight. Make a visual scan for dry, flaky skin; for skin that tents, which can relate to dehydration; or for a nonhealing wound, purpura, or bruises. As a person ages, dramatic changes in the skin occur. Sweat glands diminish in number. There is atrophy and thinning of the epithelial and fatty layers of tissue. Both collagen and elastic components of the dermis undergo degenerative changes. Collagen content of the skin decreases about 1% throughout adult life. The result is a thin, dry, and inelastic skin (59). The loss of subcutaneous fat in older clients results in frequent complaints of being cold. See Table 16.10 (33) to help identify additional problems. Figures 16.8 and 16.9 (60,61) serve as guides for the interdisciplinary team working with older adults to manage and seek solutions to nutrition problems.

TABLE 16.9. Diseases and Drugs That Alter Olfaction and Taste

	Olfaction	Taste
Central nervous system	Alzheimer's disease Head trauma Multiple sclerosis Neoplasia Parkinson's disease	Head trauma Multiple sclerosis Bell's palsy
Endocrine	Diabetes mellitus Hypothyroidism Adrenocortical insufficiency Kallman's syndrome	Diabetes mellitus Hypothyroidism Adrenocortical insufficiency Panhypopituitarism
Systemic diseases	Cirrhosis of liver Renal failure	Cirrhosis of liver Renal failure Cancer
Nutritional	Vitamin B-12 deficiency	Zinc deficiency Niacin deficiency
Local infections	Influenza Allergic rhinitis Sinusitis Sjögren's syndrome Dental problems	Influenza Glossitis Sjögren's syndrome
Iatrogenic	Laryngectomy	Radiation therapy
Drugs	Opiates Streptomycin Diltiazem	Antihistamines Allopurinol Metronidazole Amiloride Captopril/Enalapril Nifedipine/diltiazem Carbamazepine Lithium Phenytoin Metformin

Source: Reprinted with permission from Morley JE, Thomas DR, Wilson MM; Council for Nutritional Clinical Strategies in Long-Term Care. Appetite and orexigenic drugs. *Ann Long-Term Care.* 2001;9(Suppl):6. Available at: http://www.ltcnutrition.org/PDF/OrexigenicGuidelines.pdf. Accessed April 28, 2004.

TABLE 16.10. Physical Signs of Malnutrition

Signs	Possible Nutrition-Related Causes
Hair	
Dull, dry; lack of natural shine	Protein-energy deficiency
	Essential fatty acid deficiency (EFA)
Thin, sparse; loss of curl	Zinc deficiency
Color changes, depigmentation, easily plucked	Other nutrient deficiencies: manganese, copper
Eyes	
Small, yellowish lumps around eyes	Hyperlipidemia
White rings around both eyes	
Angular inflammation of eyelids, "grittiness" under eyelids	Riboflavin deficiency
Pale eye membranes	Vitamin B-12, folacin, and/or iron deficiency
Night blindness, dry membranes, dull or soft cornea	Vitamin A, zinc deficiency
Redness and fissures of eyelid corners	Niacin deficiency
Ring of fine blood vessels around cornea	General poor nutrition
Lips	
Redness and swelling of mouth	Niacin, riboflavin, iron, and/or pyridoxine deficiency
Angular fissures, scars at corner of mouth	Niacin, riboflavin, iron, and/or pyridoxine deficiency
Soreness, burning lips, pallor	Riboflavin deficiency
Gums	
Spongy, swollen, bleeds easily, redness	Vitamin C deficiency
Gingivitis	Folic acid, vitamin B-12 deficiency
Mouth	
Cheilosis, angular scars	Riboflavin, folic acid, pyridoxine deficiency
Soreness, burning	Riboflavin deficiency
Tongue	
Sores, swollen, scarlet, raw	Folacin, niacin deficiency
Soreness, burning tongue	Riboflavin deficiency
Purplish color	
Smooth with papillae (small projections)	Riboflavin, vitamin B-12, pyridoxine deficiency
Glossitis	Iron, zinc, pyridoxine deficiency
Taste	
Sense of taste diminished	Zinc deficiency
Teeth	
Gray-brown spots	Increased fluoride intake
Missing or erupting abnormally	Generally poor nutrition

continued

TABLE 16.10. Physical Signs of Malnutrition (continued)

Signs	Possible Nutrition-Related Causes
Face	
Skin color loss, dark cheeks and eyes; enlarged parotid glands, scaling of skin around nostrils	Protein-energy deficiency; specifically niacin, riboflavin, and pyridoxine deficiencies
Pallor	Iron, folacin, vitamin B-12, and vitamin C deficiencies
Hyperpigmentation	Niacin deficiency
Neck	
Thyroid enlargement	Iodine deficiency
Symptoms of hypothyroidism	Iodine deficiency
Nails	
Fragility, banding	Protein deficiency
Spoon-shaped	Iron deficiency
Skin	
Slow wound healing	Zinc deficiency
Psoriasis	Biotin deficiency
Eczema	Riboflavin deficiency
Scaliness	Biotin deficiency, pyridoxine deficiency
Black and blue marks due to skin bleeding	Vitamin C and/or vitamin K deficiency
Dryness, mosaic, sandpaper feel, flakiness	Increased or decreased vitamin A
Swollen and dark	Niacin deficiency
Lack of fat under skin or bilateral edema	Protein-energy deficiency
Yellow colored	Carotene deficiency or excess
Cutaneous flushing	Niacin
Pallor	Iron, folic acid deficiencies
Gastrointestinal	
Anorexia, flatulence, diarrhea	Vitamin B-12 deficiency
Muscular system	
Weakness	Phosphorus or potassium deficiency
Wasted appearance	Protein-energy deficiency
Calf tenderness, absent knee jerks	Thiamin deficiency
Peripheral neuropathy	Folacin, pyridoxine, pantothenic acid, phosphate, thiamin deficiencies
Muscle twitching	Magnesium or pyridoxine excess or deficiency
Muscle cramps	Chloride decreased, sodium deficiency
Muscle pain	Biotin deficiency

continued

Signs	Possible Nutrition-Related Causes
Skeletal system	
Demineralization of bone	Calcium, phosphorus, vitamin D deficiencies
Epiphyseal enlargement of leg and knee Bowed legs	Vitamin D deficiency
Nervous system	
Listlessness	Protein-energy deficiency
Loss of position and vibratory sense, decrease and loss of ankle and knee reflexes, depression, inability to concentrate, defective memory, delirium	Thiamin, vitamin B-12 deficiencies
Seizures, memory impairment, and behavioral disturbances	Magnesium, zinc deficiencies
Peripheral neuropathy, dementia	Pyridoxine deficiency

Source: Reprinted with permission from Consultant Dietitians in Health Care Facilities. *CD-HCF Pocket Resource for Nutrition Assessment, 2001 Revision.* Chicago, Ill: Consultant Dietitians in Health Care Facilities; 2001:55-59.

SUMMARY

The nutrition screening and assessment process form the basis for initiating a plan of care for the older adult. In the assisted living or home care environment, the screening process may be completed by a designated health care professional who then notifies the registered dietitian of high-risk older adults. The assessment is a comprehensive process that includes physical examination, anthropometric measurements, and laboratory values. If the condition of the older adult declines, a reassessment may be required to achieve positive outcomes.

REFERENCES

1. Identifying patients at risk: ADA's definitions for nutrition screening and nutrition assessment. Council on Practice (COP) Quality Management Committee [Correction in *J Am Diet Assoc.* 1994;94:1101]. *J Am Diet Assoc.* 1994;94:838-839.
2. Nutrition Screening Initiative. DETERMINE Your Nutritional Health Checklist. Washington, DC: Nutrition Screening Initiative; 1991. Available at: http://www.aafp.org/x17367.xml. Accessed April 15, 2004.
3. Nutrition Screening Initiative. Level I Screen. Washington, DC: Nutrition Screening Initiative; 1991.
4. Nutrition Screening Initiative. Level II Screen. Washington, DC: Nutrition Screening Initiative; 1991.
5. Gates G. Clinical reasoning: an essential component of dietetic practice. *Top Clin Nutr.* 1992;7(3):78.
6. Guigoz Y, Vellas B, Garry PJ. Assessing the nutritional status of the elderly: the Mini-Nutritional Assessment as part of the geriatric evaluation. *Nutr Rev.* 1996;54(suppl):S59-S65.
7. Cataldo CB, DeBruyne LK, Whitney EN. *Nutrition and Diet Therapy: Principles and Practices.* 4th ed. Minneapolis, Minn: West Publishing; 1995:4-6.
8. American Medical Directors Association. *Clinical Practice Guideline: Altered Nutritional Status.* Columbia, Md: AMDA; 2002.
9. Dwyer JT. *Screening Older Americans' Nutritional Health: Current Practices and Future Possibilities.* Washington, DC: Nutrition Screening Initiative; 1991.
10. Rossman I, ed. *Clinical Geriatrics.* 2nd ed. Philadelphia, Pa: Lippincott Co; 1979.
11. Chumlea WC, Roche AF, Makjerjee D. *Nutrition Assessment of the Elderly Through Anthropometry.* Columbus, Ohio: Ross Laboratories; 1990.
12. Reeves SL, Varakamin C, Henry CJK. The relationship between arm-span measurement and height with specific reference to gender and ethnicity. *Eur J Clin Nutr.* 1996;50:398-400.
13. Michels KB, Greenland S, Rosner BA. Does body mass index adequately capture the relation of body composition and body size to health outcomes? *Am J Epidemiol.* 1998;147:167-172.
14. *Report of the Dietary Guidelines Advisory Committee on the Dietary Guidelines for Americans, 2000.* Washington, DC: US Department of Agriculture, Agricultural Research Service; 2000:3.

Figure 16.8

Nursing nutritional checklist (for use in care planning). Reprinted by permission. Copyright © 2000, Programs in Medicine.

Nursing Nutritional Checklist (for use in Care Planning)

The American Dietetic Association supports the Nursing Nutritional Checklist (for use in Care Planning).
Representatives from the American Dietetic Association were instrumental in its development.

This Nursing Nutritional Checklist (for use in Care Planning) was developed by the Council for Nutrition.
A special committee of The Gerontological Society of America (GSA) served as critical reviewers and provided input and modification of the final Checklist.
While GSA does not endorse specific clinical measures, we support the principles underlying this Checklist and its potential to improve nutrition in the nursing home.

Problem List (check all that apply)	Suggested Action Plan (check when completed)
○ 1. Patient has ≥ 5% involuntary weight loss in 30 days?	○ 1-4 . Monitor weight weekly. Continue to step #5 on problem list
○ 2. Patient has ≥10% involuntary weight loss in 180 days or less.	
○ 3. BMI is ≤ 21. (703 x weight in lbs/height in inches² **or** weight in kilograms/height in meters²)	
○ 4. Resident leaves 25% or more food on tray? (in last 7 days)	
5. Quality Indicators — Does patient have:	5.
○ A. Fecal impaction in last 7 days	○ A. Implement bowel program
○ B. Infection (UTI, URI, Pneumonia, GI) in last 7 days	○ B. Get physician order for U/A
○ C. Tube feeding	○ C. Contact dietitian for assessment
○ D. Functional ADL decline	○ D. Consider OT/PT assessment
○ E. Development of pressure ulcer in low risk patient	○ E. Implement skin program
○ 6. Patient takes in ≤1500cc fluid/day for the last 7 days? Is patient on fluid restriction?	○ 6. Develop systematic plan to ensure adequate fluid intake (e.q., 300 mL with meals and 240 mL between meals)
○ 7. Available labwork completed in the last 30 days: Hgb _____ Albumin_____ Hct _____ Cholesterol _____ Serum WBC _____ U/A: Sodium _____ Urine WBC _____ Potassium _____ Spec. Gravity _____ Glucose _____ Leuk. Esterase _____ BUN _____ Other_____ Creatinine _____	○ 7. Notify physician of values
8. Nursing assessment of physical/psychological problems	8.
○ A. Skin (pressure ulcers and skin tears)	○ A. Implement skin program
○ B. Presence of fever (2° above baseline)	○ B. Implement facility protocol
○ C. Presence of diarrhea	○ C. Implement facility protocol
○ D. Presence of constipation	○ D. Implement facility protocol
○ E. Takes drugs other than multivitamins/minerals	○ E. Contact pharmacy consultant for drug review
○ F. Symptoms of depression/anxiety	○ F. Evaluate for depression/anxiety (short geriatric mini depression scale)
○ G. Loss of usual appetite	○ G. Implement care plan to increase appetite
○ H. Presence of nausea/vomiting	○ H. Implement facility protocol
○ I. Presence of dysphagia/choking	○ I. Contact dietitian for evaluation
○ J. Ill-fitting dentures, missing teeth, periodontal disease	○ J. Contact dentist or dental technician
○ 9. Not satisfied with food currently offered (for example, ethnic preferences)	○ 9. Stop therapeutic diets and provide preferred foods/food substitutions
○ 10. Patient needs meal time assistance	○ 10. Provide timely, polite assistance during dining ○ Provide tray set up ○ Provide partial assistance/supervision (evaluate resident/staff ratio and supervision by licensed professional staff) ○ Provide total assistance (consider resident/staff ratio and supervision by licensed professional staff) ○ Consider training staff to provide meal time assistance
○ 11. Patient has motor agitation, tremors, or wanders	○ 11. Consider OT evaluation ○ Provide meal time assistance ○ Provide self-help feeding devices ○ Offer finger foods
○ 12. Presence of environmental distractions or meal time environment concerns	○ 12. Minimize environmental distractions ○ Provide compatible companions
○ 13. Inadequate lighting in the dining room	○ 13. Evaluate location in dining room
○ 14. Patient needs 30–60 minutes to eat	○ 14. Implement dining program, e.g. special area to eat for impaired residents or two meal time sessions
○ 15. Patient is unable to tolerate current food consistency	○ 15. Contact dietitian for texture screen
○ 16. Supplements are given at meal time	○ 16. Give liquid supplements in a pattern that optimizes nutrient intake
○ 17. Medications are given at meal time	○ 17. Contact pharmacist for appropriate administration time
○ 18. Impaired visual acuity	○ 18. Assure resident is wearing clean glasses at meal time ○ Provide meal time assistance (see #10)
○ 19. Impaired hearing	○ 19. Ensure that hearing aid is in place and working at meal time
○ 20. Patient has a decline in taste and smell	○ 20. Season foods ○ Serve food at proper temperature

○ **When problem list is completed, contact physician, dietitian and pharmacist as appropriate with suggested action plan.**

Completed by: _____   Date: _____

Figure 16.9

New admission nutrition questionnaire. Copyright © 2001 Programs in Medicine. Reprinted by permission. Sponsored by an unrestricted educational grant from Bristol-Myers Squibb.

New Admission Nutrition Questionnaire

As a member of the professional team of caregivers you want to make sure your residents are as comfortable and healthy as possible in their new home. To ensure that they enjoy mealtimes and maintain their general nutritional health, here are some questions for you to ask new residents and their family to ensure proper nutrition and health.

Meals and Dining

Ask about the new resident's eating habits:

1. Does the resident need assistance in eating meals?   ☐ Yes   ☐ No

    If so, type of assistance given   _____

2. Does the resident have difficulty chewing or swallowing?   ☐ Yes   ☐ No

3. Does the resident have dental problems?
   (i.e. Ill fitting dentures, teeth in poor condition)   ☐ Yes   ☐ No

4. Does the resident enjoy dining with others?   ☐ Yes   ☐ No

5. Does the resident have a good appetite?   ☐ Yes   ☐ No

Food

Ask about the resident's food preferences:

6. List the resident's favorite foods   _____

7. List the resident's least favorite foods   _____

8. Does the resident like spicy foods?   ☐ Yes   ☐ No

9. List the resident's beverage choices for meals   _____

10. Does the resident snack between meals?   ☐ Yes   ☐ No

     If so, favorite snacks _____

11. Does the resident prefer 2-3 meals a day?   ☐ Yes   ☐ No

12. Does the resident prefer many small meals?   ☐ Yes   ☐ No

13. Does the resident drink a lot of fluids during the day?   ☐ Yes   ☐ No

14. The resident's usual main meal is   ☐ breakfast   ☐ lunch   ☐ dinner

15. Does the resident have religious food guidelines?   ☐ Yes   ☐ No

     Please specify _____

16. Does the resident have any known food allergies?   ☐ Yes   ☐ No

     Please specify _____

General Health

Ask about the resident's general health and needs:

17. Does the resident have bouts of sadness or crying?   ☐ Yes   ☐ No

18. Does the resident appear confused at times?   ☐ Yes   ☐ No

19. Has the resident lost/gained weight?   ☐ Yes   ☐ No

     If so, _____ lbs. x _____ time period

20. Has the resident had a decline in appetite?   ☐ Yes   ☐ No

21. Does the resident experience constipation?   ☐ Yes   ☐ No

22. Does the resident complain of diarrhea?   ☐ Yes   ☐ No

23. Does the resident complain of stomach pain?   ☐ Yes   ☐ No

24. Does the resident occasionally have nausea/vomiting?   ☐ Yes   ☐ No

25. Does the resident have less interest in meals?   ☐ Yes   ☐ No

26. Does the resident say food tastes different now?   ☐ Yes   ☐ No

15. National Institutes of Health. Calculate Your Body Mass Index. Available at: http://nhlbisupport.com/bmi/bmicalc.htm. Accessed April 20, 2004.

16. Galanos AN, Pieper CF, Kussin PS, Winchell MT, Fulkerson WJ, Harrell FE Jr, Teno JM, Layde P, Connors AF Jr, Phillips RS, Wenger NS. Relationship of body mass index to subsequent mortality among seriously ill hospitalized patients. SUPPORT Investigators. The Study to Understand Prognoses and Preferences for Outcome and Risks of Treatment. *Crit Care Med.* 1997;25:1962-1968.

17. Hebebrand J, Himmelmann GW, Herzog W, Herpertz-Dahlmann BM, Steinhausen HC, Amstein M, Seidel R, Deter HC, Remschmidt H, Schafer H. Prediction of low body weight at long-term follow-up in acute anorexia nervosa by low body weight at referral. *Am J Psychiatry.* 1997;154:566-569.

18. Galanos AN, Pieper CF, Cornoni-Huntley JC, Bales CW, Fillenbaum GG. Nutrition and function: is there a relationship between body mass index and the functional capabilities of community-dwelling elderly? *J Am Geriatr Soc.* 1994;42:368-373.

19. Greenspan SL, Myers ER, Maitland LA, Resnick NM, Hayes WC. Fall severity and bone mineral density as risk factors for hip fracture in ambulatory elderly. *JAMA.* 1994;271:128-133.

20. Mehr DR, Foxman B, Colombo P. Risk factors for mortality from lower respiratory infections in nursing home patients. *J Fam Pract.* 1992;34:585-591.

21. Rowland ML. A nomogram for computing body mass index. *Diet Curr.* 1989;16:5-12.

22. Modlesky CM, Lewis RD. Assessment of body size and composition. In: Rosenbloom C, ed. *Sports Nutrition: A Guide for the Professional Working With Active People.* 3rd ed. Chicago, Ill: American Dietetic Association; 2000:188-189.

23. Osterkamp LK. Current perspective on assessment of human body proportions of relevance to amputees. *J Am Diet Assoc.* 1995;95:215-218.

24. Himes JH. New equation to estimate body mass index in amputees [letter]. *J Am Diet Assoc.* 1995;95:646.

25. Weiss GN, Gorton TA, Read RC, Neal LA. Outcomes of lower extremity amputations. *J Am Geriatr Soc.* 1990;38:877-883.

26. Coletta EM. Care of the elderly patient with lower extremity amputation. *J Am Board Fam Pract.* 2000;13:23-34.

27. Peifer SC, Blust P, Leyson JF. Nutritional assessment of the spinal cord injured patient. *J Am Diet Assoc.* 1981;78:501-505.

28. Medical nutrition therapy for neurologic disorders. In: Mahan LK, Escott-Stump S, eds. *Krause's Food, Nutrition, and Diet Therapy.* 11th ed. Philadelphia, Pa: WB Saunders; 2003:1117.

29. Hamwi GJ. Therapy: changing dietary needs. In: Dankowski TS, ed. *Diabetes Mellitus: Diagnosis and Treatment.* New York, NY: American Diabetes Association; 1964:73-78.

30. Master AM, Laser RP, Beckman G. Tables of average weight and height of Americans aged 65 to 94 years. *JAMA.* 1960;172:658.

31. Blackburn GL, Bistrian BR, Maini BS, Schlamm HT, Smith MF. Nutritional and metabolic assessment of the hospitalized patient. *JPEN J Parenter Enteral Nutr.* 1977;1:11-22

32. Grant A, DeHoog S. *Nutrition Assessment Support and Management.* 5th ed. Seattle, Wash: Grant-DeHoog; 1999.

33. Consultant Dietitians in Health Care Facilities. *CD-HCF Pocket Resource for Nutrition Assessment, 2001 Revision.* Chicago, Ill: Consultant Dietitians in Health Care Facilities; 2001:39-45, 55-59.

34. Shronts EP, Gottschlich MM, Matarese LE. *Nutrition Support Dietetics Core Curriculum.* Silver Springs, Md: American Society for Parenteral and Enteral Nutrition; 1993.

35. Food and Agricultural Organization/World Health Organization. *Energy and Protein Requirements.* Geneva, Switzerland: World Health Organization; 1985. Technical Report Series 724.

36. Amato P, Keating KP, Quercia RA, Karbonic J. Formulaic methods of estimating caloric requirements in mechanically ventilated obese patients: a reappraisal. *Nutr Clin Pract.* 1995;10:229-230.

37. Mahar K, Escott-Stump S. *Krause's Food Nutrition and Diet Therapy.* San Diego, Calif: Elsevier Science; 2003.

38. Munro HN, Young VR. Protein metabolism in the elderly: observations relating to dietary needs. *Postgrad Med.* 1978;63:143-148.

39. Beers MH, Berkow R, eds. *Merck Manual of Geriatrics.* Whitehorse Station, NJ: Merck & Co; 2000.

40. Chidester JC, Spangler AA. Fluid intake in the institutionalized elderly. *J Am Diet Assoc.* 1997;97:23-28.

41. Lewis CW, Frongillo EA Jr, Roe DA. Drug-nutrient interactions in three long-term care facilities. *J Am Diet Assoc.* 1995;95:151-155.

42. Pronsky Z. *Food Medication Interactions.* 13th ed. Birchrunville, Pa: Food Medication Interactions; 2004.

43. Blaum CS, Fries BE, Fiatarone MA. Factors associated with low body mass index and weight loss in nursing home residents. *J Gerontol A Biol Sci Med Sci.* 1995;50:M162-M168.

44. Coulston AM, Mandelbaum D, Reaven GM. Dietary management of nursing home residents with non-insulin dependent diabetes mellitus. *Am J Clin Nutr.* 1990;51:67-71.

45. Lan SJ, Justice CL. Use of modified diets in nursing homes. *J Am Diet Assoc.* 1992;91:46-51.

46. Dorner B, Niedert KC, Welch PK. American Dietetic Association. Position paper: liberalized diets for older adults in long-term care. *J Am Diet Assoc.* 2002;102:1316-1323.

47. Sidenvall B, Ek AD. Long-term care patients and their dietary intake related to eating ability and nutritional needs: nursing staff interventions. *J Adv Nurs.* 1993;18:565-573.

48. Russell C, ed. *Dining Skills: Practical Interventions for the Caregivers of Older Adults with Eating Problems.* Chicago, Ill: Consultant Dietitians in Health Care Facilities; 2001:163-171.

49. Schiffman SS. Perception of taste and smell in elderly persons. *Crit Rev Food Sci Nutr.* 1993;33:17-26,28.

50. Hunter-Smith DG, Kessel K, Grant M, Piotrowski ZH. Association between elevated body mass index and impaired sense of smell in older people. *J Am Geriatr Soc.* 1996;44:100-101.

51. Morley JE, Thomas DR, Wilson MM; Council for Nutritional Clinical Strategies in Long-Term Care. Appetite and orexigenic drugs. *Ann Long-Term Care.* 2001;9(Suppl):1-12. Available at: http://www .ltcnutrition.org/PDF/OrexigenicGuidelines.pdf. Accessed April 28, 2004.

52. Katz IR, Beaston-Wimmer P, Parmelee P, Friedman E, Lawton MP. Failure to thrive in the elderly: exploration of the concept and delineation of psychiatric components. *J Geriatr Psychiatry Neurol.* 1993;6:161-169.

53. Kahn R. Weight loss and depression in a community nursing home. *J Am Geriatr Soc.* 1995;43:83.

54. Dumford M. Nutrition and Alzheimer's disease. *Today's Dietitian.* 2003(June):12-15.

55. Roubenoff R, Roubenoff RA, Cannon JG, Kehayias JJ, Zhuang H, Dawson-Hughes B, Dinarello CA, Rosenberg IH. Rheumatoid cachexia: cytokine-driven hypermetabolism accompanying reduced body cell mass in chronic inflammation. *J Clin Invest.* 1994;93:2379-2386.

56. Anand A, Bashey B, Mir T, Glatt AE. Epidemiology, clinical manifestations, and outcome of Clostridium difficile-associated diarrhea. *Am J Gastroenterol.* 1994:89:519-523.

57. Portnoi VA. Helicobacter pylori infection and anorexia of aging. *Arch Intern Med.* 1997;157:269-272.

58. Schiffman SS. Smell. In: Maddox GL, ed. *Encyclopedia of Aging.* New York, NY: Springer Publishing; 1987:618-619.

59. Maklebust J, Sieggreen M. *Pressure Ulcers: Guidelines for Prevention and Nursing Management.* 2nd ed. Springhouse, Pa: Springhouse Corp; 1996:9-10.

60. Council for Nutrition Clinical Strategies in Long-Term Care. Nursing nutritional checklist (for use in care planning). 2000. Available at: http://www.ltcnutrition .org/PDF/clinicalMalnutritionGuide.pdf. Accessed April 28, 2004.

61. Council for Nutrition Clinical Strategies in Long-Term Care. New admission nutrition questionnaire. 2001Available at: http://www.ltcnutrition.org/PDF/ Admission_English.pdf. Accessed April 28, 2004.

ADDITIONAL RESOURCES

Apelgren KN, Wilmore DW. Nutritional care of the critically ill patient. *Surg Clin North Am.* 1993;63:497-507.

Long CL, Schaffel N, Geiger JW, Schiller WR, Blakemore WS. Metabolic response to injury and illness: estimation of energy and protein needs from indirect calorimetry and nitrogen balance. *JPEN J Parenter Enteral Nutr.* 1979;3:452-456.

Preventing Pressure Sores. Evansville, Ind: Mead Johnson Enteral Nutritionals, Bristol Myers Squibb; 1989.

Wilmore DW. *The Metabolic Management of the Critically Ill.* New York, NY: Plenum Medical Book Co; 1977:34-36.

CHAPTER 17

Laboratory Assessment

Nutrition assessment determines whether the body can convert food into body components. Nutrition screening is the process of identifying characteristics known to be associated with nutrition problems. Historically, nutrition screening and assessment have primarily emphasized anthropometric data and dietary intake, especially in nursing facilities. However, laboratory assessment is an essential tool to assess nutritional status, to evaluate nutrition intervention programs, and to predict medical outcomes (1).

National trends indicate that a declining number of laboratory tests are being ordered in all areas of health care. This trend is a reflection of cost-reduction programs nationwide. Assessment of physical and nutritional status is done primarily through physical assessment and observed dietary intake. Clinical signs and symptoms must be identified in order to justify the request for laboratory tests. Facility protocols or clinical pathways form the infrastructure for ordering more laboratory tests.

IMPLICATIONS OF SELECTED LABORATORY TESTS

All requests for laboratory tests must be justified by the health care team. It is important to remember that no single laboratory test evaluates a client's short-term response to medical nutrition therapy (MNT). In addition, not all tests are appropriate for all clients. For example, creatinine excretion cannot be used to evaluate muscle mass in clients with renal failure because the test assumes normal renal function. Remember that the overall medical condition of older adults and the current pharmacological intervention strategies must be considered in the interpretation of laboratory tests (1).

CHANGES IN NUTRITIONAL STATUS

One laboratory test may or may not reflect improved nutritional status once an MNT intervention program has begun. Changes in hydration status significantly impact laboratory results. Hydration status is commonly overlooked (2). To evaluate hydration status, a variety of laboratory tests, recent dietary history, and physical assessment will need to be used. Table 17.1 lists laboratory tests that can be used to evaluate hydration status (1). As the older adult's hydration and dietary intake changes, more than one laboratory test will be required to accurately document changes in nutritional status. A review of support data (such as physical findings, changes in anthropometric data, reported symptoms, and nutrition intake) will increase confidence in laboratory results (3).

EFFECT OF STRESS

When interpreting laboratory test results, one must consider the effect of stress on the older adult. A change in laboratory values is often seen in those who have short-term emotional stress or physical stress from surgery or an infection. For example, an unexpected hospitalization of an older adult because of a fall may result in an elevated fasting blood glucose. Two fasting blood glucose levels above 126 mg/dL are one of the criteria for a diagnosis of non-insulin-dependent diabetes (4). If the elevated fasting blood glucose is due to stress, it will return to normal once the stressful situation is resolved (5). Unfortunately, some older adults are not reevaluated after an appropriate time interval and will have a diagnosis of non-insulin-dependent diabetes as a permanent part of their medical records.

TABLE 17.1. Laboratory Screening for Hydration Status

Laboratory Test	Normal Values	Dehydration	Overhydration
Osmolality	Adults: 285-295 mOsm/kg H_2O	> 295 mOsm/kg H_2O	< 285 mOsm/kg H_2O
Serum sodium	136-145 mEq/L 136-145 mmol/L	> 145 mEq/L	< 130 mEq/L
Albumin	3.5-5.0 g/dL 35-50 g/L	Higher than normal	Lower than normal
Urea nitrogen	10-20 mg/dL 3.6-7.1 mmol/L	Elevated	Lower than normal
BUN:Creatinine ratio	10:1	> 25:1	< 10:1

Abbreviation: BUN, blood urea nitrogen.

Source: Adapted with permission from Litchford MD. *Practical Applications in Laboratory Assessment of Nutritional Status.* Greensboro, NC: CASE Software; 2002.

EFFECT OF OTHER MEDICAL INTERVENTIONS

Laboratory tests done before admission to an extended-care facility may not reflect the true nutritional status of an older adult. For example, if a hospitalized older adult has a very poor iron status, he/she might receive a blood transfusion to improve the iron status, in order to shorten the length of stay in the hospital. However, the laboratory tests taken after the blood transfusion reflect the nutritional status of the blood donor, not the person who received the transfusion. This is a short-term solution that increases the iron levels while the body begins to use nutrients from food. The initial assessment must consider the impact of blood products, the withdrawal of fluids, and other medical procedures that may change the short- and long-term nutritional status of the older adult (3).

REFERENCE STANDARDS

Standard laboratory reports are referenced using suggested normal or age-appropriate values. Remember that most reference standards were developed on the basis of clinical research using primarily young and middle-aged adults. Clinical research on the very young and the very old is lim-

ited. Reference standards may not apply to these age groups. This is of particular concern in assessing older adults, because their norms appear to be slightly lower or higher than the standards. However, acceptable differences have yet to be defined. Dietetics professionals must consider how the standards were developed.

Laboratory assessment of nutritional status must be viewed in the unique context of each client. The frequency of tests; the technology used; and the age, disease state, and stress level of the client must be considered. Laboratory tests are an essential tool for improving health outcomes and reducing costs.

EQUIPMENT

Changes in nutritional status are measured most accurately by using laboratory test results from the same laboratory. Comparing laboratory test results from different institutions can be like comparing apples with oranges. Each institution establishes reference standards and laboratory procedures for each test, as suggested by the equipment manufacturer. Other sources of variation include equipment used, the degree of equipment calibration, and the skill of the technician (1).

CONSIDERATIONS FOR REQUESTING LABORATORY TESTS

As a member of the health care team, the dietetics professional should consider the following questions when requesting additional laboratory tests:

1. *Will the outcome actually change the nutrition care plan?*

   Example: The care of a client with acquired immunodeficiency syndrome (AIDS) is being directed by a hospice nurse. The client is not eating and is losing weight. The protein status is likely declining. The client is receiving comfort measures only. Requesting a prealbumin test will not change the nutrition care plan. Knowing the degree to which the protein status is declining will not change the plan of care. In other words, the client would most likely not receive additional oral nutritional supplements or enteral or parenteral support as a means to improve nutritional status.

2. *Is the test cost effective?* Managed care mandates cost effectiveness. Laboratory tests must be cost effective.

   Example: Albumin and prealbumin tests indicate both early depletion of protein stores and repletion of protein stores once an intervention program has begun. The half-life of prealbumin is 2 to 3 days; for albumin, it is 18 to 21 days. It takes at least 3 weeks in adults, and longer in older adults, after an MNT intervention program has begun, to see an improvement in the albumin (6). In managed care with an expected short-term stay, the prealbumin may be a more cost-effective measure, because it identifies the change in protein status earlier than the albumin. With the extended-care client, the primary concern is to reduce the risk of pressure ulcers, with early risk assessment and appropriate nursing and nutrition intervention.

3. *Is the nutrition goal for the client consistent with treatment goals and advance directives?*

   Example: An 85-year-old woman with a hemoglobin level of 9 g/dL may not be interested in improving her iron status through an MNT intervention program followed by a reevaluation of her iron status. The low iron status may be secondary to anemia of chronic disease. In anemia of chronic disease, the body is unable to use dietary or supplemental iron. In this case, the iron supplement would be neither nutritionally nor cost effective. Putting the client on an oral daily supplement for 3 months and then rechecking the iron level in 90 days may not be consistent with treatment goals.

CLINICAL LABORATORY VALUES

The system for reporting clinical data is in transition. Most health care professionals learned the conventional units for each laboratory test. Many laboratories continue to use conventional units in their summary reports. Laboratory values may be converted from one system to another by using the unique conversion factor for each laboratory test.

The preferred method for reporting clinical laboratory data is in terms of International Units (SI units). "SI units" is an abbreviation for le Systeme International d'Unites, or International System. The reason for the change to SI units is to have an international standard for reporting research and medical data. Laboratory values are provided in both conventional and SI units.

LABORATORY TESTS USED FOR NUTRITION ASSESSMENT

Commonly used laboratory tests ordered to evaluate nutritional status are included. Summary charts for laboratory test results reflecting protein status, anemias, and risk for chronic diseases are found in Tables 17.2, 17.3, and 17.4 (1,5). Values listed for "adults" typically refer to persons 25 to 59 years of age. Values listed for "older adults" refer to individuals older than 60 years.

Alanine Aminotransferase

Normal Values (5)

- Adult: 4-36 IU/L; 4-36 U/L (SI)
- Older adult: slightly higher than adults

Nutritional Significance

Alanine aminotransferase (ALT; formerly called SGPT) is an enzyme found primarily in the liver and to a lesser degree in the kidneys, heart, and skeletal muscle. Injury to the liver results in elevated levels of ALT. Serum aspartate aminotransferase (AST) levels are often compared with ALT. The AST:ALT ratio > 1.0 is seen in alcoholic cirrhosis, liver congestion, and metastatic tumor of the liver. The

TABLE 17.2. Laboratory Screening for Protein Status

Laboratory Test	Normal Values	PEM	AIR	Infection
Prealbumin	15-36 mg/dL 150-360 mg/L	Low	Very low	Low
Albumin	3.5-5.0 gm/dL 35-50 g/L	Low	Very low	Low
Cholesterol	< 200 mg/dL < 5.2 mmol/L	Lower than usual or < 160 mg/dL	Unchanged	Unchanged

Abbreviations: AIR, acute inflammatory response; PEM, protein-energy malnutrition.

Source: Adapted with permission from Litchford MD. *Practical Applications in Laboratory Assessment of Nutritional Status.* Greensboro, NC: CASE Software; 2002.

TABLE 17.3. Guide to Anemias

Laboratory Test	Normal Values	Iron Deficiency Anemia	Megaloblastic Anemia (Folate Deficiency)	Pernicious Anemia (B-12 Deficiency)	Anemia of Chronic Disease
Hgb (g/dL)					
Females	12-16	< 12	< 12	< 12	< 12
Males	14-16	< 14	< 14	< 4	< 14
Hct (%)					
Females	37-47	< 37	< 37	< 37	< 37
Males	42-52	< 42	< 42	< 42	< 42
MCV (μm^3)	80-95	< 80	> 95	> 95 or normal	Normal
Serum Fe (g/dL)	60-160	< 60	> 160	> 160	< 60
TIBC (g/dL)	250-460	> 460	Normal	Normal	< 250
Serum B-12 (pg/mL)	160-950	Normal	Decreased	Decreased	Normal
Folate (g/mL)	5-25	Normal	< 5	> 25	Normal or decreased

Abbreviations: Hgb, hemoglobin; Hct, hematocrit; MCV, mean corpuscular volume; TIBC, total iron binding capacity.

Source: Adapted with permission from Litchford MD. *Practical Applications in Laboratory Assessment of Nutritional Status.* Greensboro, NC: CASE Software; 2002.

TABLE 17.4. Laboratory Screening for Other Chronic Diseases

Laboratory Test	Normal Values	CHD	ESRD	DM	LD
Cholesterol	< 200 mg/dL < 5.20 mmol/L	> 200 mg/dL	N/A	> 200 mg/dL	Rapidly declining levels
HDL	> 40 mg/dL > 60 mg/dL	< 35 mg/dL	N/A	< 35 mg/dL	N/A
AST (SGOT)	0-35 IU/L 0.58 µKat	elevated with MI	N/A	N/A	Elevated
ALT (SGPT)	4-36 UI/L 4-36 U/L	N/A	N/A	N/A	Elevated
Blood urea nitrogen	10-20 mg/dL 3.6-7.1 mmol/L	Elevated with MI	Elevated	Normal or elevated	Declining value
Potassium	3.5-5.0 mEq/L 3.5-5.0 mmol/L	Normal	Elevated	Normal or elevated	Normal
Creatinine	0.6-1.2 mg/dL 44-97 µmol/L	Normal	Elevated	Normal or elevated	Normal
Glucose	70-110 mg/dL 3.9-6.1 mmol/L	Elevated with MI	N/A	> 126 mg/dL	Shifts dramatically

Abbreviations: ALT, alanine transaminase; AST, aspartate aminotransferase; CHD, coronary heart disease; DM, diabetes mellitus; ESRD, end-stage renal disease; HDL, high-density lipoprotein; LD, liver disease; MI, myocardial infarction; N/A, not applicable; SGOT, serum glutamic-oxaloacetic transaminase; SGPT, serum glutamic-pyruvic transaminase.

Source: Data are from references 1 and 5.

AST:ALT ratio < 1.0 is seen in acute hepatitis, viral hepatitis, and infectious mononucleosis (1).

ALT levels increase with

- Hepatocellular disease:
  - Hepatitis
  - Cirrhosis or necrosis
  - Tumor
- Cholestasis

The following drugs may increase ALT levels (1):

- Acetaminophen
- Allopurinol
- Aspirin
- Cephalosporins
- Clofibrate
- Codeine
- Indomethacin
- Isoniazid (INH)
- Methotrexate
- Tetracycline

Aspartate Aminotransferase

Normal Values (5)

- Adults: 0-35 IU/L; 0-0.58 µKat/L (SI)
- Older adults: slightly higher than adults

Nutritional Significance (1)

Aspartate aminotransferase (AST; formerly called serum glutamic-oxaloacetic transaminase [SGOT]) is an enzyme primarily found in the heart, liver, and skeletal muscle cells and to a lesser degree in the kidneys and pancreas. AST enzyme is one of the enzymes tested in the cardiac enzyme series, along with creatinine phosphokinase (CPK) and lactic dehydrogenase (LDH). AST levels rise within 6 to 10 hours of a myocardial infarction (MI), peak between 12 and 48 hours, and return to normal in 3 to 4 days, unless more cardiac injury occurs. AST levels may be monitored to estimate the time of the MI. Other laboratory tests are also used in conjunction with AST.

AST levels increase with

- MI
- Cardiac catheterization and angioplasty
- Hepatitis
- Hepatic cirrhosis or necrosis
- Acute pancreatitis
- Skeletal muscle trauma
- Burns
- Acute renal failure

AST levels decrease with

- Beriberi
- Diabetic ketoacidosis
- Chronic renal failure

The following drugs may increase AST levels:

- Aspirin
- Antihypertensives
- Cholinergic agents
- Anticoagulants
- Digitalis
- Erythromycin
- Isoniazid
- Methyldopa

Blood Urea Nitrogen

Normal Values (5)

- Adults: 10-20 mg/dL; 3.6-7.1 mmol/L (SI)
- Older adults: slightly higher than for adults

Nutritional Significance (1,2,5)

The blood urea nitrogen (BUN) level is directly related to the metabolic function of the liver and excretory function of the kidney. BUN increases as the kidney's function declines. Slightly higher values of BUN seen in older adults are often the result of an inability to concentrate urine or dehydration. If the BUN continues to increase, it may indicate that the kidney function is declining. The BUN is interpreted in conjunction with the creatinine test, to assess kidney excretory function. A BUN > 100 mg/dL usually indicates serious kidney problems.

The BUN also increases in individuals on a high-protein diet or who have gastrointestinal bleeding. Both result in excess amounts of protein in the hepatic circulation, and elevated BUN levels result. Dehydration also creates a temporary elevation of BUN. BUN is often used as a measure of hydration status after surgery.

In clients with both kidney disease and liver disease, the BUN may be elevated and may then return to normal. This is not a reflection of improved renal excretory function but rather an indication that the liver is unable to form urea. As the liver continues to decline, the blood ammonia levels will rise, while the BUN may remain normal or slightly elevated.

BUN levels increase with

- Increased protein catabolism:
  - Hemorrhage into GI tract
  - Acute MI
  - Stress
  - Starvation
  - Diabetes
  - Fever
  - Burns
- Impaired renal function
- CHF
- Urinary obstruction
- Dehydration
- Very-high-protein diet

BUN levels decrease with

- Severe liver damage:
  - Drugs
  - Poisoning
  - Hepatitis
- Impaired absorption:
  - Celiac disease
- Low-protein, high-carbohydrate diet
- Overhydration

The following drugs may increase BUN levels:

- Allopurinol
- Aminoglycosides
- Cephalosporins
- Furosemide
- Guanethidine
- Indomethacin
- Methotrexate
- Methyldopa
- Aspirin
- Bacitracin
- Carbamazepine
- Neomycin
- Penicillamine
- Propranolol
- Spironolactone
- Tetracyclines
- Rifampin

The following drugs may decrease BUN levels:

- Chloramphenicol
- Streptomycin

Creatinine

Normal Values (5)

- Men: 0.6-1.2 mg/dL; 53-106 µmol/L (SI)
- Women: 0.5-1.1 mg/dL; 44-97 µmol/L (SI)
- Older adults: slightly decreased

Nutritional Significance (1)

Creatinine is a by-product of the metabolism of muscle creatinine phosphate to form ATP. It is produced at a constant rate determined by the individual's muscle mass and excretory function of the kidney. Often creatinine levels are slightly lower in older adults because of decreased muscle mass.

An elevated creatinine level suggests rapid muscle loss from trauma or surgery. Elevated levels also indicate possible renal failure. Critical values > 4 mg/dL indicate serious impairment in renal function. However, a normal creatinine does not always mean unimpaired renal function. Creatinine level is interpreted in conjunction with BUN. Unlike the BUN, creatinine is not significantly affected by dehydration, malnutrition, or hepatic function.

Hydration status can be evaluated using the BUN:creatinine ratio. The normal ratio is 10:1. Ratios more than 25 suggest dehydration; ratios less than 10 suggest overhydration. For information on creatinine clearance, see Chapter 8.

Creatinine levels increase with

- Rapid muscle loss
- Surgery, trauma
- Impaired renal function
- Azotemia
- Chronic nephritis
- Obstruction of urinary tract
- Reduced renal blood flow
- Shock, dehydration
- CHF
- Diabetes
- Rhabdomyolysis

Creatinine levels decrease with

- Muscular dystrophy
- Debilitation

The following drugs may increase creatinine levels:

- Cimetidine
- Aminoglycosides
- Cephalosporins
- Heavy metal chemotherapeutic agents

Folate

Normal Values (5)

- 5-25 ng/mL; 11-57 nmol/L (SI)

Nutritional Significance (1)

Folate levels are used to evaluate hemolytic disorders and to detect megaloblastic anemia. Decreased folate levels are associated with megaloblastic anemia, hemolytic anemia, malnutrition, malabsorption syndromes, liver disease, and celiac disease. Elevated levels are often seen in pernicious anemia.

Folate supplementation may mask a B-12 deficiency; however, the level at which this occurs is not well documented. Recent studies using folate supplements to reduce elevated homocysteine levels recommend supplementing B-12 when a folate supplement is ordered.

Folate levels increase with

- Pernicious anemia

- Vegetarianism

Folate levels decrease with

- Megaloblastic anemia

- Hemolytic anemia

- Protein-energy malnutrition

- Malabsorption syndromes

- Cancer

- Alcoholism

- Liver disease

The following drugs may decrease folate levels:

- Alcohol

- Aminopterin

- Ampicillin

- Antimalarials

- Chloramphenicol

- Erythromycin

- Estrogens

- Methotrexate

- Para-aminosalicylic acid (PAS)

- Penicillin

- Phenobarbital

- Phenytoin

- Tetracycline

Glucose, Blood

Normal Values (5)

- Adults: 70-110 mg/dL; 3.9-6.1 mmol/L (SI)
- Older adults: increased slightly

Critical Values (5)

- 400 mg/dL (renal threshold is about 180 mg/dL)
- < 50 mg/dL in men; < 40 mg/dL in women

Nutritional Significance

The serum glucose level is a test used to diagnose many metabolic diseases. Serum glucose levels must be elevated at different times of day for an accurate diagnosis. There are a number of factors, including stress, infection, caffeine, and smoking, that can elevate fasting blood glucose levels. Elevated blood glu-cose levels often give falsely low serum sodium values (1). One formula to correct serum sodium values is as follows:

Corrected Na = [(Glucose/6) x 2] + Measured Na

The most common diagnosis associated with an elevated blood glucose level is diabetes mellitus. A fasting blood glucose test is performed on serum or plasma rather than on whole blood. Values will likely vary from the whole-blood glucose tests performed on capillary blood using the finger-stick method. Laboratory values using whole blood are likely 10% to 15% higher than capillary values (5).

In the 2002 *Standard of Medical Care for Patients with Diabetes Mellitus* (4), the diagnostic criteria for diabetes are as follows:

- Categories using fasting glucose levels:

  - Fasting plasma glucose (FPG) < 110 mg/dL = normal fasting glucose

  - FPG ≥ 110 mg/dl/L and < 126 mg/dL = impaired fasting glucose (IFG)

  - FPG ≥ 126 mg/dL = provisional diagnosis of diabetes

- Categories using oral glucose tolerance test (OGTT):

  - 2h postload glucose (2hPG) < 140 mg/dL = normal glucose tolerance

  - 2hPG ≥ 140 and < 200 mg/dL = impaired glucose tolerance

  - 2hPG ≥ 200 mg/dL = provisional diagnosis of diabetes

Diagnostic Criteria (4)

1. Signs and symptoms of diabetes plus a casual plasma glucose concentration ≥ 200 mg/dL

   OR

2. FPG ≥ 126 mg/dL (7.0 mmol/L) after an 8-hour fast

   OR

3. 2hPG ≥ 200 mg/dL (11.1 mmol/L) during oral glucose tolerance test (75-g load)

Diabetes is seen in about 10% of the clients older than 65 years (4). There are currently no long-term studies to demonstrate the benefits of tight glycemic control in older adults. Individuals who are active, cognitively intact, and expect to live 10 to 20 years should be encouraged to control the disease process with diet, exercise, and medications. Individuals with advanced diabetes complications, other comorbidities, or cognitive or functional impairments are less likely to benefit from tight glycemic control. Reasonable glycemic goals for these individuals are fasting glucose < 140 mg/dL and postprandial glucose < 200-220 mg/dL (4).

Blood glucose levels increase with (1)

- Diabetes
- Cystic fibrosis
- Cushing's syndrome (due to increased glucocorticoids)
- Hyperthyroidism
- Pituitary adenoma
- Acute pancreatitis
- Adenoma of pancreas
- Dehydration, stress, trauma
- Chronic liver disease
- Hemochromatosis
- General anesthesia
- Cerebral vascular accident (CVA)
- MI

Blood glucose levels decrease with (1)

- Liver disease
- Poisoning
- Hepatitis
- Cirrhosis
- Metastatic tumor
- Pancreatic disorders
- Glucagon deficiency
- Islet cell carcinoma
- Enzyme diseases
- Von Gierke's disease
- Galactosemia
- Maple syrup urine disease
- Fructose intolerance
- Endocrine disorders
- Addison's disease
- Hypothyroidism
- Water overload
- Insulin overdose
- Alcoholism

The following drugs may increase blood glucose levels (1):

- Antidepressants
- Beta blockers
- Caffeine
- Corticosteroids
- Dextrothyroxine
- Diazoxide
- Diuretics
- Epinephrine
- Estrogen
- Isoniazid
- Lithium
- Pentamidine
- Phenothiazines
- Phenytoin

The following drugs may decrease blood glucose levels (1):

- Acetaminophen
- Alcohol
- Anabolic steroids
- Clofibrate
- Disopyramide
- Gemfibrozil
- Insulin
- Monamine oxidase inhibitor (MAOI)
- Pentamidine
- Propranolol
- Tolazamide
- Tolbutamide

Glycosylated Hemoglobin (A$_{1C}$)

Normal Values (4)

- Adults: 4% to 6%
- Good diabetic control: 7% or less
- Fair diabetic control: > 7.01% to < 8%
- Poor diabetic control: > 8%

Nutritional Significance (1)

Glycosylated hemoglobin (GHb A$_{1C}$) is a test that provides an accurate 2- to 3-month index of average blood glucose levels. GHb A$_{1C}$ is a valuable test because the sample can be drawn at any time. In addition, recent food intake, exercise, stress, hypoglycemic agents, or patient/resident cooperation do not affect the values. It is used to evaluate the success of diabetic therapy, especially when new strategies for care are implemented. GHb A_{1C} has been used to determine the duration of hyperglycemia in newly diagnosed diabetics as well as in those with impaired glucose tolerance. It is helpful to differentiate between short-term hyperglycemia and diabetes.

GHb A_{1C} levels increase with

- Newly diagnosed or poorly controlled diabetes
- Impaired glucose tolerance
- Hyperglycemia
- Iron-deficiency anemia
- Hemodialysis
- Acute stress response
- Corticosteroid therapy

GHb A_{1C} levels decrease with

- Hemolytic anemia (sickle cell)
- Chronic renal failure
- Vitamin E supplementation
- Chronic blood loss

Hematocrit

Normal Values (5)

- Women: 37%-47%; 0.37-0.47 (SI)
- Men: 42%-52%; 0.42-0.52 (SI)
- Older adults: values may be slightly decreased

Nutritional Significance (1)

Hematocrit is the percentage of red blood cells in total blood volume and is used, along with hemoglobin, to evaluate iron status. Usually the hematocrit percentage is three times the hemoglobin concentration in grams per deciliter. This will not be the case if the red blood cells are of abnormal size or hemoglobin concentration.

The hematocrit value is affected by extremely high white blood cell count and hydration status. It should be evaluated in light of other laboratory values. Individuals living in high altitudes often have increased values. It is common for individuals older than 50 years to have slightly lower levels than younger adults. Individuals with anemia of chronic disease will not be able to maintain normal hematocrit levels, because the body lacks the ability to use stored iron.

Hematocrit levels increase with

- Dehydration
- Erythrocytosis
- Shock
- Surgery
- Trauma
- Burns
- High altitudes

Hematocrit levels decrease with

- Acute blood loss
- Overhydration
- Anemias
- Iron deficiency
- Anemia of chronic disease
- Pernicious anemia
- Megaloblastic anemia
- Bone marrow failure
- Hyperthyroidism
- Hodgkin's disease
- Leukemia
- Multiple myeloma
- AIDS
- Cirrhosis

The following drugs may decrease hematocrit levels:

- Chloramphenicol
- Penicillin

Hemoglobin

Normal Values (5)

- Women: 12-16 g/dL; 7.4-9.9 mmol/L (SI)
- Men: 14-18 g/dL; 8.7-11.2 mmol/L (SI)

Nutritional Significance (1)

The hemoglobin concentration is a measure of the total amount of hemoglobin in the peripheral blood and is a more direct measure of iron deficiency than hematocrit. Changes in hydration status affect hemoglobin. Overhydration decreases the concentration, and dehydration increases the concentration. Living in high altitudes may cause higher hemoglobin values.

Hemoglobin concentration increases with

- Dehydration
- Polycythemia
- Chronic obstructive pulmonary disease (COPD)
- CHF
- High altitudes
- Severe burns

Hemoglobin concentration decreases with

- Anemias
  - Iron-deficiency anemia
  - Anemia of chronic disease
  - Pernicious anemia
  - Megaloblastic anemia
  - Sickle cell anemia
- Hypertension
- Cirrhosis
- Systemic diseases
  - Leukemia
  - Lymphoma
  - Erythematous
  - Hodgkin's disease
  - Sarcoidosis
  - Systemic lupus
- Overhydration
- Kidney disease
- Chronic hemorrhage
- Splenomegaly
- AIDS

The following drugs may increase hemoglobin levels:

- Gentamicin
- Methyldopa

The following drugs may decrease hemoglobin levels:

- Sulfonamides
- Antibiotics
- Aspirin
- Antineoplastic
- Indomethacin
- Rifampin

Iron Level: Serum Fe, Total Iron-Binding Capacity

Normal Values (5)
Serum Fe:

- Women: 60-160 µg/dL; 11-29 µmol/L (SI)
- Men: 80-180 µg/dL; 11-29 µmol/L (SI)

Total Iron-Binding Capacity (TIBC):

- 250-460 µg/dL; 45-73 µmol/L (SI)

Nutritional Significance (1)
Most of the iron in the body is found in the hemoglobin of the red blood cells. Dietary iron is absorbed in the small intestine and transported to the plasma. In the plasma, iron is bound to transferrin and transported to the bone marrow for production of hemoglobin. The remaining iron is stored as ferritin and hemosiderin in the liver and other tissues for future use. The serum iron reflects the amount of iron bound to transferrin. TIBC is a direct measure of transferrin. When TIBC is not available, transferrin can be directly measured.

Serum Fe levels increase with

- Pernicious anemia
- Aplastic anemia
- Hemolytic anemia
- B-6 deficiency
- Acute hepatitis
- Repeated transfusions
- Nephritis
- Excessive iron therapy
- Hemosiderosis, hemochromatosis
- Iron poisoning
- Hepatic necrosis
- Lead toxicity

Serum Fe levels decrease with

- Iron-deficiency anemia
- Acute and chronic infection
- Cancer
- Protein-energy malnutrition
- Nephrosis
- Insufficient dietary iron
- Chronic blood loss
- Inadequate absorption of iron
- Neoplasia

- Chronic gastrointestinal blood loss
- Chronic hematuria

The following drugs may increase serum Fe levels:

- Chloramphenicol
- Dextran
- Estrogen
- Ethanol
- Methyldopa

The following drugs may decrease serum Fe levels:

- Cholestyramine
- Colchicine
- Corticotropic hormone (ACTH)
- Deferoxamine
- Methicillin
- Testosterone

TIBC levels increase with

- Iron-deficiency anemia
- Polycythemia vera

TIBC levels decrease with

- Hypoproteinemia
- Inflammatory diseases
- Cirrhosis
- Hemolytic, pernicious, and sickle cell anemias

Fluoride may increase TIBC levels. Corticotropic hormone and chloramphenicol may decrease TIBC levels.

Osmolality, Serum

Normal Values (5)

- Adults, older adults: 285-295 mOsm/kg water

Critical Values
- 320 mOsm/kg water

Nutritional Significance (1,5)
Osmolality measures the concentration of particles in a solution. Serum osmolality is increased with dehydration and decreased with overhydration. When serum osmolality increases, the antidiuretic hormone is secreted, which causes more water reabsorption, a more concentrated urine, and a less concentrated serum. When osmolality is low, the body decreases water reabsorption and excretes large amounts of dilute urine.

Serum osmolality is used to evaluate fluid and electrolyte imbalance, seizures, liver disease, hydration status, and acid-base balance.

Serum osmolality increases with

- Hypernatremia
- Dehydration
- Hyperglycemia
- Mannitol therapy
- Azotemia
- Uremia
- Ingestion of ethanol, methanol, ethylene, or glycol
- Hyperosmolar nonketotic hyperglycemia
- Diabetes insipidus
- Hypercalcemia
- Renal tubular necrosis
- Severe pyelonephritis
- Ketosis
- Shock

Serum osmolality decreases with

- Hyponatremia
- Overhydration
- Syndrome of inappropriate antidiuretic hormone (ADH) secretion
- Paraneoplastic syndromes associated with lung carcinoma
- Excess fluid intake

Potassium, Serum

Normal Values (5)

- Adults: 3.5-5.0 mEq/L; 3.5-5.0 mmol/L (SI)

Nutritional Significance (1)
The normal potassium levels within cells are approximately 150 mEq/L, compared with 3.5-5.0 mEq/L in serum. The level of potassium found outside the cells is the level measured by this laboratory test. As a positively charged ion, potassium is involved in regulating the osmolality of the extracellular fluid by exchanging with sodium. Its level is essential to maintain the transmembrane electrical potential between the intracellular fluid and the extracellular fluid.

Potassium levels increase with

- Renal failure
- Excessive intake

- Cell damage
  - Burns
  - Surgery
  - Crushing injuries
  - Chemotherapy
- Acidosis
- Addison's disease
- Internal hemorrhage
- Uncontrolled diabetes
- Dehydration

Potassium levels decrease with

- Protein-energy malnutrition
- Malabsorption
- Diarrhea
- Severe vomiting
- Renal tubular acidosis
- Diuretic therapy
- Liver disease with ascites
- Chronic stress
- Chronic laxative abuse
- Cushing's syndrome
- IV fluids without adequate potassium

The following drugs may increase potassium levels:

- Aminocaproic acid
- Antibiotics
- Antineoplastic drugs
- Captopril
- Epinephrine
- Heparin
- Histamine
- Isoniazid
- Lithium
- Mannitol
- K-sparing diuretics
- K-supplements

The following drugs may decrease potassium levels:

- Acetazolamide
- Aminosalicylic acid

- Amphotericin B
- Carbenicillin
- Insulin
- Laxatives
- Aspirin
- K-wasting diuretics

Clinical Signs of Hypokalemia and Hyperkalemia
The following are clinical signs of hypokalemia:

- Muscle weakness
- Cramps
- Hypoflexia
- Paresthesia
- Decreased bowel motility
- Hypotension
- Cardiac arrhythmia
- Drowsiness
- Lethargy
- Coma

The following are clinical signs of hyperkalemia:

- Confusion
- Irritability
- Nausea
- Vomiting
- Intestinal colic
- Paresthesia
- Abdominal cramps
- Muscle paralysis

Protein, Blood: Prealbumin
Normal Values (5)

- 15-36 mg/dL; 150-360 mg/L (SI)

Degree of Depletion (5)

- Mild: 10-15 mg/dL
- Moderate: 5-10 mg/dL
- Severe: < 5 mg/dL

Nutritional Significance (1,6)
Prealbumin (PAB) is in a class of proteins having rapid turnover with short half-lives (2-3 days). PAB is also called "transthyretin" and "thyroxine-binding prealbumin." PAB is a sensitive indicator of protein deficiency and of improvement in pro-

tein status with refeeding. When malnutrition is significant, the serum PAB will usually fall below 11 mg/dL. Serum PAB is not greatly affected by mild renal or liver disease, by fluid compartment shifts, or in clients receiving exogenous albumin. However, as renal and liver disease become more significant, the levels are decreased. In addition, iron deficiency does not significantly impact its level.

Serum PAB increases when more than 60% of basal energy expenditure (BEE) needs are met and decreases when less than 45% are met or when there is no oral intake. A reasonable goal of a refeeding program in extended care is to increase serum PAB by at least 2.0 to 3.0 mg/dL in 1 week.

PAB levels increase with dehydration. Corticosteroids may increase PAB levels.

PAB levels decrease with

- Overhydration
- Acute catabolic stress
- Stress
- Infection
- Postsurgery
- AIDS

Protein, Blood: Serum Albumin

Normal Values (5)

- 3.5-5.0 g/dL; 35-50 g/L (SI) (values vary depending on assay method used)

Degree of Depletion (1)

- Mild: 3.0-3.5 g/dL
- Moderate: 2.1-3.0 g/dL
- Severe: < 2.1 g/dL

Nutritional Significance

Albumin and globulin constitute most of the protein within the body and are measured as total protein. Albumin is synthesized in the liver at a rate of 8 to 14 g/day. It makes up approximately 60% of the total protein. Albumin provides approximately 80% of colloidal osmotic pressure of the plasma. When albumin decreases, the water in plasma moves to the interstitial compartment. The loss of plasma fluid results in hypovolemia, which in turn triggers renal retention of water and sodium. Albumin also serves as a carrier of metals, ions, fatty acids, amino acids, metabolites, bilirubin, enzymes, hormones, and drugs (1).

Nonnutritional factors can determine albumin levels. Albumin level is dependent on hepatocyte function. With age and declining liver function, the liver can lose its ability to synthesize albumin. Because the half-life of albumin is 12 to 21 days, significant changes in liver function specific to albumin synthesis may go undetected until after that point. Severely malnourished individuals have greatly decreased levels of serum albumin. However, because of its long half-life, albumin is a poor indicator of early malnutrition (1,6-9).

When albumin levels are low, the serum calcium level is also low. When the serum albumin is elevated, the serum calcium is elevated (5).

Albumin levels increase with dehydration (1). Albumin levels decrease with (1)

- Overhydration
- Decreased absorption
  - Pancreatic insufficiency
  - Malabsorption
- Inadequate intake
- Impaired synthesis
  - CHF
  - Cirrhosis
  - Acute stress
- Increased need
  - Hyperthyroidism
- Increased loss
  - Edema
  - Ascites
  - Burns
  - Pressure ulcers
  - Hemorrhage
  - Nephrotic syndrome
  - Crohn's disease
  - Sprue
  - Whipple's disease
- AIDS
- Protein dilution secondary to excessive IV fluids
- Increased capillary permeability
- Increased breakdown
  - Cancer
  - Trauma
- Infection

The following drugs may increase albumin levels (1):

- Anabolic steroids
- Androgens
- Corticosteroids
- Dextran
- Growth hormone
- Insulin
- Phenazopyridine
- Progesterone

The following drugs may decrease albumin levels (1):

- Ammonium ions
- Estrogens
- Hepatotoxic drugs

Mean Corpuscular Volume

Normal Values (5)

- 80-95 μm^3; 80-95 fL (SI)

Nutritional Significance (1,10)

Mean corpuscular value (MCV) is a measure of the average volume of a single red blood cell. MCV is determined by dividing the hematocrit by the total red blood cell count. An increased MCV suggests that the red blood cells are macrocytic. Megaloblastic anemia (B-12 and folic acid deficiency) are associated with elevated MCV. A low MCV suggests that the red blood cells are microcytic. Iron-deficiency anemia and thalassemia are associated with decreased MCV.

MCV increases with

- Liver disease
- Folate deficiency
- B-12 deficiency
- Excess alcohol intake
- Sprue
- Early pernicious anemia

MCV decreases with

- Advanced iron deficiency
- Chronic blood loss
- Iron malabsorption
- Excessive iron requirements

- Thalassemia
- Lead poisoning

Serum B-12

Normal Values (5)

- 160-950 pg/mL; 118-701 pmol/L

Nutritional Significance

Serum B-12 is a measure used to identify pernicious anemia and megaloblastic anemia in older adults. Low levels may reflect poor intake or lack of intrinsic factor. Some studies suggest that a serum B-12 of < 350 pg/mL should be considered a deficiency state and treated accordingly (11).

Serum B-12 levels increase with (1)

- Liver disease
- Chronic myelocytic leukemia
- Polycythemia urea

Serum B-12 levels decrease with (1)

- Zollinger-Ellison syndrome
- B-12 deficiency
- Hypothyroidism
- Folate deficiency
- Alcoholism
- Aplastic anemia
- Myeloma
- Megadoses of vitamin C
- HIV
- Transcobalamin I deficiency

The following drugs may decrease serum B-12 levels (1):

- Antibiotics
- Aspirin
- Cimetidine
- Chlorpromazine
- Ranitidine
- Cholestyramine
- Antifolate drugs
- Extended-release K preparations

Sodium, Serum

Normal Values (5)

- 136-146 mEq/L; 136-145 mmol/L (SI)

Nutritional Significance

The serum sodium level reflects the relationship between total body sodium and extracellular fluid volume. The concentration of sodium serves as a major determinant of extracellular osmolality. A decreased serum sodium level also results in a decreased extracellular osmolality. An elevated serum sodium level results in increased extracellular osmolality. Elevated osmolality stimulates secretion of the antidiuretic hormone, which in turn increases tubular reabsorption of water.

Clinical signs of hypernatremia include dehydration, thirst, agitation, restlessness, hyperflexia, mania, tachycardia, dry mucous membranes, lethargy, hyperactive reflexes, and seizures. As the fluid shifts to compensate for excessive levels of sodium, the serum becomes more dilute. Other laboratory values associated with hypernatremia include urine-specific gravity > 1.015 and serum osmolality > 295 mOsm/kg (1,5).

All laboratory values will appear less concentrated when hyponatremia is present. The body compensates for hyponatremia by increasing water loss. As water is lost, the serum sodium, as well as other laboratory values, becomes more concentrated.

Other laboratory values associated with hyponatremia include urine-specific gravity < 1.010 and serum osmolality < 285 mOsm/Kg. Clinical signs of hyponatremia include muscle cramps, muscle twitching, headache, dizziness, lethargy, confusion, convulsions, stupor, and coma. The changes in the central nervous system are due to fluid shifts, from the extracellular spaces to the intracellular spaces, which cause the cells to swell (1).

Serum sodium levels increase with (1)

- Excessive intake
- Primary aldosteronism
- Dehydration
- Excessive sweating
- Diabetes insipidus
- Hypercalcemic nephropathy
- Hypokalemic nephropathy
- Cushing's disease

Serum sodium decreases with (1)

- Decreased intake
- Severe diarrhea
- Excessive water intake
- Overhydration
- Vomiting
- Excessive use of IVs of non-electrolyte fluids
- Cirrhosis with ascites
- Inappropriate secretion of antidiuretic hormone
- Hyperglycemia
- Hyperproteinemia
- Addison's disease

The following drugs may increase serum sodium levels (1):

- Anabolic steroids
- Antibiotics
- Clonidine
- Corticosteroids
- Laxatives
- Methyldopa

The following drugs may decrease serum sodium levels (1):

- Carbamazepine
- Diuretics
- Sulfonylureas
- Triamterene
- Vasopressin

Total Serum Cholesterol, Low-Density Lipoprotein, and High-Density Lipoprotein

Normal Values (1,12)

- Adults—cholesterol: < 200 mg/dL; < 5.20 mmol/L (SI)
- Adults—low-density lipoprotein (LDL): 60-160 mg/dL; < 3.37 mmol/L (SI)
- Adults—high-density lipoprotein (HDL): > 40 mg/dL, < 60 mg/dL; > 0.66 mmol/L, < 1.0 mmol/L

Nutritional Significance

Elevated serum cholesterol has been associated with increased risks for arteriosclerotic vascular disease in young and middle-aged adults. The most accurate results are from a fasting blood cholesterol test. Current research suggests that arteriosclerotic vascular disease is a multifactorial condition. Dietary cholesterol may not be as important as once believed, especially for older women with no history of heart disease, hypertension, or diabetes. For older adults with no history of heart disease, an elevated cholesterol is probably not justification for a cholesterol-lowering diet (13-15).

Cholesterol is used as an indicator of malnutrition. When cholesterol levels decline along with other indicators of protein status, nutrition needs are probably not being met, and the risk for skin breakdown increases. In older adults, the problem may be chronic failure to thrive, very low intake, or overall declining status. Cholesterol of less than 160 mg/dL may be an indicator of malnutrition and may be a predictor of mortality. Historic cholesterol levels must be considered in evaluating the risk for malnutrition (1,13-15).

Total serum cholesterol levels increase with (1)

- Hypercholesterolemia
- Hyperlipidemia
- Hypothyroidism
- Uncontrolled diabetes
- Nephrotic syndrome
- Stress
- High-cholesterol diet
- Xanthomatosis
- Hypertension
- MI
- Atherosclerosis
- Nephrosis
- Biliary cirrhosis

Total serum cholesterol levels decrease with (1)

- Malabsorption
- Protein-energy malnutrition
- Hyperthyroidism
- Pernicious anemia
- Hemolytic anemia
- Sepsis
- Stress
- Liver disease
- AIDS

The following drugs may increase total serum cholesterol levels (1):

- ACTH
- Anabolic steroids
- Beta blockers
- Corticosteroids
- Epinephrine
- Dilantin
- Sulfonamides
- Thiazide diuretics
- Vitamin D

The following drugs may decrease total serum cholesterol levels (1):

- Allopurinol
- Androgens
- Bile-salt binding agents
- Captopril
- Chlorpropamide
- Clofibrate
- Colchicine
- Erythromycin
- Cytomel
- Isoniazid
- Mevacor
- Neomycin
- Niacin

HDL levels increase with (1)

- Frequent exercise
- Liver disease
- Moderate alcohol intake

HDL levels decrease with (1)

- High alcohol intake
- Smoking
- AIDS

LDL and very low-density lipoproteins (VLDL) levels increase with (1)

- Hyperlipidemia
- High-fat diet

LDL and VLDL levels decrease with (1)

- Malnutrition
- Malabsorption
- AIDS

The following drugs may increase LDL and VLDL levels (1):

- Aspirin
- Phenothiazines
- Steroids
- Sulfonamides

Triglycerides

Normal Values (5)

- < 150 mg/dL; < 1.69 mmol/L (SI)

Nutritional Significance (1)

Triglycerides are a form of fat found in the bloodstream. They are transported in the blood by VLDL and LDL. Excess levels of triglycerides are seen in individuals consuming a high-fat diet; high levels of alcohol; and very-low-fat, high-carbohydrate diets.

Triglyceride levels increase with

- Glycogen storage disease
- Hyperlipidemias
- Hypertension
- MI
- Hypothyroidism
- High-carbohydrate diet or high-fat diet
- Poorly controlled diabetes
- Nephrotic syndrome
- Alcoholic cirrhosis
- Alcohol

Triglyceride levels decrease with

- Malabsorption
- Protein-energy malnutrition
- Hyperthyroidism
- AIDS

Cholestyramine may increase triglyceride levels. The following drugs may decrease triglyceride levels:

- Ascorbic acid
- Asparaginase
- Clofibrate
- Colestipol

CASE STUDIES

Case Study 1

An 89-year-old woman is admitted to an extended-care facility secondary to inability to care for herself any longer. She has a history of rheumatoid arthritis, constipation, and mild dementia. Her diet order is regular. Her medications include enteric-coated aspirin and milk of magnesia every 3 days. She provides a history of weight being stable at 140 lb until the last month. She has lost weight to her present 136 lb.

Current laboratory values include the following: Na, 149 mEq/L; K, 4.0 mEq/L; BUN, 24 mg/dL; Creat, 0.8 mg/dL; Glu, 120mg/dL; Alb, 3.4 g/dL; Hgb, 10.1 g/dL; Hct, 30.3%; MCV, 90 μm^3; serum Fe, 45 μg/dL ; TIBC, 198 μg/dL; ferritin, 120 ng/dL; Osm, 302 mOsm/kg water.

Information generated from the laboratory test results for the dietetics professional's nutrition assessment includes mild dehydration. The client's sodium, BUN, and osmolality are all elevated, consistent with dehydration. Physical examination will help to support this conclusion. Often the albumin level can be falsely high, depending on hydration status. This client's albumin is borderline normal. One could consider, with the recent weight loss and decline in the activities of daily living including meal preparation, that mild protein calorie malnutrition may be the cause of her lower albumin level. The albumin will be falsely high until rehydration is completed. Improved nutritional intake, including meal supervision, will help to replete albumin levels. The client has low hemoglobin, hematocrit, and serum iron levels, with normal MCV and ferritin levels. Anemia of chronic disease is the most likely rationale. The body stores of iron are normal; however, there is impaired release of these stores for heme synthesis. Providing iron supplementation would be of little benefit for this client, either from a monetary standpoint or from a nutritional perspective, and could further aggravate her constipation.

Case Study 2

An 85-year-old man was transferred to an extended-care facility after hospitalization for rehabilitation after a fractured left hip. He has a history of CHF and HTN. He has had an 8-lb weight loss from pre-hospitalization to admission to the extended-care facility. His diet is no-added-salt. His current medications include bumetanide, clonidine, warfarin, Niferex, and famotidine.

Values from his laboratory tests, taken before discharge from the hospital, include the following: Na, 140 mEq/L; K, 3.2 mEq/L; BUN, 25 mg/dL; Glu, 112 mg/dL; Alb, 2.8 g/dL; Hgb, 11.3 g/dL; Hct, 34%; MCV, 78 μm^3; ferritin, 11 ng/dL; PAB, 15 mg/dL.

This client has hypokalemia and depleted visceral proteins secondary to stress and surgery. He is on a diuretic, bumetanide, which is a potassium depleter. The dietetics professional should review the menu for potassium content and evaluate the client's actual intake. If dietary sources are inadequate, potassium supplementation should be considered. The acute-phase reactants were preferentially produced in the liver, as opposed to nutritional proteins. If quick initial response to nutrition therapy is desired, serum prealbumin levels should be checked, because of their more rapid repletion, secondary to the shorter half-life. The client also has iron-deficiency anemia, most likely a result of blood loss from surgery. He is being treated with Niferex, and an adequate diet is also recommended. Repeat testing of Hgb and Hct should be recommended, so that timely discontinuation of the iron supplement can be achieved.

Case Study 3

A 79-year-old man is admitted to an extended-care facility with chronic renal failure, type 2 diabetes, hypertension, and peripheral vascular disease. He lived with his wife until his disease progressed to the point where she could no longer manage his care. He has been eating fairly well, with no change in his dry weight of 152 lb. His medications at admission include calcium carbonate, Epogen (at dialysis), Nephrocaps, diltiazem HCl, and pentoxifylline.

Values from his laboratory tests, sent from dialysis at admission, include the following: Na, 142 mEq/L; K, 5.2 mEq/L; BUN, 75 mg/dL; Creat, 6.8 mg/dL; Glu, 155 mg/dL; CO_2, 19 mEq/L; Cl, 104 mEq/L; Alb, 3.5 g/dL; Hgb, 12.7 g/dL; Hct, 38.1%; Ca, 8.4 mg/dL; PO_4, 6.0 mg/dL.

This client's end-stage renal disease (ESRD) and medication administration must be evaluated to accurately interpret the laboratory test results. His elevated BUN and creatinine are consistent with ESRD. The hyperkalemia is mild and should be addressed with diet, so that it does not continue to increase and lead to cardiac arrhythmia. The low Hgb and Hct are also consistent with ESRD. Further workup is not recommended, because the client is on Epogen provided at dialysis for his ane-

mia. Mild hyperglycemia is present. Blood draw in relationship to meal time needs to be considered. This client may have eaten breakfast before dialysis, and this may be representative of a 2-hour postprandial result. If this is the case, adequate control is present at this time. A fasting glucose level can be suggested, as two consecutive fasting blood sugars of 126 are needed before diabetes can be diagnosed. Evaluation of this client's diet history for high phosphorus foods and administration of the phosphorus binder, calcium carbonate, is recommended, because of the hyperphosphatemia and hypocalcemia. If evaluation of the diet history reveals low to moderate phosphorus intake, then the administration of the binder should be considered. If the binder was not taken with meals, this could be the cause of the abnormal laboratory values. The registered dietitian should instruct caregivers in more effective administration of the calcium carbonate. The albumin level is borderline. Adequate protein intake can help prevent future decline.

REFERENCES

1. Litchford MD. *Practical Applications in Laboratory Assessment of Nutritional Status.* Greensboro, NC: CASE Software; 2002.

2. Chidester JC, Spangler AA. Fluid intake in the institutionalized elderly [Erratum in: *J Am Diet Assoc.* 1997;97:584]. *J Am Diet Assoc.* 1997;97:23-28,29-30.

3. DeHoog S, Grant A. *Nutrition Assessment Support and Management.* 5th ed. Seattle, Wash: Ann Grant, Susan DeHoog; 1999:44-54.

4. American Diabetes Association. Standards of medical care for patients with diabetes mellitus. *Diabetes Care.* 2002;25:213-229.

5. Pagana KD, Pagana TJ. *Mosby's Diagnostic and Laboratory Test Reference.* St. Louis, Mo: Mosby; 2002.

6. Mears E. Prealbumin and nutritional assessment. In: *Dietetic Currents.* Columbus, Ohio: Ross Products Division, Abbott Laboratories; 1994.

7. Puskarich-May CL, Sullivan DH, Nelson CL, Stroope HF, Walls RC. The change in serum protein concentration in response to the stress of total joint surgery: a comparison of older persons versus younger patients. *J Am Geriatr Soc.* 1996;44:555-558.

8. Baumgartner RN, Koehler KM, Romero L, Garry PJ. Serum albumin is associated with skeletal muscle in elderly men and women. *Am J Clin Nutr.* 1996;64:552-558.

9. Cederholm T, Jagren C, Hellstrom K. Outcome of protein-energy malnutrition in elderly medical patients. *Am J Med.* 1995;98:67-74.

10. Stabler SP. Screening the older population for cobalamin (vitamin B12) deficiency. *J Am Geriatr Soc.* 1995;43:1290-1297.

11. Pennypacker LC, Allen RH, Kelly JP, Matthews LM, Grigsby J, Kaye K, Lindenbaum J, Stabler SP. High prevalence of cobalamin deficiency in elderly outpatients. *J Am Geriatr Soc.* 1992;40:1197-1204.

12. National Institutes of Health. ATP III At-A-glance: quick desk reference. 2001. Available at: http://www.nih.gov/guidelines/cholesterol/atglance.htm. Accessed May 31, 2001.

13. Iribarren C, Reed DM, Burchfiel CM, Dwyer JH. Serum total cholesterol and mortality: confounding factors and risk modification in Japanese-American men. *JAMA.* 1995;273:1926-1932.

14. Verdery RB, Goldberg AP. Hypocholesterolemia as a predictor of death: a prospective study of 224 nursing home residents. *J Gerontol Med Sci.* 1991;46:M84-M90.

15. Corti MC, Guralnik JM, Salive ME, Harris T, Field TS, Wallace RB, Berkman LF, Seeman TE, Glynn RJ, Hennekens CH. HDL cholesterol predicts heart disease mortality in older persons. *JAMA.* 1995;274:539-544.

ADDITIONAL RESOURCES

Carmel R. Prevalence of undiagnosed pernicious anemia in the elderly. *Arch Intern Med.* 1996;156:1097.

Chermecky C, Berger B. *Laboratory Tests and Diagnostic Procedures.* Philadelphia, Pa: Saunders; 1997.

Coulter JS. Red blood cell distribution width and mean corpuscular volume: clinical applications. *Adv Clin Care.* 1991;6(6):13.

Gallagher-Allred CR, Voss AC, Finn S, McCamish MA. Malnutrition and clinical outcomes: the case for medical nutrition therapy. *J Am Diet Assoc.* 1996;96:366-369.

Hine RJ. What practitioners need to know about folic acid. *J Am Diet Assoc.* 1996;96:451-452.

Joosten E, vandenBerg A, Riezler R, Naurath HJ, Lindembaum J, Stabler SP, Allen RH. Metabolic evidence that deficiencies of vitamin B-12 (cobalamin), folate, and vitamin B-6 occur commonly in elderly people. *Am J Clin Nutr.* 1993;58:468-476.

Kee JL, Hayes ER. Assessment of patient laboratory data in the acutely ill. *Nurs Clin North Am.* 1990;25:751-759.

Koehler KM, Pareo-Tubbeh SL, Romero LJ, Baumgartner RN, Garry PJ. Folate nutrition and older adults: challenges and opportunities. *J Am Diet Assoc.* 1997;97:167-173.

Paradiso C. *Fluids and Electrolytes.* Philadelphia, Pa: Lippincott; 1995.

Shine JW. Microcytic anemia. *Am Fam Physician.* 1997;55:2455-2462.

Yao Y, Yao S-L, Yao S-S, Yao G, Lou W. Prevalence of vitamin B12 deficiency among geriatric outpatients. *J Fam Pract.* 1992;35:524-528.

Drug-Nutrient Interactions

Drug-nutrient interactions can be described as the influence that drugs have on the nutritional status of an individual or, conversely, as the influence that food has on medication. The direct effect that a drug may have on nutrient absorption, metabolism, or excretion can have a detrimental effect on the nutritional status of older adults taking the medication. In addition, the indirect influence that a medication may have on altering food intake may have a significant impact on nutritional status.

Most drug-nutrient interactions are caused by food-induced changes in drug bioavailability. ("Bioavailability" refers to the extent to which the unaltered active ingredient of a drug enters the general circulation.) This can lead to a loss of therapeutic efficacy or toxic effects of drug therapy. Of significant relevance to dietetics professionals are adverse drug side effects that influence dietary intake.

Vulnerability of drug-induced nutritional deficiencies is greatest in older adults, chronically ill persons, and anyone with marginal or inadequate nutrient intake. At special risk are those individuals who are on polypharmacy and/or long-term drug therapy. Without proper nutrition management, these high-risk individuals may be subject to nutrient depletion or altered drug response.

DRUG-NUTRIENT ADVERSE SIDE EFFECTS

Technically, any drug effect other than the intended therapeutic effect can be classified as an adverse reaction. Mild but predictable adverse reactions are known as adverse side effects. Drowsiness is an example of a mild, relatively benign adverse side

effect. An adverse side effect is often tolerated, because the benefits of a drug outweigh the risk of the adverse side effect. However, an adverse side effect may prove to be unacceptably harmful and necessitate discontinuation of a drug. Adverse effects may diminish or disappear with continued drug administration because of tolerance.

Adverse drug side effects that can influence the nutritional status of older adults include appetite changes, weight changes, edema, altered taste, thirst, dry mouth, increased risk of dental problems, gastrointestinal (GI) distress, nausea/vomiting, diarrhea, constipation, blood pressure changes, and drowsiness. In addition, dietetics professionals must understand a medication's influence on electrolytes, its consequences for nutritionally significant laboratory tests, and whether it should be taken with food, alcohol, or caffeine.

Even if a drug is identified in clinical trials to have a potential for an adverse side effect, an individual taking the drug may or may not experience the side effect. Many factors, such as medical status; nutritional status; polypharmacy; concurrent use of over-the-counter medications, herbals, or nutritional supplements; and non-drug factors, may contribute to or cause adverse side effects.

FOOD-DRUG INTERACTIONS

In addition to a drug's potential adverse side effects and its influence on the nutritional status of older adults, the alert dietetics professional is aware of the influence that food and nutrients have on the pharmacokinetics of a drug. Pharmacokinetics includes the absorption, distribution, conversion to active form, and elimination of medication. Individuals taking vitamins, minerals, and other food supplements concurrently with medication use are at increased risk for nutrient-induced alterations in pharmacokinetics (1).

The presence of food, vitamin, mineral, and other dietary supplements has the ability to alter the pH and the osmolality of the GI tract. These changes can alter the absorption of drugs as a result of alterations in drug ionization, stability, solubility, and transit time. Food can also affect drug absorption, because of physical or chemical interactions between the food and the drug itself. Table 18.1 describes potential drug interactions with vitamins, minerals, and other food supplements (2).

DRUG-NUTRIENT INTERACTIONS AND OLDER ADULTS

Older adults are at particular risk for drug-nutrient interactions. Several factors contribute to this heightened risk, including drugs, pathological factors, geriatric factors, and nutrition.

Drug-Associated Factors

Medications are prescribed to older adults to treat the multiple pathologic processes associated with aging, as well as memory loss, confusion, and altered sleep patterns. Older adults living at home typically take three or more different prescribed medications per day (3). In addition, they may take nonprescription drugs, such as analgesics, antacids, and antihistamines, as well as nutritional herbal remedies and supplements. This polypharmacy pattern in older adults leads to difficulty with compliance and greatly increases the risk for drug-nutrient and drug-drug interactions (3). In fact, although older adults comprise 13% of the population of the United States, they consume more than 40% of all prescription drugs and experience 30% of the adverse drug reactions reported to the Food and Drug Administration (4,5).

Other drug-associated factors contributing to increased risk of drug-nutrient interactions besides polypharmacy include the dosage, the duration, and the frequency of prescribed medications. The physical changes associated with aging (see Geriatric Factors) could contribute to drug efficacy, and, if the dosage is not adjusted, potential drug toxicity. Drug duration and frequency also need to be monitored, especially in those individuals on "inherited therapy" from drugs started in middle age (2).

Pathological Factors

Older adults are more likely than young or middle-aged adults to have disease conditions, such as cardiovascular disease, GI malabsorption, liver disease, and/or renal disease. The presence of these disease states may have an adverse effect on the pharmacokinetics of a medication (2,6,7).

Geriatric Factors

Regardless of the presence of disease states that could be risk factors for drug-induced nutrient deficiencies, certain age-related factors still put any person older than 65 years at significant risk for drug-induced nutritional deficiencies. Anyone older than 75 years is at even higher risk, and those older than 85 years are at the greatest risk for drug-induced nutrient deficiencies (7). Age-related GI factors include a decrease in gastric emptying, splanchnic (visceral) blood flow, and intestinal motility, and thus a decrease in the absorption of the drug (2). Age-related changes in the kidney and liver affect drug metabolism and excretion (2,7). In addition, age-related body composition changes, such as increased adipose tissue and loss of skeletal muscles, can impact drug distribution (2). Furthermore, drug receptors and tissue sensitivity are affected by age (2). Thus, age-related factors contribute to alterations in drug efficacy and drug toxicity among older adults.

Nutrition-Related Factors

An individual consuming a poor-quality diet or one with compromised nutritional status is more likely to experience nutrition-related side effects associated with drug-nutrient interactions than is a person whose nutritional status is adequate. The older adult often consumes a diet that is not adequate in energy, protein, calcium, and B vitamins and thus is at risk for side effects resulting from the deficiency of these nutrients (5,7,8).

ENTERAL FEEDINGS AND DRUG-NUTRIENT INTERACTIONS

Drug-nutrient incompatibilities associated with enteral feeding can be classified as physical, pharmaceutical, pharmacologic, physiologic, and pharmacokinetic.

Physical Incompatibilities

Physical incompatibilities are the changes in formulas that occur when certain medications mix with enteral formulas. Physical incompatibilities include changes

TABLE 18.1. Food Supplements and Drug Interactions

Supplement	Drug	Effect
Vitamins		
Vitamin A	Aluminum hydroxide	Drug-induced precipitated bile acids may decrease vitamin absorption.
	Cholestyramine	Concurrent use may impair vitamin absorption.
	Mineral oil	Concurrent use may interfere with vitamin absorption.
	Warfarin	Megadoses may induce anticoagulant activity.
Vitamin D	Digoxin	Vitamin D–induced hypercalcemia may sensitize the client to toxic effects of the drug.
	Mineral oil, aluminum hydroxide, cholestyramine	Concurrent use may decrease vitamin absorption.
Vitamin E	Warfarin	Megadoses may enhance anticoagulant activity.
	Mineral oil, aluminum hydroxide, cholestyramine	Concurrent use may decrease vitamin absorption.
Vitamin K	Warfarin	Concurrent use inhibits hypoprothrombic effect of drug.
	Mineral oil, aluminum hydroxide, cholestyramine	Concurrent use may decrease vitamin absorption.
Ascorbic acid	Estrogen	Megadoses may increase (serum) drug serum levels.
	Haloperidol	Concurrent use may enhance antipsychotic effect of drug.
	Warfarin	Megadoses may decrease prothrombin time.
B-12 (cobalamin)	Cimetidine, Neomycin	Concurrent use may reduce absorption of vitamin.
Folacin	Phenytoin	Vitamin replacement in folate-deficient clients may increase drug metabolism.
Thiamin	Aluminum hydroxide	Inactivated by drug
Pyridoxine	Levodopa	Concurrent use reverses anti-Parkinsonian effect.
	Phenytoin	Large doses may reduce anticonvulsant activity.
	Hydralazine, isoniazid, penicillamine	Concurrent use may reverse drug-induced peripheral neuropathy.
Minerals		
Calcium	Digitalis	Concurrent use with vitamin D may result in hypercalcemia and may enhance toxic effects of drug.
	Hydrochlorothiazide	Concurrent use with vitamin D may result in hypercalcemia.
	Laxatives (abuse)	Reduced absorption
	Phenytoin	Concurrent use may decrease both drug and calcium.
	Verapamil	Concurrent use with vitamin D may counter the antidysrhythmic effect of drug.

continued

Minerals *(continued)*

Copper	Penicillamine	May induce mineral depletion
Iron	Penicillamine	Concurrent use may decrease drug effectiveness.
	Non-narcotic analgesic (aspirin, indomethacin)	May aggravate or contribute to iron deficiency anemia. (405 g daily in long-term use causes 308 mL fecal blood loss.)
	Calcium carbonate	Concurrent use may impair iron absorption.
Magnesium	Ethanol	Reduces absorption
Phosphorus	Antacids	Reduces absorption
Potassium	Furosemide, hydrochlorothiazide, spironolactone	Monitor for abnormal levels.
	Ethanol	Reduces absorption
Zinc	Penicillamine	Reduces absorption
	Ethanol	Reduces absorption

Other supplements

Protein or amino acids	Levodopa, methyldopa	Concurrent use may potentially inhibit drug absorption/action.
	Theophylline	Concurrent use may potentially decrease plasma half-life of drug.
Tryptophan	Fluoxetine	Concurrent use may intensify agitation, restlessness, and GI problems.
	Monoamine oxidase inhibitors (MAOI)	Concurrent use may result in confusion, a deterioration in mental status, headaches, agitation, and other adverse effects.
	Tricyclic antidepressants	Variable results are observed when used to augment antidepressant effects.

Source: Adapted with permission from Morley JE, Glick Z, Rubenstein L, eds. *Geriatric Nutrition: A Comprehensive Review.* 2nd ed. New York: Raven Press Ltd; 1995.

in formula texture (granulation or gel formation), flow rate, viscosity, separation, precipitation, or breaking of an emulsion. In general, avoiding acidic medication syrups reduces the risk for physical incompatibilities (9). Formulas with intact protein are also more likely to break the emulsion than are peptide or free amino-acid–based enteral products (9).

Pharmaceutical Incompatibilities

Pharmaceutical incompatibility occurs when the form of a medication is changed on administration, resulting in alteration in the potency, efficiency, or tolerance of the medication or enteral formula. The classic example of pharmaceutical incompatibility is the crushing of enteric-coated tablets or the opening of slow-release capsules in an effort to administer the medication through the tube. A list of medications that should not be crushed is published regularly in the journal *Hospital Pharmacy* (10). The following summarizes medications that should not be crushed:

- *Enteric-coated medications.* These products are designed to pass through the stomach intact, with the drug being released in the intestines, in order to (*a*) prevent destruction of the drug by stomach acids, (*b*) prevent stomach irritation, and (*c*) delay onset of action.

- *Extended-release medications.* These products are designed to release the drug over an extended period of time. Such products include (*a*) multiple-layered tablets that release the drug as each level is dissolved, (*b*) mixed-release pellets that dissolve at different time intervals, and (*c*) special (inert) matrixes that contain and slowly release the active drug.

- *Sublingual medications.* These are designed to dissolve quickly in oral fluids for rapid absorption by the abundant blood supply of the mouth.

- *Miscellaneous.* These drugs irritate the oral mucosa, are extremely bitter, or contain dyes or substances that could stain teeth and mucosal tissue.

Pharmacologic Incompatibilities

Pharmacologic incompatibility is the most common drug-nutrient interaction. Pharmacologic incompatibilities include enteral feeding intolerance caused by the drug's mechanism of action, antagonistic activity between a drug and a nutrient, and biochemical alterations associated with drug use.

Enteral feeding intolerance may be manifested by nausea, vomiting, GI distention, or diarrhea. The dietetics professional should review all medications for these potential GI side effects. This is especially significant when the formula is suspect for causing the intolerance.

A common antagonistic relationship between a drug and a nutrient is the incompatibility between vitamin K and warfarin. Serum vitamin K levels should not be excessive and need to remain constant in order for the anticoagulation therapy to be stable. Excessive vitamin K decreases the drug's effect, whereas low vitamin K levels increase the drug efficacy and thus decrease blood-clotting times (11).

The dietetics professional should review the vitamin K content of the enteral formula for those individuals on anticoagulation therapy. It is best to avoid formulas containing more than 75 to 80 mg of vitamin K per 1,000 kcal (9). In addition, when enteral formulas are initiated, changes in vitamin K levels as the enteral formula is being progressed toward the goal rate should be considered, and prothrombin time should be monitored (9,11).

The final example of pharmacologic incompatibility is the altered biochemical levels associated with medication prescribed for enterally fed clients. Table 18.2 lists some of the more frequently seen biochemical alterations and the medications associated with these abnormalities (12). Those alterations classified as pharmacologic incompatibility are also indicated.

Physiologic Incompatibilities

Physiologic incompatibility involves the nonpharmacologic actions of medication that result in enteral feeding intolerance. Diarrhea related to increased osmolality is the most common physiologic incompatibility (9,11,13-16). Changing from medications with high osmolalities to medications with lower osmolalities or simply diluting the medication with water before administration through the feeding tube are methods to use to avoid physiologic incompatibilities (9,11).

Another form of physiologic incompatibility is intolerance caused by additives used in the production of medications. These additives, such as sorbitol, mannitol, lactose, saccharin, sucrose, flavorings, and dyes, may not be included in product information. Dietetics professionals should be aware of the additive content of medications, to avoid adverse reactions such as diarrhea, hives, itching, asthma, belching, nausea, or even anaphylactic shock in susceptible individuals (17,18).

Pharmacokinetic Incompatibilities

Pharmacokinetic incompatibility occurs when the enteral formula alters the absorption, distribution, metabolism, or elimination of the drug or, conversely, when the drug alters nutrient kinetics. One of the most extensively studied of the pharmacokinetic incompatibilities associated with enteral feeding is phenytoin. As a result, it has been recommended that enteral feedings occur 1 to 2 hours before and after the phenytoin dose (9,11,19-23). Other approaches include providing the phenytoin intravenously or in capsule form, to enhance absorption and frequent monitoring of the serum levels of phenytoin and to adjust doses to maintain therapeutic levels (9).

TABLE 18.2. Common Biochemical Abnormalities Associated With Medications Prescribed for Enterally Fed Patients

Abnormality	Medications
Serum Glucose	
• Hyperglycemia	• Morphine, phenytoin, thiazides,* corticosteroids,* estrogen,* phenothiazine,* probenecid,* clonidine,* chemotherapeutic agents
• Hypoglycemia	• Acetaminophen,* monoamine oxidase inhibitors,* sulfonamides,* phenylbutazone,* propranolol, barbiturates
Serum potassium	
• Hyperkalemia	• Spironolactone,* penicillin G potassium
• Hypokalemia	• Ampicillin, carbenicillin, piperacillin, ticarcillin, amphotericin,* thiazides,* furosemide,* diuretics,* laxatives*
Serum sodium	
• Hypernatremia	• Penicillin G sodium, medications with large volume, normal saline
• Hyponatremia	• Laxatives,* diuretics,* probenecid,* amphotericin, potassium-sparing diuretics,* thiazides, furosemide*
Serum magnesium	
• Hypermagnesemia	• Magnesium-containing antacids in patients with renal dysfunction
• Hypomagnesemia	• Amphotericin, cyclosporine, thiazides,* furosemide,* cisplatin, ciprofloxacin, probenecid, carbenicillin, pentamidine
Serum phosphorus	
• Hyperphosphatemia	• Chemotherapeutic agent-induced cell lysis,* excess glucose administration with medications
• Hypophosphatemia	• Sucralfate, corticosteroids, furosemide,* thiazide*
• Calcium losses	• Furosemide,* triamterene,* probenecid, corticosteroids, indomethacin
Serum lipids	
• Hypertriglyceridemia	• Cyclosporine,* corticosteroids, thiouracil, chlorpromazine

*Classified as pharmacologic incompatibility.

Source: Reprinted from Rombeau JL, Roandelli RH, eds. *Clinical Nutrition: Enteral and Tube Feeding.* 3rd ed. Philadelphia, Pa: WB Saunders Co; 1997, with permission from Elsevier.

ALCOHOL

Many older adults consume alcohol on a regular basis and may not consider the effect that alcohol can have on nutritional status and on medications. Older adults have a lower tolerance for alcohol, because aging is associated with lower total body water and, therefore, blood alcohol becomes more concentrated in the older adult (24).

The physical effects of alcohol may affect several nutrients. One consequence of long-term alcohol abuse, Wernicke-Korsakoff syndrome, is associated with thiamin deficiency (24). Absorption or utilization of vitamins B-6, B-12, and C is affected by regular alcohol intake (24). In addition, increased iron absorption and decreased zinc absorption may occur (24).

Box 18.1   Pressor Amines Guidelines

Drug-Nurtrient Interaction Issues

Altered pressor amine levels may occur with

- Classic nonselective MAOIs prescribed for depression
- Amphetamines
- Decongestants
- Cold medications
- Caffeine
- Phenelzine
- Procarbazine
- Selegiline

Non-Drug-Nutrient Interaction Causes of Elevated Pressor Amines

- Cardiovascular disease
- Chronic alcoholism/liver disease

Clinical Signs/Symptoms of Excess Pressor Amines

- High blood pressure (hypertension)
- Neck stiffness or soreness

- Nausea/vomiting
- Severe headaches
- Flushing/sweating (sometimes with fever)
- Increased or decreased heart rate (tachycardia or bradycardia)
- Light sensitivity
- Severe hypertensive crisis (sudden severe increase in blood pressure to a level > 200/120)
- Intracranial hemorrhage (possibly fatal in severe hypertensive crisis)

Interventions

- Avoid foods high in tyramine and other pressor amines.
- Monitor blood pressure frequently.
- Monitor individual for signs of pressor response (ie, report of frequent headaches, palpitation).
- Physician will discount MAOI as appropriate.

Source: Adapted with permission from *Clinical and Nutrient Guidelines: Part of the Drug-Nutrient Intervention System.* © 2001, Roche Dietitians LLC. 708/442-0123.

Because alcohol is distributed throughout the body and is able to cross all membrane barriers, its likelihood to interact with a drug's mechanism of action is great. For all medications, dietetics professionals should review warnings to restrict or avoid alcohol, and they should always be aware of the alcohol content of drugs.

PRESSOR AMINES

Amines are nitrogen-containing organic compounds that are naturally present in foods. Some amines are biologically active. Monoamines are called pressor amines, or vasoactive amines, because of their action of constricting blood vessels. Examples of pressor amines include tyramine, histamine, dopamine, serotonin, and norepinephrine. Biologically active amines do not normally pose a health hazard, because they are broken down by oxidases. Certain drugs, however, inhibit the work of the oxidases in the body. These

drugs are called oxidase inhibitors. Monoamine oxidase inhibitors (MAOIs) are a group of drugs that interfere with the work of monoamine oxidase (MAO). MAO is found in the liver, the GI tract, and adrenergic nerve endings. It metabolizes (oxidizes) tyramine, histamine, and other pressor amines before they reach the systemic circulation. MAOIs block MAO activity, causing an increase in the concentration of unoxidized pressor amines, such as tyramine, in the body. The presence of unoxidized pressor amines causes constriction of the blood vessels, which results in abnormal elevation of blood pressure, headaches, mood elevations, and possible death. When a drug with known MAOI activity is taken, foods high in pressor amines, such as tyramine, need to be avoided (25) (see Boxes 18.1 and 18.2).

CAFFEINE

Caffeine stimulates the central nervous system and may cause nervousness, irritability, and insomnia. Most individuals are aware of the amount of caffeine they can tolerate before experiencing jitters, insom-

Box 18.2   Patient Education Guide for Pressor Amines

- MAO inhibitors (MAOIs) block MAO activity, causing an increase in the concentration of unoxidized pressor amines (monoamines), such as tyramine, in the body. The presence of unoxidized pressor amines constricts the blood vessels, which results in abnormal elevation of blood pressure, headaches, mood elevations, and possibly death.

- When a drug with known MAOI activity is taken, foods high in pressor amines, such as tyramine, need to be avoided.

- Generally, high-protein foods that have been aged (ie, dried, fermented, pickled, and/or smoked) should be eliminated from the diet.

- When purchasing foods, be sure to select only fresh foods. Prolonged storage and food spoilage will increase the tyramine content of foods. Therefore, freeze or discard any high-protein foods that have not been cooked or eaten within 24 hours of purchase or refrigeration.

- Talk to your physician. Make sure he or she is aware of *all* medications you are taking. Report any medication side effects, unusual symptoms, or feelings immediately.

Foods to Avoid Because High in Tyramine and Other Pressor Amines

Dry fermented sausages
- Summer sausage
- Pepperoni

- Salami
- Pastrami
- Mortadella

Smoked or pickled fish
- Herring
- Lox
- Caviar

Salted dry cod
Aged game or meats
Nonfresh meat or poultry
Any leftover foods containing meat, fish, or poultry
Protein dietary supplements
Aged processed cheeses
Blue cheese
Anchovies
Tuna
Chinese pea pods/ snow peas

Fava (Italian broad) beans
Sauerkraut/kim chee
Fermented soybean products
Overripe fruits/ banana peel
Meat extracts (broths, bouillons, gravies)
Yeast extracts
Herbal teas
Malt beverages (including beer, ale)
Chianti
Burgundy, red, and white wines
Port
Sherry
Vermouth

In addition, do not consume more than 1 small serving (1/4 cup or 2 oz) per day of any of the following: avocado, peanuts, raspberries, soy sauce, chocolate, yogurt, cream, or any unpasteurized dairy products.

Limit caffeine to less than 500 mg per day. Caffeine acts as a weak pressor agent.

Avoid alcohol entirely. The consumption of alcohol, especially the beverages listed, significantly increases risk of a hypertensive crisis.

Adapted with permission from *Clinical Indications of Drug-Nutrient Interactions and Herbal Use: A Guideline for Practitioners.* © 2001, Roche Dietitians, LLC. 708/442-0123.

---

nia, or heart palpitations. However, medications may interact with caffeine to enhance its effects. Some medications slow the elimination of caffeine; others, like bronchodilators, whose mechanism of action (dilating airways) is similar to caffeine, increase elimination. Caffeine intake, along with bronchodilators, could have a multiplying effect on the drug, similar to an overdose. When limiting caffeine in the diet, it is important to consider over-the-counter (OTC) medication that may be high in caffeine, such as appetite suppressants, caffeine pills, analgesics, and allergy/cold relief tablets (4). Box 18.3 outlines the

drug-nutrient interaction issues associated with caffeine, as well as signs and symptoms of clinical excesses and withdrawal (25).

GRAPEFRUIT JUICE

Grapefruit juice contains the flavonoids naringenin, quercetin, and kaempferol. Naringenin appears to interfere with liver enzymes that facilitate the metabolism of certain drugs, including calcium-channel blockers. For example, felodipine (Plendil) was investigated by assessing the drug levels after administration with water, orange juice, and grapefruit juice. Although neither water nor orange juice had a measurable effect on blood levels of felodipine, grapefruit juice tripled the serum levels of the

Box 18.3 Caffeine: Clinical Guidelines

Drug-Nutrient Interaction Issues

Caffeine may enhance the adverse effects of the following drugs:

- Cardiac regulators: calcium-channel blockers, antihypertensives, H_2 antagonists
- Anti-psychotics/antidepressants/antianxiety medications
- Anti-ulcer agents
- Diuretics
- Insulin/oral hypoglycemics
- Bronchodilators
- Stimulants/sedatives
- Anticonvulsants
- NSAIDs
- Pain relievers
- Decongestants
- Potassium supplements

Clinical Excess Signs/Symptoms

- Increased heartbeat
- Irritability

- Nervousness
- Insomnia
- Increased urination
- Hyperglycemia in individuals with diabetes
- Decreased calcium absorption
- Decreased iron absorption
- Increased gastric acid secretion/gastrointestinal irritation
- Increased free fatty acid concentrations
- Pressor activity

Clinical Withdrawal Signs/Symptoms

- Nausea
- Vomiting
- Headache
- Irritability

Source: Adapted with permission from *Clinical and Nutrient Guidelines: Part of the Drug-Nutrient Intervention System.* © 2001, Roche Dietitians, LLC. 708/442-0123

drug. This increase in felodipine is associated with headaches, flushing, and light-headedness (26). Other drugs associated with increased bioavailability when taken with grapefruit juice include calan (Verapamil), nifedipine (Procardia), terfenadine (Seldane), and cyclosporine (Sandimmune) (27).

ALTERNATIVE THERAPIES

Herbal and nutritional supplement use among older adults is increasing. In a recent study, 8% of older adults used herbal therapies and 5% used megavitamins. Six percent of older adults surveyed were taking both herbs and prescription drugs (28). The majority of older patients who use alternative medicine make no mention of it to their physician (28,29).

The use of herbal remedies, food supplements, and nonprescription hormones should be taken very seriously. Concurrent use of herb and dietary supplements may mimic, magnify, or oppose the effects of a drug or the side effects of the drug (30), and

OTC herbal remedies, food supplements, and nonprescription hormones add to an already dangerous situation. It is prudent to proceed with caution and be very certain of the validity of the information about alternative therapies. A number of these therapies may not be successful and, in fact, may be questionable. The lack of supportive research data to validate claims is a concern, but research is now becoming available on herbal remedies and medication interactions.

REGULATORY COMPLIANCE

Federal Guidelines

Federal Omnibus Budget Reconciliation Act (OBRA) guidelines specify 10 types of drugs that contribute to nutritional deficiencies (31).

- Antacids
- Anti-inflammatory
- Anticonvulsants
- Antineoplastic drugs
- Cardiac regulators (antiarrhythmics)

- Diuretics

- Laxatives (chartics)

- Oral hypoglycemics (antidiabetics)

- Phenothiazines

- Psychotropic drugs (psychotherapeutic agents)

Joint Commission on the Accreditation of Healthcare Organizations

The Joint Commission on the Accreditation of Healthcare Organizations (JCAHO) requires that all clients receive education on drug-nutrient interactions and that this education be documented in the client's medical record. This is true across the continuum of care, including home care, long-term care, subacute care, and acute care (32).

Dietetics professionals should be part of the interdisciplinary team that determines which medications will be addressed in client education. Furthermore, dietetics professionals should be instrumental in developing or selecting the materials that are used for education. However, dietetics professionals do not need to complete the client instruction on drug-nutrient interactions. It is often more efficient for nursing or pharmacy personnel to complete client education at discharge, because these departments often provide discharge counseling on other issues. This type of team effort meets the interdisciplinary vision of JCAHO standards and improves the quality of client care.

REFERENCES

1. Gurley BJ, Hagan DW. Herbal and dietary supplement interactions with drugs. In: McCabe BJ, Wolfe JJ, Frankel EH, eds. *Handbook of Food-Drug Interactions.* Boca Raton, Fla: CRC Press; 2003.

2. Blumberg J, Coris R. Pharmacology, nutrition and the elderly: interactions and implications. In: Chernoff R, ed. *Geriatric Nutrition. A Handbook for Health Professionals.* 2nd ed. Gaithersburg, Md: Aspen Publishers; 1999:342-365.

3. Stewart RB, Moore M, May FE, Marks RO, Hale WE. A longitudinal evaluation of drug use in an ambulatory elderly population. *J Clin Epidemiol.* 1991;44:1353-1359.

4. Diehl M, Lago D, Ahern F, Smyer MA, Hermanson S, Rabatin V. Examination of priorities for therapeutic drug utilization review. *J Geriatr Drug Ther.* 1992;6:65-85.

5. Barrocas A, Jastram CW, McCabe BJ. Nutrition and drug regimens in older persons. In: McCabe BJ, Wolfe JJ, Frankel EH, eds. *Handbook of Food-Drug Interactions.* Boca Raton, Fla: CRC Press; 2003.

6. Campbell WW, Crim MC, Dallal GE, Young VR, Evans WJ. Increased protein requirements in elderly people: new data and retrospective reassessments. *Am J Clin Nutr.* 1994;60:501-509.

7. Saltzman E, Mason J. Enteral nutrition in the elderly. In: Rombeau JL, Rolandelli RH, eds. *Clinical Nutrition: Enteral and Tube Feeding.* 3rd ed. Philadelphia, Pa: WB Saunders Co; 1997:385-402.

8. US Dept of Health and Human Services. *Tracking Healthy People 2010.* Washington, DC: U.S. Government Printing Office, November 2000. Available at: http://www.healthypeople.gov/Publications. Accessed May 3, 2004.

9. Thomson CA, Rollins CJ. Nutrient-drug interactions. In: Rombeau JL, Rolandelli RH, eds. *Clinical Nutrition: Enteral and Tube Feeding.* 3rd ed. Philadelphia, Pa: WB Saunders Co; 1997.

10. Mitchell JF. Oral dosage forms that should not be crushed: 2000 Update. *Hosp Pharm.* 2000;35:553-567.

11. Strausburg KM. Drug interaction in nutrition support. In: McCabe BJ, Wolfe JJ, Frankel EH, eds. *Handbook of Food-Drug Interactions.* Boca Raton, Fla: CRC Press; 2003.

12. Rombeau JL, Roandelli RH, eds. *Clinical Nutrition: Enteral and Tube Feeding.* 3rd ed. Philadelphia, Pa: WB Saunders Co; 1997.

13. Bowling TE, Silk DB. Diarrhea and enteral nutrition. Rombeau JL, Roandelli RH. *Clinical Nutrition: Enteral and Tube Feeding.* 3rd ed. Philadelphia, Pa: WB Saunders Co; 1997.

14. Guenter PA, Settle RG, Perlmutter S, Marino PL, DeSimone GA, Rolandelli RH. Tube feeding related diarrhea in acutely ill patients. *JPEN J Parenter Enteral Nutr.* 1991;15:277-280.

15. Fuhrman PM. Diarrhea and tube feeding. *Nutr Clin Pract.* 1999;14:83-84.

16. Williams MS, Harper RA, Magnuson BL, Loan TD, Kearney PA. Diarrhea management in enterally fed patients. *Nutr Clin Pract.* 1998;13:225-229.

17. Miller SJ, Oliver AD. Sorbitol content of selected sugar-free liquid medications. *Hosp Pharm.* 1993;28:741-744.

18. Lutomski DM, Gora ML, Wright SM, Martin JE. Sorbitol content of selected oral liquids. *Ann Pharmacother.* 1993;27:269-274.

19. Bauer LA. Interference of oral phenytoin absorption by continuous nasogastric feedings. *Neurology.* 1982;32:570-572.

20. Au Yeung SC, Ensom MH. Phenytoin and enteral feedings: does evidence support an interaction? *Ann Pharmacother.* 2000;34:896-905.

21. Fleisher D, Sheth N, Kou JH. Phenytoin interaction with enteral feedings administered through nasogastric tubes. *JPEN J Parenter Enteral Nutr.* 1990;14:513-516.

22. Rodman DP, Stevenson TL, Ray TR. Phenytoin malabsorption after jejunostomy tube delivery. *Pharmacotherapy.* 1995;15:801-805.

23. Doak KK, Haas CE, Dunnigan KJ, Reiss RA, Reiser JR, Huntress J, Altavela JL. Bioavailability of phenytoin acid and phenytoin sodium with enteral feedings. *Pharmacotheraphy.* 1998;18:637-645.

24. Light KB, Hakkak R. Alcohol and nutrition. In: McCabe BJ, Wolfe JJ, Frankel EH, eds. *Handbook of Food-Drug Interactions.* Boca Raton, Fla: CRC Press; 2003:168-189.

25. Roche-Dudek M, Roche-Klemma K. *Clinical and Nutrient Guidelines: Part of the Drug Nutrient Intervention System.* Riverside, Ill: Roche Dietitians, LLC; 2001.

26. Yamreudeewong W, Henann NE, Fazio A, Lower DL, Cassidy TG. Drug-food interactions in clinical practice. *J Fam Pract.* 1995;40:376-384.

27. *Drug Facts and Comparison.* St Louis, Mo: Facts and Comparison; 2001.

28. Foster DF, Phillips RS, Hamel MB, Eisenberg DM. Alternative medicine use in older Americans. *J Am Geriatr Soc.* 2000;48:1560-1565.

29. Stupay S, Sivertsen L. Herbal and nutritional supplement use in the elderly. *Nurs Pract.* 2000;25:56-58, 61-62, 64 passim.

30. Fugh-Berman A. Herb-drug interactions [erratum in *Lancet* 2000;355:1020]. *Lancet.* 2000;355:134-138.

31. Centers for Medicare & Medicaid Services. State Operations Manual. 2003. Available at: http://www.cms.hhs.gov/manuals/pub07pdf/AP-P-PP.pdf. Accessed May 3, 2004.

32. Joint Commission on Accreditation of Healthcare Organizations. *1996 Comprehensive Accreditation Manual for Hospitals.* Oak Brook Terrace, Ill: Joint Commission on Accreditation of Healthcare Organizations; 1995.

CHAPTER 19

Complementary and Alternative Medicine

Complementary and alternative medicine (CAM) encompasses the diverse approaches to health care that are outside the realm of conventional medicine as practiced in the United States. Although there is new interest in CAM among conventional Western practitioners, most CAM therapies and practices have not been studied through traditional scientific research. This lack of empirical research data on the safety and efficacy of CAM has slowed down its integration into general American medical practices and has limited its reimbursement by insurance companies.

The term "complementary medicine" refers to practices that are used in conjunction with conventional medicine. An example of complementary therapy is the use of acupuncture to relieve postsurgical discomfort. The same practice, acupuncture, can be used as an "alternative medicine" therapy when it is used in place of conventional medicine—for example, when acupuncture is used instead of prescription medication to treat hypertension.

The blending of traditional medicine and CAM is "integrative medicine." In integrative medicine, mainstream medical practitioners combine conventional treatments with CAM therapies for which there is some high-quality scientific evidence of safety and efficacy.

CAM THERAPY CATEGORIES

The National Center for Complementary and Alternative Medicine (NCCAM), a component of the National Institutes of Health (NIH), is the federal government's lead agency for scientific research on CAM. The NCCAM classifies CAM therapies into five categories, or domains, as follows (1):

1. *Alternative medical systems.* Alternative medical systems are built on complete systems of theory and practice. Often, these systems have evolved apart from and earlier than the conventional medical approach used in the United States. Examples of alternative medical systems that have developed in the Western cultures include homeopathic medicine and naturopathic medicine. Examples of systems that have developed in non-Western cultures include traditional Chinese medicine and Ayurveda.

2. *Mind-body interventions.* Mind-body medicine uses a variety of techniques designed to enhance the mind's capacity to affect bodily function and symptoms. Some techniques that were considered CAM in the past have become mainstream (for example, patient support groups and cognitive-behavioral therapy). Other mind-body techniques are still considered CAM, including meditation, prayer, mental healing, and therapies that use creative outlets, such as art, music, or dance.

3. *Biologically based therapies.* Biologically based therapies in CAM use substances found in nature, such as herbs, foods, and vitamins. Some examples include dietary supplements, herbal products, and the use of other so-called "natural" but as yet scientifically unproven therapies (for example, using shark cartilage to treat cancer).

4. *Manipulative and body-based methods.* Manipulative and body-based methods in CAM are based on manipulation and/or movement of

one or more parts of the body. Some examples include chiropractic or osteopathic manipulation and massage.

5. *Energy therapies.* Energy therapies involve the use of energy fields. They are of two types:

- Biofield therapies are intended to affect energy fields that purportedly surround and penetrate the human body. The existence of such fields has not yet been scientifically proven. Some forms of energy therapy manipulate biofields by applying pressure and/or manipulating the body by placing the hands in or through these fields. Examples include qi gong, Reiki, and Therapeutic Touch.

- Bioelectromagnetic-based therapies involve the unconventional use of electromagnetic fields, such as pulsed fields, magnetic fields, or alternating-current or direct-current fields.

COMMON TERMS AND DEFINITIONS

The NCCAM provides definitions of many commonly used terms in CAM (1), such as the following:

- *Aromatherapy* involves the use of essential oils (extracts or essences) from flowers, herbs, and trees, to promote health and well-being.

- *Ayurveda* ("ah-yur-VAY-dah") is a CAM alternative medical system that has been practiced primarily in the Indian subcontinent for 5,000 years. Ayurveda includes diet and herbal remedies and emphasizes the use of body, mind, and spirit in disease prevention and treatment.

- *Chiropractic* is a CAM alternative medical system that focuses on the relationship between bodily structure (primarily that of the spine) and function, and how that relationship affects the preservation and restoration of health. Chiropractors use manipulative therapy as an integral treatment tool.

- *Electromagnetic fields* (EMFs; also called electric and magnetic fields) are invisible lines of force that surround all electrical devices. The earth also produces EMFs: electric fields are produced when there is thunderstorm activity, and magnetic fields are believed to be produced by electric currents flowing from the earth's core.

- *Homeopathic* medicine is a CAM alternative medical system based on the belief that "like cures like," meaning that small, highly diluted quantities of medicinal substances are given to cure symptoms, whereas the same substances given at higher or more concentrated doses would actually cause those symptoms.

- *Massage* therapists manipulate muscle and connective tissue, to enhance function of those tissues and to promote relaxation and well-being.

- *Naturopathic* medicine is a CAM alternative medical system in which practitioners work with natural healing forces within the body, with a goal of helping the body heal from disease and attain better health. Practices may include dietary modifications, massage, exercise, acupuncture, minor surgery, and various other interventions.

- *Osteopathic* medicine is a form of conventional medicine that, in part, emphasizes diseases arising in the musculoskeletal system. There is an underlying belief that all of the body's systems work together, and disturbances in one system may affect function elsewhere in the body. Some osteopathic physicians practice osteopathic manipulation, a full-body system of hands-on techniques to alleviate pain, restore function, and promote health and well-being.

- *Qi gong* ("chee-GUNG") is a component of traditional Chinese medicine that combines movement, meditation, and regulation of breathing to enhance the flow of qi in the body (qi is an ancient term given to what is believed to be vital energy), to improve blood circulation, and to enhance immune function.

- *Reiki* ("RAY-kee") is a Japanese word representing "universal life energy." Reiki is based on the belief that when spiritual energy is channeled through a Reiki practitioner, the patient's spirit is healed, which in turn heals the physical body.

- *Therapeutic touch* is derived from an ancient technique called laying-on of hands. It is based on the premise that it is the healing force of the therapist that affects the patient's recovery. Healing is promoted when the body's energies are in balance; by passing their hands over the patient, healers can identify energy imbalances.

NUTRITION AND CAM

Nutrition plays a significant role in CAM as both a complementary and an alternative therapy. In many CAM practices, food acts as a foundation of medicine. Food as well as herbal preparations are recognized as a healing force (2,3). A balanced lifestyle, exercise, rest, sleep, and emotional tranquility are considered prerequisites for a state of health. Unprocessed, whole foods without toxins, pesticides, or additives are emphasized. Selecting foods low on the food chain is recommended. Wellness is encouraged beyond just a neutral stage where disease is absent (3,4).

DIETARY SUPPLEMENTS AND CAM

NCCAM defines dietary supplements as follows (1):

> Congress defined the term "dietary supplement" in the Dietary Supplement Health and Education Act (DSHEA) of 1994. A dietary supplement is a product (other than tobacco) taken by mouth that contains a "dietary ingredient" intended to supplement the diet. Dietary ingredients may include vitamins, minerals, herbs or other botanicals, amino acids, and substances such as enzymes, organ tissues, and metabolites. Dietary supplements come in many forms, including extracts, concentrates, tablets, capsules, gel caps, liquids, and powders. They have special requirements for labeling. Under DSHEA, dietary supplements are considered foods, not drugs.

Because government regulation of dietary supplements is not as stringent as regulation of drugs, dietetics professionals should take special care to follow the latest scientific findings regarding safety and efficacy of these products and clients should be educated regarding potential benefits, adverse effects, and interactions with medications. Table 19.1 provides an overview of supplements clients may use or be interested in using.

DIETETICS PROFESSIONALS AND CAM

The scope of CAM is vast. The use of these therapies by the general population is growing exponentially. Dietetics professionals need ongoing education in complementary and alternative nutrition interventions (5).

There are many good sources of information on alternative medicine and alternative nutrition. The best source of information is the ADA dietetic practice group Nutrition in Complementary Care (3). Box 19.1 lists additional resources (2).

REFERENCES

1. National Center for Complementary and Alternative Medicine Web site. National Institutes of Health. Available at: http://www.nccam.nih.gov. Accessed April 26, 2004.
2. Burke PK, Roche-Dudek M, Roche-Klemma K. *Clinical Indications of Drug-Nutrient Interactions and Herbal Use: A Guideline for Practitioners*. 2nd ed. Riverside, Ill: Roche Dietitians; 2001.
3. Pitchford P. *Healing With Whole Foods, Oriental Traditions, and Modern Nutrition*. Berkeley, Calif: North Atlantic Books; 1993.
4. Goldberg B. *Alternative Medicine: The Definitive Guide*. Tiburon, Calif: Future Medicine Publishing; 1997.
5. Nutrition in Complementary Care: A Dietetic Practice Group of the American Dietetic Association Web site. Available at: http://www.ComplementaryNutrition.org. Accessed March 11, 2004.

TABLE 19.1. Common Herbal/Supplement Therapies

Supplement	Health Claim/Action	Dosage	Notes/Safety/Side Effects
Alfalfa *Medicago sativa* *Type:* Herb, food (sprouts) *Active ingredients:* 2%–3% saponins (leaves); also flavones, isoflavones, sterols, coumarin derivatives	• Blocks absorption of cholesterol and prevents atherosclerotic plaque. • Appetite stimulant. • Estrogenic effect. • Anticoagulant effect. Used to treat high cholesterol, atherosclerosis, anorexia, menopausal symptoms.	Available as bulk herb, tablets, capsules, liquid extract. 500–1000 mg dried leaf/d. OR 1–2 mL/tincture 3 times/d.	• Contains protein, vitamins A, B-1, B-6, C, E, K; calcium, potassium, iron, zinc. • Moderate use is considered safe. • Ingestion of large amounts of saponins may cause red blood cell damage. • Ingestion of large amounts of seeds or sprouts has been linked to onset of SLE secondary to presence of canavanine. Should not be used by individuals with SLE or history of SLE. • Do not use with corticosteroids, cyclosporine, NSAID, anticoagulant drugs. • Avoid > 400 IU vitamin E/d.
Aloe *Aloe ferox* *Aloe barbadensis* *Aloe vera* *Type:* Herb, topical gel *Active ingredients:* Anthraquinone glycosides (aloe latex) polysaccharides (gel)	• Latex used for acute constipation or as a cathartic laxative. • Topical gel used for anti-inflammatory effects and promotion of wound healing (ie, minor burns). • Antibacterial effect.	Available as capsules, juice, gel. Latex as laxative: 50–200 mg capsule/d. Internal juice ingestion: 30 mL 3 times/d. Gel as topical: Apply to affected area 3–5 times/d.	• Safe and effective laxative for acute constipation per Food and Drug Administration. • May cause GI distress, diarrhea. • For short-term use only; do not use for chronic constipation; do not use over long term (> 7 d). • Long-term use may cause electrolyte imbalance (especially decreased potassium), renal damage. • Should not be used by individuals with GI disorders. • May alter drug absorption; do not use with medications. • All of the above do not apply to topical usage. • Lethal dose is 1 g/d × several days. • Injection of aloe vera products or chemical components for cancer is not recommended and has been associated with fatalities.

Angelica Chinese angelica, Dong quai *Angelica sinensis* *Type:* Herb *Active ingredients:* Specific chemical not identified, possible coumarin derivatives	• Anticoagulant effect. Used for gynecological disorders, menstrual disorders, menopausal symptoms, anemia, headache, backache, osteoporosis, asthma, hay fever, poor peripheral circulation	Available as fluid extract, tincture, essential oil, root (cut, dried, or powdered). No consensus on dosing; 3-4 g/d has been reported as a standard dose.	• Adverse effects include photosensitivity, photodermatitis, hypotension. • Do not use with anticoagulant drugs. • Avoid > 400 IU vitamin E/d.
Bilberry *Vaccinum myrtillus* *Type:* Herb *Active ingredients:* Anthocyanosides (bioflavonoid)	• Antioxidant. • Supports normal connective tissue formation. • Strengthens capillaries and systemic blood flow. Used to treat night blindness, retinopathy, cataracts, macular degeneration, diabetes mellitus, atherosclerosis, bruising, varicose veins.	Available in tablets, capsules, liquid, tincture, fluid extract, root (dried), leaves, berries. Standardized products containing 25% anthocyanide content are recommended. For night vision: 60-120 mg/d (orally). For other visual, circulatory disorders: 240-480 mg/d in 2-3 divided doses.	• Use with caution if taking anticoagulant drugs. • Long-term use at high dosage can be poisonous. • **>1.5g/kg/d may be fatal.** • Avoid > 400 IU vitamin E/d.
Black cohosh *Cimicifuga racemosa* *Type:* Herb *Active ingredients:* Triterpene glycosides (eg, acetin, cimicifugoside), isoflavones (eg, formonoetin)	• Reduces hot flashes associated with decreased estrogen (menopause) via action of formonoetin, as isoflavones, binding to estrogen receptor sites. • Benefits also due to reducing luteinizing hormone secretion as a result.	Available as crude, dried root or rhizome, dry powdered extract, tincture. Standardized extracts containing 1 mg deoxycytidinu/tablet are available. 300-2000 mg/d root/rhizome. Powdered extract: 250 mg 3 times/d. Standardized extract: 40 mg 2 times/d.	• Contains aromatic acids, tannins, resins, fatty acids, starches, sugars. • Consult with doctor if currently on estrogen replacement therapy. • Not for long-term use (> 6 mo). • May cause GI distress at high doses. • Potential herb-drug interaction with medicinal iron; possible decreased iron absorption due to formation of tannin-iron complex.

continued

TABLE 19.1. Common Herbal/Supplement Therapies (continued)

Supplement	Health Claim/Action	Dosage	Notes/Safety/Side Effects
Capsicum Cayenne, capsaicin *Capsicum annuum* *Type:* Herb, food	• Temporarily relieves pain (associated with neuralgia, arthritis, diabetes mellitus, neuropathy, postsurgical recovery, refractory pruritis) and itching by stimulating neurotransmitter release to depletion. • Antioxidant. • Decreases platelet aggregation.	Available as cream, gel, lotion. Generally: 0.025%–0.075% applied topically 3-5 times/d	• Adverse effects include burning pain (skin, eyes), tearing of eyes, GI discomfort (ie, as food, especially if seeds are eaten). Avoid direct contact. • Do not use with MAOIs, ACE inhibitors (ie, captopril).
Cat's Claw Samento, una de gato, life-giving vine of Peru *Uncaria tomentosa* *Type:* Herb *Active ingredients:* Oxyindole alkaloids, glycosides	• Stimulates immune system function. • Anti-inflammatory. • Antioxidant. • Antitumor activity (in vitro). • Decreases platelet aggregation. • Decreases SNS activity. • Antiviral activity. Used to treat arthritis, rheumatism, GI disorders.	Available as tablets; capsules; teas; tincture; and cut, dried or powdered bark, roots, leaves. Tea: add 1 g root bark to 250 mL boiling water, steep for 10-15 min., cool and strain. 1 cup 3 times/d. Tincture: 1-2 mL 2 times/d. Standardized extract: 20-60 mg/d or up to 500-1000 mg 3 times/d also reported.	• Adverse effects may include hypotension; do not use with antihypertensive medications. • Do not use with anticoagulation drugs; should not be taken by individuals with coagulation disorders. • Should not be taken by individuals with autoimmune disorders. • Commonly used by patients with cancer or human immunodeficiency virus but there is no evidence of efficacy. • Avoid > 400 IU vitamin E/d.
Chamomile *Matricaria recutita* *Type:* Herb *Active ingredients:* Alpha-bisabolol and its oxides A and B; matricin (usually converted to chamazulene), bioflavonoid, apignen, luteolin, quercetin	• Anti-inflammatory. • Anti-allergenic. • Antidiuretic. • Antibacterial. • Antifungal. • Sedative (mild). • Digestive aid (anti-ulcer). • May lower serum urea levels. • Stimulates liver regeneration. • Anti-tumor activity (in vitro).	Available as tablets, capsules, tincture, teas. Tea: 3-4 cups/d between meals OR Tablets/capsules: 2-3 g/d OR	• Associated with allergic reactions including conjunctivitis, anaphylaxis, contact dermatitis. • Do not take with anticoagulation medications. • Do not take with other medications; may decrease absorption. • Potential herb-drug interaction with medicinal iron; possible decreased iron absorption due to formation of tannin-iron complex.

Name / Type	Uses	Forms / Dosage	Cautions
Chasteberry Chaste tree, agnuscastus, monk's pepper *Vitex agnus-castus* *Type:* Herb *Active ingredients:* Whole fruit extract components (ie, agnuside)	Used for GI distress, insomnia, migraine, menstrual disorders, skin irritation, hemorrhoids, mouthwash. • Nonhormonal regulatory effect on the pituitary gland, which aids to restore a more normal estrogen-progesterone balance (via luteinizing hormone, increases production of progesterone to help regulate menstrual cycle). • Regulates prolactin secretion. Used for premenstrual syndrome, menstrual or hormonal disorders, hot flashes associated with menopause or low estrogen levels, infertility, fibroid cysts in smooth muscle tissue or body cavities, acne in teenagers.	Tincture: 4-6 mL 3 times/d between meals. External use as bath or rinse. Available as tablets, capsules, liquid, extract. For premenstrual syndrome use for 4-6 mo. For amenorrheal infertility use for 12-18 mo. Tablets/capsules: 15 mg 3 times/d. Standardized liquid extract: 40 drops in 1 glass water daily, in morning.	• Emphasis on long-term hormonal balance; effects are not immediate. • Adverse effects include minor GI distress, skin rash. • Avoid > 400 IU vitamin E/d.
Dong quai (see Angelica)			
DHEA *Debydroepiam drosterone* *Type:* Hormone *Active ingredients:* Same	• Anti-aging (improves memory, cardiovascular function). • Increases libido. • Stimulates immune system (ie, lupus, AIDS). • Antitumor. • Aids in weight loss. • Antidepressant.	Available as synthetic hormone supplement as tablets, capsules, liquid, and in sublingual form. 2-50 mg/d.	• Increases risk of prostate, breast, endometrial cancers. • May promote masculinization. • Some product claims of "natural" DHEA precursors (ie, wild yam) are not convertible to DHEA in vivo (are based on in vitro conversion). • **Use is controversial due to potential dangers associated with inappropriate hormonal use.**

continued

TABLE 19.1. Common Herbal/Supplement Therapies (continued)

Supplement	Health Claim/Action	Dosage	Notes/Safety/Side Effects
Echinacea Coneflower, black susan, Indian head *Echinacea purpura, Echinacea angustifolia, Echinacea pallida* *Type:* Herb *Active ingredients:* Unknown but contains polysaccharides, volatile oil, caffeic acid derivatives, isobutylanides, polyenes, polyines	• Stimulates immune system function. • Antibacterial. • Local anesthetic and anti-inflammatory. • Antitumor activity. • Stimulates adrenal cortex activity. • Antiviral. • Promotes wound healing. Used to treat colds, flu, sore throat, mouth ulcers, ear infections, yeast infections, Crohn's disease, burns, external wounds.	Available as extracts, juice, glycerite, lozenges, tinctures, capsules, tablets, tea. Juice: 6–9 mL/d. Capsules, tablets: 900–1000 mg 3 times/d. Tincture: 0.75–1.5 mL 2–5 times/d OR 60 drops 3 times/d. Tea: Add 4 g (2 tsp) coarse powder to 250 mL boiling water. Steep for 10 min.	• Adverse effects include allergic reactions. • Long-term or excessive use associated with immunosuppression. • Do not use for long term (> 8 wk); 10–14 days is adequate. • Do not use for autoimmune illness or progressive disease without medical supervision. • Do not use with corticosteroids, cyclosporine. • Tea is not recommended due to decreased activity (water-insoluble compounds).
Ephedra Ma huang, desert herb *Ephedra sinica, Ephedra intermedia, Ephedra equisetina* *Type:* Herb *Active ingredients:* Alkaloids (ephedrine, pseudoephedrine, norephedrine, norpseudoephedrine). Stem contains 1%–3% total alkaloids, 30%–90% as ephedrine.	• Stimulates central nervous system (SNS: elevated blood pressure and heart rate). • Bronchodilator. • Decongestant. • Appetite suppressant. • Marked peripheral vasoconstriction.	**BANNED BY FOOD AND DRUG ADMINISTRATION.**	• On December 30, 2003, the FDA ruled that "dietary supplements containing ephedrine alkaloids present an unreasonable risk of illness or injury" and banned sale of products containing ephedra.

Evening primrose oil (EPO) King's cure all *Type:* Herb *Active ingredients:* GLA	• GLA converts to PGE-1 with associated anti-inflammatory, anticoagulant, and vasodilatory effects. Used to treat asthma, GI disorders, multiple sclerosis, respiratory disorders, skin disorders, premenstrual syndrome, diabetes mellitus, neuropathy, rheumatoid arthritis, high cholesterol, hypertension. Rationale for supplement: • Western diet deficient. • Conversion of linoleic acid often compromised by disease, aging, saturated/hydrogenated oil intake, glucose intolerance, and/or inadequate intake magnesium, zinc, B vitamins (cofactors in conversion).	Available primarily as supplement in tablets, gel caps. Based on a standardized gamma linolenic acid 8%. 320 mg–8 g/d. Poultices have been used to promote wound healing.	• GLA also found in black currant seed oil and borage oil. • Avoid > 400 IU vitamin E/d. • Possible side effects include headache, thrombosis, epilepsy, nausea, rash, inflammation, immunosuppression with long-term use (> 1 yr). • Should not be used by individuals with schizophrenia, seizure, or history of such conditions. Do not use with phenothiazide, anticonvulsant medications, warfarin.
Fennel Carosella, fenchel, fenouil *Foeniculum vulgare, Focniculum officinalis* *Type:* Herb (as essential oil) or spice (whole seed) *Active ingredients:* In the volatile oil, anethole and other terpenoids	• Stimulant. • Antiflatulent. • Combined with methyl paraben inhibits growth of *Salmonella enteritides* and *Listeria monocytogenes*. Used to increase milk secretion, facilitate birth, promote menses, increase libido due to estrogen-like activity.	Available as volatile oil in water (2%), as sweet fennel (4%), and as bitter fennel, or as flower, whole seed, tea, tincture. Oil: 0.1–0.6 mL/d. Fruit: 5–7 g/d. Seed: Add 1/2 tsp crushed to 250 mL boiling water. Steep 10–15 min, cool and strain. 1 cup 3 times/d. Tincture: 2–4 mL 3 times/d.	• Adverse effects include GI distress (nausea, vomiting), seizures, pulmonary edema, contact dermatitis, photodermatitis, tumors. • Individuals with allergies to celery, carrots, mugwort (*umbelliferae* family) should use with caution. • Avoid long-term or excessive intake (effect unknown). • Avoid excessive exposure to sunlight. • Should not be used by individuals with estrogen-dependent cancer. • Use with caution if taking with other medications, hormones.

continued

TABLE 19.1. Common Herbal/Supplement Therapies (continued)

Supplement	Health Claim/Action	Dosage	Notes/Safety/Side Effects
Flax (seed) Linseed, lintbells, linum *Type:* essential fatty acid, omega-3 oil *Active ingredients:* Alpha-linolenic acid, lignans	• Decreases total and LDL cholesterol. • Decreases platelet aggregation. • Lignans may have weak estrogenic, anti-estrogenic and corticosteroid-like effects. Used to lower risk of breast, hormone-dependent cancers; treat benign prostatic hyperplasia; constipation, colon function disorders due to laxative abuse, irritable bowel syndrome, diverticulitis.	Available as whole seeds, powder, capsules (soft gel), oil. Seeds/oil: 15-30 mL/d in 2-3 divided doses. Oil: 1 Tbsp/d or 5 capsules/d. Poultices have been used topically to treat local areas of inflammation.	• Overdose symptoms include shortness of breath, cyanosis, tachypnea, weakness, unstable gait, progressing to paralysis and seizures. • Avoid immature pods (which have increased toxicity). • Do not use with laxatives, stool softeners (flax increases their effects). • Do not use with oral medications (flax decreases absorption). • Maintain adequate fluid. • Should not be used by individuals with ileus, prostate cancer. • Avoid > 400 IU vitamin E/d.
Garlic Stinking rose, dasuan *Allium sativum* *Type:* Herb, food *Active ingredients:* Sulfur compound allicin, when crushed (chewed) produces ajoene, allyl sulfides, vinyldithiins	• Supports cardiovascular system by lowering blood cholesterol and triglycerides, decreasing platelet aggregation, increasing fibrinolysis, lowering blood pressure. • Antioxidant. • Antibacterial. • Antiviral. • Antifungal. • Lowers risk of GI cancer. • Antitumor activity in breast, skin. • Hypoglycemic effect. Used to treat asthma, diabetes mellitus, inflammation, athlete's foot, heavy metal poisoning, constipation, AIDS, CHF, hypertension, recurrent yeast and ear infections; used to improve serum lipid profile.	Available as capsules, tablets, fresh bulb, antiseptic oil, fresh extract, powder, essential oil. Standardized allicin potential: 400-500 mg 2 times/d. Tincture: 2-4 mL 3 times/d. Oil: 8 mg/d. Fresh: 4 g/d.	• Adverse effects include GI distress, dizziness, diaphoresis, body odor (deodorized formula available). • Do not use with anticoagulant medications. • Decreases hemoglobin and red blood cell lysis with long-term use or high dose. • Avoid > 400 IU vitamin E/d.

Herb	Actions/Uses	Dosage	Adverse Effects/Cautions
Ginger Zingiber *Zingiber officinale* *Type:* Herb *Active ingredients:* Volatile oils, aromatic principles include bisabolene, zingiberene; pungent principles shogaols, gingerols	• Antiemetic, antinausea (pungent factors) by uncertain means. • Supports GI function and integrity (stimulates digestion, intestinal muscle tone to support peristalsis, protective against ethanol and NSAIDs, ulcers). • Supports cardiovascular function (decreased platelet aggregation). • Often added to herbal formulas to aid digestion and enhance activities of other herbs. Used to treat migraine, morning/motion sickness, atherosclerosis, arthritis, chemotherapy support.	Available as root, extract, liquid, powder, capsules, tablets, tea, topical. Root: 2–4 g/d. Tincture: 1.5–3 mL 3 times daily. Capsules/tablets: 250 mg 4 times/d. For motion sickness, take 2–3 days prior to planned trip. Topical: burn remedy.	• Adverse effects include GI distress. • Individuals with history of gallstones should use with caution. • Do not use with anticoagulant drugs. • Overdose associated with central nervous system depression, arrhythmia. • Avoid > 400 IU vitamin E/d.
Gingko biloba Maidenhair tree *Gingko biloba* *Type:* Herb *Active ingredients:* Group 1: gingko flavone glycosides; Group 2: terpene lactones; both contain bioflavonoid, gingkolides, bilobalide	• Antioxidant. • Decreases platelet aggregation. • Increases systemic circulation (large and small vessels). • CNS supportive, regenerative, protective effect. • Increases serum insulin. Used to enhance memory, treat Alzheimer's disease, atherosclerosis, congestive heart failure, depression, diabetes mellitus, male impotence/infertility, migraine, macular degeneration, arthritis, cerebrovascular accident (stroke), vertigo, hearing loss.	Available as capsules, tablets, spray, concentrated ethanol extract (standardized). 120–240 mg extract/d in 2–3 divided doses. Tincture: 0.5 mL 3 times daily. Medical benefits of extract dependent on balance of bioflavenoids (24% flavones, 6% terpenes).	• Adverse effects include GI distress, headache, contact dermatitis. • Do not use with anticoagulant drugs. • Avoid > 400 IU vitamin E/d. • Fruit pulp/seeds contain urushiols. • Effect not immediate, may take 8–12 wk. • Use with caution if coadministering anti-diabetes mellitus agent. • Do not take with over-the-counter drugs containing aspirin. • Do not take with NSAID, trazodone.

continued

TABLE 19.1. Common Herbal/Supplement Therapies (continued)

Supplement	Health Claim/Action	Dosage	Notes/Safety/Side Effects
Ginseng Asian, Korean, Chinese ginseng *Panax ginseng* *Type:* Herb *Active ingredients:* Ginsenosides (> 13 variations), panaxans, polysaccharides	• Compounds exert opposing effects. • Tonic or adaptogenic used as both relaxant and stimulant. • Enhances intellectual and physical performance. • Hypoglycemic effect. Used to treat diabetes mellitus, Alzheimer's disease, atherosclerosis, fibromyalgia, cold, flu, sore throat; to increase stress tolerance; to enhance immune function; to lower cancer risk; to improve well-being; to aid weak, debilitated older adults; for chemotherapy support; to support male reproductive function.	Available as standardized/non-standardized extracts (require higher intake). Root: 0.4–0.8 g/d. Dried Root: 0.5–2.0 g/d. Extract: 200–600 mg/d.	• General recommendation is to use for 2-to 3-wk time period with 1-2 week rest period cycle. • Adverse effects include headache, insomnia, nervousness, epistaxis, increased blood pressure, palpitations, GI distress. • Avoid excessive caffeine • Ginseng abuse syndrome (with high doses, combined with other psycho-motor stimulants such as tea or coffee) includes hypertension, diarrhea, insomnia, skin eruptions, depression, decreased appetite, euphoria, edema. • Long-term, uninterrupted use may cause menstrual abnormalities, impotence. • Use with caution if individual has cardiovascular disease, hypertension, hypotension, or diabetes mellitus, or is taking corticosteroid medications. • Do not use with MAOI, loop diuretics, anticoagulants. • Siberian (Russian), wild red (Russian), and wild American ginseng are not true ginseng. • Avoid > 400 IU vitamin E/d.
Glucosamine chondroitin Glucosamine sulfate, chondroitin sulfate *Type:* Supplement *Active ingredients:* Glycosaminoglycans, mucopolysaccharides (both compounds structurally similar)	• Promotes bone healing. • Promotes restoration of joint cartilage by providing structure. • Allows adequate movement of water and nutrients for proper function (no blood supply exists to cartilage). • Presence in lining of blood vessels and urinary bladder aids movement and prevents excessive blood clotting.	Available as tablets, capsules. 500 mg 3 times/d.	• Not found in food. Glucosamine is derived from seashells, chondroitin from animal cartilage; supplemental form is combination of both sulfates and beneficial effect dependent on synergy. • Contains sulfur. • Major constituent of cartilage. • Considered safe. • Minor GI distress with high dose (> 10 g/d). • Avoid form processed with sodium chloride if on sodium-restricted diet.

	Uses/Effects	Forms/Dosage	Cautions
	• Hypocholesterolemia. • Promotes wound healing. Used to treat osteoarthritis, tendonitis, bursitis, atherosclerosis, renal stones, sports-related injury to tendons or ligaments.		
Green tea *Camellia sinensis* *Type:* Herb, tea *Active ingredients:* Polyphenols, including EGCG	• Antioxidant. • Protects against cardiovascular disease by decreasing total cholesterol, improving LDL/HDL ratio, decreased platelet aggregation, decreasing blood pressure. • Protects against cancer. • Stimulates immune system function. • Antibacterial. Used to treat gingivitis, high cholesterol, hypertension, high triglycerides, infection.	Available as tablets, capsules, tea. Tea: 1 tsp green tea leaves in 250 mL boiling water, steep for 5 min. 1 cup 3 times daily (240–320 mg polyphenols). Standardized extracts of polyphenol (especially EGCGs) are available (some decaffeinated) with < 97% polyphenol content (equivalent to 4 cups of tea).	• All teas (green, black, oolong) are derived from same plant. Green tea is not fermented. • Do not take with warfarin, anticoagulant drugs. • Adverse effects include insomnia, nervousness with high intake of caffeinated tea (also contains caffeine). • Avoid > 400 IU vitamin E/d.
Hawthorn *Crataegus laevigata, Crataegus oxyacantha, Crataegus monogyna* *Type:* Herb *Active ingredients:* bioflavenoids: oligomeric procyanidins, vitexin, quercetin, hyperoside, rutin, orientin, vicenin-1, tyramine	• Benefits heart and blood vessels by improving coronary artery blood flow and heart contractibility. • May inhibit ACE and reduce production of angiotensin II (vasoconstrictor) to reduce resistance (arterial), thereby improving peripheral circulation. • Antioxidant. • May mildly decrease blood pressure. • Mild sedative.	Available as dried form for decoction, liquid, dry extract, capsules, tablets, standardized dry extract (2.2% for total bioflavonoid content OR 18.75% oligomeric procyanidines). Capsules/tablets: 80–300 mg 2–3 times/d. Tincture: 4–5 mL 3 times/d. Traditional berry preparations > 4–5 g/d.	• Do not take with digoxin (in Germany, often coadministered). • Treatment minimum ≥ 6 wk. • Protect product from light. • May decrease absorption of medicinal iron due to formation of tannin-iron complex. • Individuals with diabetes mellitus should use with caution; may affect blood glucose levels.

continued

TABLE 19.1. Common Herbal/Supplement Therapies (continued)

Supplement	Health Claim/Action	Dosage	Notes/Safety/Side Effects
	Used to treat congestive heart failure, angina pectoris, atherosclerosis, hypertension, decrease in cardiac output (NYHA Stage II).		
Kava Kava kava, ava, awa, kawa, kew, sakau, tonga yagona *Pipermethysticava* *Type:* Herb *Active ingredients:* Kavalactones, also known as kava pyrones	• Pain reliever. • Anti-anxiety. • Increased mental acuity, memory, sensory perception. • Anticonvulsant. • Muscle relaxant. • Effects thought to be due to direct influence on the limbic system.	Available as drink, tablets, capsules, extract (30%–70% = 60–120 mg kava-lactones). Extract: 140–330 mg/d. Tincture: 1–3 mL 3 times/d. Drink: 400–900 g/wk.	• Adverse effects include mild GI distress, yellowed skin (with high doses or long-term use), allergic skin reaction, visual disturbance. • Absorption increased with food. • Do not use with other agents that affect the central nervous system (ie, etoh, barbiturate, antidepressants, antipsychotics [eg, levodopa, alprazolam]) • Chronic abuse associated with red eyes, decreased platelet and lymphocyte counts, weight loss, shortness of breath, pulmonary hypertension, dopamine antagonist. • FDA issued a consumer advisory (3/25/02) concerning 11 reports of liver failure from Kava use.
Licorice root *Glycyrrhiza glabra, Glycyrrhiza uralensis* *Type:* Herb *Active ingredients:* triterpenes, beta-sitosterol	• Anti-inflammatory (inhibits cortisol breakdown). • Antiviral by decreased growth of several DNA/RNA viruses and inactivates herpes simplex particles irreversibly. • Antioxidant. • Hepatoprotective. • Promotes healing of GI mucosal cells.	Available as deglycyrrhizinated licorice (DGL) as well as glycyrrhizin (G) form. DGL for GI remedies: 200–300 mg tablet 3 times/d. DGL for mouth ulcers: 200 mg DGL powder mixed with 200 mL warm water, swish and spit. DGL tincture: 2–5 mL 3 times/d.	• Not for long-term use without medical supervision. • G form may increase blood pressure. • G form associated with fluid retention. • Do not use with corticosteroids (ie, prednisone), cyclosporine, digoxin, MAOIs, potassium-sparing diuretics, anticoagulant drugs. • Avoid > 400 IU vitamin E/d.

	Uses	Forms/Dosage	Cautions
	Used to treat asthma, bronchitis, herpes simplex, canker sores, fibromyalgia, GI distress, pelvic inflammatory disease, chronic fatigue syndrome	G form for respiratory infection, chronic fatigue syndrome or topically for herpes. G capsules: 5–6 g/d. G tea: add 1/2 oz root to 250 mL water, boil 15 min. 1 cup 2–3 times/d. G topically as cream or gel: 3–4 times/d.	

Ma huang (see Ephedra)

Melatonin *Melatonin* *Type:* Hormone *Active ingredients:* melatonin	• Aids regulation of sleep-wake schedule ("biological clock"). • Antioxidant. • Stimulates immune system function. • Supplementary goal to enhance natural melatonin levels that decline with age. • May decrease ocular pressure. Used to treat jet lag, insomnia.	Available as tablets, capsules (time-release). 1–3 mg; take 1–2 hr before bedtime.	• Do not take during day (or awake hours). • Adverse effects include grogginess upon waking, drowsiness, disorientation, sleepwalking. • Do not use with fluvoxamine (increases effects). • Should not be used by individuals with depression, schizophrenia, autoimmune disorders. • Long-term effects are unknown.
Milk thistle Holy thistle, lady's thistle *Silybum marianum* *Type:* Herb *Active ingredients:* Bioflavonoid silymarin, which has 3 components: silibinin (most active), silidianin, silicristin	• Hepatoprotective by blocking entry of toxins and aiding elimination of toxins from liver cells. • Antioxidant. • Aids in regeneration of damaged liver cells. Used as liver "cleaner," to treat acute and chronic liver disease (including hepatitis C), and to blunt toxicity due to psychotic drug-induced liver damage, gallstones, psoriasis.	Available as seeds and standardized extract (70%–80% silymarin). Seeds: 12–15 g ground and eaten or made into tea (prophylaxis, not therapeutic). Extracts: for use by individuals with liver disease, 420 mg/d for 8–12 wk (when improvement noted) then decreased to 280 mg/d (prophylaxis dose also).	• History of use as an antidote to Amanita phalloides and other poisonous mushrooms. • Standardized extracts have mild laxative effect. • Uterine stimulant. • Monitor liver function tests. • Allow 8–12 wk to see improvement.

continued

TABLE 19.1. Common Herbal/Supplement Therapies (continued)

Supplement	Health Claim/Action	Dosage	Notes/Safety/Side Effects
Nettle *Irtica dioica* *Type:* Herb *Active ingredients:* Polysaccharides, lectins	• Anti-inflammatory (by blocking PGE synthesis). • Diuretic (by increasing urine volume and decreasing systolic blood pressure). • Stimulates uterine contractions. • Extract reduces urine flow, nocturia, and residual urine. • Affects sex hormone transport. Used to treat hay fever, benign prostatic hyperplasia, asthma, rheumatism, tuberculosis, hypertension, diabetes mellitus, gout, cancer, eczema, heart failure.	Available as tablets, capsules, dried leaf, root extract, tincture. Tablets/capsules: 150–300 mg 2–3 times/d. Tincture: 2–4 mL 3 times/d.	• Adverse effects include edema, rash (from direct contact with herb), GI distress, dysuria. • For benign prostatic hyperplasia, may be combined with saw palmetto or pygeum. • Individuals older than 65 years should not take with diuretics. • Maintain adequate potassium intake. • Individuals with benign prostatic hyperplasia or edema should not take without medical supervision. • Potential for decreased absorption of medicinal iron due to formation of tannin–iron complex.
Psyllium*, psyllium seed†, plantain‡ Buckhorn, flea seed, chimney-sweeps *Plantago afra†, Plantago ispaghula*†, Plantago lanceolata‡, Plantago ovata*†* *Type:* Herb, over-the-counter laxative	• Promotes/regulates intestinal peristalsis. • Bulk-forming laxative: husk swells upon contact with water to form a gelatinous, soft, hydrated stool (mucilage). • Hypocholesterolemic effect. • Hypoglycemic effect. • Plantain has astringent, anti-bacterial effects.	Available as whole or ground seed, liquid extract, juice, powder: 5–30 g/d.	• Should not be taken by individuals with GI constriction, obstruction, ileus, labile diabetes mellitus. • Adverse effects include hypersensitivity/allergic reactions. • *Must* be taken w/adequate water to avoid choking, bowel obstruction. • Use with caution if taking medications; may delay absorption.

Reprinted by permission of Roche Dietitians, LLC. Copyright © Roche Dietitians, LLC.

Active ingredients: Mucilage (mostly drabinoxylans), 10%–30%, soluble fiber, iridide monotepenes: aucubin (rhinantin), catalpol‡; flavonoids, caffeic acid esters‡; tannins‡, hydroxy-coumarin‡, silicic acid‡	Used to treat chronic constipation, irritable colon, diabetes mellitus, diarrhea, high cholesterol, high triglycerides, atherosclerosis. Plantain also used to treat GI inflammation, respiratory conditions (cold, flu, cough, bronchitis), psoriasis.		• Do not use with carbamazepine, digoxin, lithium. • Potential for decreased absorption of medicinal iron due to formation of iron-tannin complex.
Red clover Purple clover, wild clover, trefoil *Trifolium pratense* *Type*: Herb *Active ingredients*: Isoflavones, genistein, biochanin A, volatile oils, coumarin derivatives, cyanogenic glycosides	• Weak estrogenic effects. • Cancer prevention (breast, prostate). • Antispasmodic effects. • Expectorant effects. • Anticoagulant effects. Used to treat respiratory conditions (particularly whooping cough), menopausal symptoms, chronic skin conditions (eg, psoriasis, eczema).	Available as capsules, tablets, tea, dried, tincture. Tea: add 2-3 tsp dried herb to 250 mL boiling water, steep 10-15 min. Up to 1 cup 3 times/d. Capsules/tablets: 2-4 g/d. Tincture: 2-4 mL 3 times/d.	• Use only nonfermented form; avoid fermented form. • Do not take with aspirin, estrogens, oral contraceptives, warfarin, anticoagulation drugs. • Avoid > 400 IU vitamin E/d.
Saw palmetto American dwarf palm tree, cabbage palm, IDS 89, LSESR, sabal *Serenoa repens, Sabal serrulata* *Type*: Herb *Active ingredients*: Lipophilic (fat-soluble) extract provides sterols (betasitosterol) and fatty acids (caproic, lauric, palmitic)	• Reduces prostate dihydrotestosterone levels. • Inhibits inflammatory substances that contribute to benign prostatic hyperplasia. • Inhibits prolactin and growth factor induced prostate cell proliferation. Used to treat benign prostatic hyperplasia, chronic urinary tract infections; as a mild diuretic; to increase breast size; to increase sperm production; to enhance sexual performance.	Available as tablets/capsules, teas, fresh or dried berries, liquid extract. Capsules/tablets: 160 mg 2 times/d. Tea: 1.5-6 g/d (dried or fresh). Liquid extract: 5-6 mL/d.	• Adverse effects include headache, hypertension, GI distress, dysuria, urine retention, impotence, decreased libido, back pain. • Obtain baseline PSA prior to treatment for benign prostatic hyperplasia, as false-positive PSA results from herb intake is possible. Benign prostatic hyperplasia diagnosis must be made by a physician. Caution with use other than benign prostatic hyperplasia diagnosis. • Do not use with estrogens, oral contraceptives. • Potential for decreased absorption of medicinal iron due to formation of tannin-iron complex. • Allow 4-6 wk for results.

continued

TABLE 19.1. Common Herbal/Supplement Therapies (continued)

Supplement	Health Claim/Action	Dosage	Notes/Safety/Side Effects
Soy Tofu, tempeh, textured and hydrolyzed vegetable protein, miso *Type:* Supplement, food *Active ingredients:* Phytoestrogens: isoflavones (genistein, daidzein, and others), lignins, saponins, phytosterols, protein (essential amino acids)	• Cancer prevention (breast, prostate). • Enhances immune function. • Hypocholesterolemic effects. • Antioxidant. • Estrogenic effects. • Hormonal regulation effect. • Decreases adverse effects compared with estrogen replacement therapy. Used to treat menopausal symptoms including hot flashes, high cholesterol; provides protein source of non-animal origin and less total fat.	Wide variety of food sources available. As supplement powder, tablets, capsules: 40–80 mg isoflavones.	• Adverse effects include allergic reactions. • Some constituents of soy may affect thyroid function. • Phytic acid component may alter mineral absorption. • Food sources are optimal recommended sources. • Avoid supplemental form if taking tamoxifen, toremifene, taloxifene, estrogens, or oral contraceptives.
St John's wort Amber, goat weed, devil's scourge, klamath weed *Hypericin perforatum* *Type:* Herb *Active ingredients:* Hypericum pseudohypericin, xanthines, flavonoids, phenolic carboxylic acids, alkanes, phytosterols	• Antidepressant. • Psychotropic. • Antiviral. • Antibacterial. • Promotes wound healing. • Inhibits stress-induced increase in cortisol. Used to treat moderate depression, recurrent ear infection, vitiligo, sleep disorders, HIV/AIDS, hypothyroid, bronchial inflammation, cancer, insect bites and stings, wounds, skin diseases (topical).	Available as capsules, tablets, tincture, standardized extract (0.3% hypericin): 500 mg/d. Topical for psoriasis, warts, Kaposi's sarcoma.	• Adverse effects include photosensitivity, GI distress, possible allergic reaction or hypersensitivity. • Do not take with tricyclic antidepressants. • Allow 3–4 wk for response. • Avoid foods high in tyramine. • Avoid alcohol. • Do not take with MAOIs, anticoagulant medications, oral contraceptives, protease inhibitors (eg, indinavir), serotonin re-uptake inhibitors (eg, Paroxetine), cyclosporine, digoxin, theophylline. • Potential for decreased absorption of medicinal iron due to formation of tannin-iron complex.

	Actions	Dosage	Cautions
			• Avoid > 400 IU vitamin E/d. • Avoid long-term use (> 6 mo). • Has been used in Germany for depression.
Valerian root Amantilla, all heal, herbal benedicta *Valeriana officinalis* *Type:* Herb *Active ingredients:* Essential oils, valepotriates, valeric acid, choline, flavonoids, sterols, alkaloids (actinidine, valerianine, valerine, chatinine), caffeic acid derivatives	• Sedative. • Anticonvulsant. • Antidepressant. • Antispasmodic to GI smooth muscle. • Coronary dilator. • Anti-arrhythmic activity. • Antibiotic. Used to treat insomnia, restlessness, anxiety, sleep disorders, nervous tension, stress.	Available as capsules, tablets, teas, tinctures (2%), juice, standardized extract (0.8% valerenic acid). Capsules/tablets: 300–500 mg/d, before bedtime. Tincture: 5 mL/d before bedtime. Tea: 2–3 g 3 times/d. Juice: 1 Tbsp 3 times/d.	• Adverse effects include hypersensitivity with allergic reactions, drowsiness, grogginess upon waking, GI distress. • Avoid alcohol. • Hepatotoxicity is associated with overdose or long-term use. • Should not be used by individuals with decreased liver function; monitor liver function tests with long-term use. • Avoid tincture form (contains alcohol). • Do not take with central nervous system depressants. • Potential for decreased absorption of medicinal iron due to formation of tannin-iron complex.

Abbreviations: ACE, angiotensin-converting enzyme; CNS, central nervous system; EGCG, epigallocatechin gallate; GI, gastrointestinal; GLA, gamma linolenic acid; HDL, high-density lipoprotein; LDL, low-density lipoprotein; MAOI, monoamine oxidase inhibitor; NSAID, nonsteroidal anti-inflammatory drugs; NYHA, New York Heart Association classification; PGE, prostaglandin E; PSA, prostate-specific antigen; SLE, systemic lupus erythematosus; SNS, sympathetic nervous system.

• Tincture forms generally contain alcohol and can result in disulfiram-like reactions with certain medications (including disulfiram). Avoid tincture form when alcohol intake is contraindicated.

• Health claims, usage, and dosage have not necessarily been validated by documented scientific research and should not be considered an endorsement.

• Actions, dosages, and side effects may be different for children or pregnant or lactating women. For these populations, special caution regarding supplement use should be exercised.

Source: Compiled by Paula K. Burke, RD. Copyright © Roche Dietitians, LLC. Clinical and Nutrient Guidelines: Part of the Drug-Nutrient Intervention System Riverside, Ill: Roche Dietitians, LLC 2001.

Box 19.1   Sources for Additional Information

The Health Professional's Guide to Popular Dietary Supplements, 2nd edition (2003)
By Allison Sarubin Fragakis, MS, RD
American Dietetic Association
To order: http://www.eatright.org

Center for Mind/Body Studies
5225 Connecticut Ave,
 NW, Suite 414
Washington, DC 20015
202/966-7338
http://www.healthy.net/scr/
 center.asp?centerid=1

College of Maharishi Ayurveda Health Spa
PO Box 282
Fairfield, IA 52556
515/472-5866
http://www.theraj.com

Food and Drug Administration
5800 Fishers Lane
Rockville, MD 20857
800/332-0178
http://www.fda.gov

Herb Research Foundation
4140 15th St
Boulder, CO 80304
303/449-2265 (office)
800/748-2617 (voicemail)
303/449-7849 (fax)
http://www.herbs.org

Institute of Noetic Sciences
101 San Antonio Road
Petaluma, CA 94952
707/775-3500
http://www.noetic.org

The Interfaith Health Program
Rollins School of Public Health
1256 Briarcliff Rd, NE
Building A, Suite 107
Atlanta, GA 30306
404/727-5246
http://www.ihpnet.org

International Association of Yoga Therapists/Yoga Research and Education Center
PO Box 426
Manton, CA 96059
530/474-5700
http://www.iayt.org

Med Watch
800/332-1088
http://www.fda.gov/medwatch

National Association for Holistic Aromatherapy
4509 Interlake Ave N, #233
Seattle, WA 98103-6773
888/ASK-NAHA or 206/547-2164
206/547-2680 (fax)
http://www.naha.org/

National Center for Complementary and Alternative Medicine (NCCAM)
National Institutes of Health
Bethesda, MD 20892 USA
http://altmed.od.nih.gov

NCCAM Clearinghouse
PO Box 7923
Gaithersburg, MD 20898
888/644-6226
http://altmed.od.nih.gov/health/
 clearinghouse/index.htm

National Certification Commission for Acupuncture and Oriental Medicine
11 Canal Center Plaza, Suite 300
Alexandria, VA 22314
703/548-9004
http://www.nccaom.org

Nurse Healers — Professional Associates International
3760 S Highland Dr, Suite 429
Salt Lake City, UT 84106
801/273-3399
http://www.therapeutic-
touch.org/default.asp

CHAPTER
20
Skin Integrity

Human skin is the largest organ in the body, covering more than 20 square feet in an average adult. Skin thickness varies from one fiftieth of an inch over the eyelids to one third of an inch on the palms of the hands and soles of the feet. The pH of the skin ranges from 4.5 to 5.5, which provides the protective acid mantle of the skin that maintains the skin's normal flora (1).

SKIN CONDITIONS
Skin Integrity

The loss of skin elasticity, moisture, and reduced feeling in susceptible areas places older clients at risk for impaired skin integrity. Nutritional factors that contribute to skin breakdown include protein deficiency, which creates a negative nitrogen balance; anemia, which inhibits the formation of red blood cells; and dehydration, which causes dry, fragile skin. Dehydration can also result in an increase in the blood glucose level and can slow the healing process.

When conducting a nutrition audit, note the temperature and color of the skin. Hot skin may indicate increased blood flow due to inflammation or infection. Cool or cold skin with a white or pale color usually indicates decreased blood flow and impaired circulation. Wrinkled, withered, or dry skin is a sign of dehydration. Taut and shiny skin may indicate edema.

When assessing the skin, note that the presence of moisture contributes to the development of pressure ulcers. Someone who is incontinent is at risk, because of the skin's increased exposure to bacteria and toxins in both urine and feces. Excessive perspiration also may render the person at risk. Causes of excessive perspiration may be heavy clothing or bedding, or an elevated temperature. Breaks in the skin, as well as blemishes, rashes, lesions, and discolored areas, are warning signs of irritation or trauma and

should also be noted. Decreased skin response to temperature, pain, and pressure also occurs with advancing age. This affects the skin's elasticity and the healing process (1).

Pressure Ulcers

In 1994 the federal government published guidelines for the prevention and treatment of pressure ulcers. *Pressure Ulcers in Adults: Prediction and Prevention* and *Treatment of Pressure Ulcers in Adults* was produced by the Agency for Health Care Policy and Research (AHCPR) (2).

The AHCPR guidelines recommended the identification of at-risk clients using a systematic, validated, risk assessment tool (3). The Braden Scale (Figure 20.1) is an example of a risk assessment.

Pressure ulcers usually occur over bony prominences and are graded or staged to classify the degree of tissue damage observed. They are the only type of wound whose origin is a result of external forces of pressure, shear, friction, and maceration.

Stage I

Stage I is characterized by an observable pressure-related alteration of intact skin whose indicators, as compared with the adjacent or opposite area on the body, may include changes in one or more of the following: skin temperature (warmth or coolness), tissue consistency (firm or boggy feel), and sensation (pain, itching). In lightly pigmented skin, the ulcer appears as a defined area of persistent redness; in darker skin tones, the ulcer may appear with persistent red, blue, or purple hues (4).

Stage II

Stage II is characterized by partial-thickness skin loss involving the epidermis and/or the dermis. The ulcer is superficial and appears as an abrasion, a blister, or a shallow crater.

Figure 20.1

Braden scale for predicting pressure sore risk. Braden scale or other appropriate risk assessment scale is completed by nursing in most settings. Form is included as a reference. Copyright © Barbara Braden and Nancy Bergstrom, 1988. Reprinted with permission. All rights reserved.

Patient's Name: **Evaluator's Name:**   **Date of Assessment:**

Sensory perception Ability to respond meaningfully to pressure-related discomfort	**1. Completely limited** Unresponsive (does not moan, flinch, or gasp) to painful stimuli due to diminished level of consciousness or sedation. *OR* Limited ability to feel pain over most of body surface.	**2. Very limited** Responds only to painful stimuli. Cannot communicate discomfort except by moaning or restlessness. *OR* Has sensory impairment which limits the ability to feel pain or discomfort over one-half of the body.	**3. Slightly limited** Responds to verbal commands but cannot always communicate discomfort or need to be turned. *OR* Has some sensory impairment which limits ability to feel pain or discomfort in 1 or 2 extremities.	**4. No impairment** Responds to verbal commands. Has no sensory deficit which would limit ability to feel or voice pain or discomfort.				
Moisture Degree to which skin is exposed to moisture	**1. Constantly moist** Skin is kept moist almost constantly by perspiration, urine, etc. Dampness is detected every time patient is moved or turned.	**2. Moist** Skin is often but not always moist. Linen must be changed at least once a shift.	**3. Occasionally moist** Skin is occasionally moist, requiring an extra linen change approximately once a day.	**4. Rarely moist** Skin is usually dry. Linen requires changing only at routine intervals.				
Activity Degree of physical activity	**1. Bedfast** Confined to bed.	**2. Chairfast** Ability to walk severely limited or nonexistent. Cannot bear own weight and/or must be assisted into chair or wheelchair.	**3. Walks occasionally** Walks occasionally during day but for very short distances with or without assistance. Spends majority of each shift in bed or chair.	**4. Walks frequently** Walks outside the room at least twice a day and inside room at least once every 2 hours during waking hours.				
Mobility Ability to change and control body position	**1. Completely immobile** Does not make even slight changes in body or extremity position without assistance.	**2. Very limited** Makes occasional slight changes in body or extremity position but unable to make frequent or significant changes independently.	**3. Slightly limited** Makes frequent though slight changes in body or extremity position independently.	**4. No limitations** Makes major and frequent changes in position without assistance.				

continued

Nutrition	1. Very poor	2. Probably inadequate	3. Adequate	4. Excellent				
Usual food intake pattern	Never eats a complete meal. Rarely eats more than 1/3 of any food offered. Eats two servings or less of protein (meat or dairy products) per day. Takes fluids poorly. Does not take a liquid dietary supplement. *OR* Is NPO* and/or maintained on clear liquids or IV** for more than 5 days.	Rarely eats a complete meal and generally eats only about 1/2 of any food offered. Protein intake includes only three servings of meat or dairy products per day. Occasionally will take a dietary supplement. *OR* Receives less than optimum amount of liquid diet or tube feeding.	Eats over half of most meals. Eats a total of four servings of protein (meat, dairy products) each day. Occasionally will refuse a meal, but will usually take a supplement if offered. *OR* Is on a tube feeding or TPN† regimen which probably meets most nutrition needs.	Eats most of every meal. Never refuses a meal. Usually eats a total of four or more servings of meat and dairy products. Occasionally eats between meals. Does not require supplementation.				
Friction and Shear	**1. Problem**	**2. Potential problem**	**3. No apparent problem**					
	Requires moderate to maximum assistance in moving. Complete lifting without sliding against sheets is impossible. Frequently slides down in bed or chair, requiring frequent repositioning with maximum assistance. Spasticity, contractures, or agitation leads to almost constant friction.	Moves feebly or requires minimum assistance. During a move skin probably slides to some extent against sheets, chair, restraints, or other devices. Maintains relatively good position in chair or bed most of the time but occasionally slides down.	Moves in bed and in chair independently and has sufficient muscle strength to lift up completely during move. Maintains good position in bed or chair at all times.					
				TOTAL SCORE				

* NPO: Nothing by mouth

** IV: Intravenously

† TPN: Total parenteral nutrition

Stage III

Stage III is characterized by full-thickness skin loss involving damage or necrosis of subcutaneous tissue that may extend down to, but not through, underlying fascia. The ulcer presents clinically as a deep crater, with or without undermining of adjacent tissue.

Stage IV

Stage IV is characterized by full-thickness skin loss with extensive destruction; tissue necrosis; or damage to muscle, bone, or supporting structures (eg, tendon or joint capsule). Undermining and sinus tracts may also be associated with Stage IV pressure ulcers.

Staging definitions recognize that when eschar is present, accurate staging of the pressure ulcer is not possible until the eschar has sloughed or the wound has been debrided (2).

The Centers for Medicare & Medicaid Services (CMS) has determined that the development of a pressure ulcer for a person who is at low risk is a sentinel event. See Box 20.1 for definition of high risk (5).

Box 20.1   Definition of High Risk for Pressure Ulcer Development

- Impaired mobility or transfer
- End-stage renal disease
- Malnutrition
- Comatose

Clinical conditions that are the *primary risk factors* for developing pressure sores include, but are not limited to, resident immobility and

1. *The resident has two or more of the following diagnoses:*
   a. Continuous urinary incontinence or chronic voiding dysfunction
   b. Severe peripheral vascular disease
   c. Diabetes
   d. Severe COPD
   e. Chronic bowel incontinence
   f. Paraplegia
   g. Quadriplegia
   h. Sepsis
   i. Terminal cancer
   j. Chronic end-stage renal, liver, and/or heart disease
   k. Disease or drug-related immunosuppression
   l. Full body cast

2. *The resident receives two or more of the following treatments:*
   a. Steroid therapy
   b. Radiation therapy
   c. Chemotherapy
   d. Renal dialysis
   e. Head of bed elevated the majority of the day due to medical necessity

Source: Data are from reference 5.

GUIDELINES FOR CARE

The following guidelines address the issue of pressure ulcers and the best practice guidelines for care.

Guideline 1

Clients who are at risk for pressure ulcers will be identified and assessed for risk factors.

Immobility and inactivity are primary risk factors for pressure ulcer development. Diagnosis or conditions that increase risk for development of pressure ulcers may include urinary and/or fecal incontinence; peripheral vascular disease; cerebral vascular accident; diabetes mellitus; chronic obstructive pulmonary disease; sepsis; chronic or end-stage renal, liver, and/or heart disease; disease-related immunosuppression; malnutrition; hip fractures; and spinal cord injury. Dietetics professionals should consider each disease diagnosed in relationship to the individual's nutrition intake. The disease may be a contributing factor to pressure ulcers.

Medical treatments and medications that may contribute to risk for pressure ulcers, including anti-kinetic drugs (such as antidepressants and sleeping pills; drugs related to immunosuppression; steroid therapy; radiation therapy; chemotherapy; and renal dialysis). As a member of the health care team, the dietetics professional reviews the nutritional side effects of medications.

Malnutrition, dehydration, or unintentional weight loss (greater than 5% in 1 month, 7.5% in 3 months, or 10% in 6 months), whether secondary to poor appetite or another disease process, places the client at risk for tissue breakdown and poor healing. Poor oral intake is a frequent cause of malnutrition and can be caused by chewing or swallowing problems (ie, dysphagia), ill-fitting dentures, loss of ability to self-feed, restrictive diet orders, and/or polypharmacotherapy. The in-depth nutrition assessment targets these areas, and a care plan is developed to address each problem area.

Guideline 2

Clients at risk for pressure ulcers will be monitored at appropriate intervals.

The client's nutritional status is monitored at a minimum of every 3 months for those at mild nutritional risk and a minimum of monthly for those clients identified to be at high risk or malnourished. Some clients may require more frequent evaluation and documentation. Weight maintenance is one of the best indicators of nutritional adequacy. Laboratory values indicative of malnutrition include serum albumin below 3.5 g/dL; weight loss of more than 5% in 1 month, 7.5% in 3 months, or 10% in 6 months; serum transferrin level (< 180 mg/dL) or prealbumin (< 17 mg/dL); hemoglobin (< 12 mg/dL) and hematocrit (< 33%); serum cholesterol (< 160 mg/dL); and hydration parameters (serum osmolality of < 295 mOsm/L). Biochemical assessment data must be used with caution, because they can be altered by medications and changes in metabolism. It is best to use the standards established by the laboratory that conducts the tests. Parameters for evaluating hydration status should include assessing urine output (I/Os), weight, BUN:creatinine ratio > 10:1, and skin turgor (see Box 20.2) (2,6-8).

Guideline 3

Clients will receive appropriate care from a multidisciplinary team to prevent and treat pressure ulcers and to prevent infection.

Adequate nutrition, including energy, protein, fluid, and vitamins/minerals, is provided to meet the clients' needs. A daily high-potency multiple vitamin/mineral supplement, meeting 100% of the RDA, is given if energy intake is substantially below required or vitamin and mineral deficiencies are confirmed by laboratory assessment. Supplements should not be more than 10 times the RDA. See Boxes 20.3 and 20.4 for further information (8-22).

Oral dietary intake and supplementation with food and nutrition supplements are the first interventions. When dietary intake is inadequate, impractical, or impossible through oral intake alone, nutrition support (compatible with the desires of the older adult and/or family) is initiated to achieve a positive nitrogen balance. See Figure 20.2 (2).

Guideline 4

Pressure ulcers are systematically monitored for improvement or deterioration.

Pressure ulcer healing is determined by the appearance of the replaced tissue. Pressure ulcer staging has been used inappropriately to denote pressure ulcer healing. No data indicate a natural progression of an ulcer from Stage I to Stage IV nor a natural regression from Stage IV to Stage I during healing. The use of pressure ulcer stages in reverse order is histologically incorrect, because the original tissue layers destroyed by a pressure ulcer are not replaced with the same kinds of tissue. Instead, the ulcerated area is filled with granulation tissue, composed primarily of endothelial cells, fibroblasts, and an extracellular matrix produced by fibroblasts. Stage IV and Stage III pressure ulcers progress to scar, which is primarily collagen, and it never possesses the characteristics of unbroken skin. The National Pressure Ulcer Advisory Panel (NPUAP) has developed the Pressure Ulcer Scale

---

Box 20.2 Laboratory Values Indicative of Increased Risk for Delayed Wound Healing

Serum transferrin < 180 mg/dL

Prealbumin < 17 mg/dL

Serum albumin < 3.5 mg/dL with normal hydration status

Hemoglobin < 12 g/dL

Hematocrit < 33%

Serum cholesterol < 160 mg/dL

Total lymphocyte count < 1800/mm

Serum osmolality > 295 mOsm/L

BUN/Creatinine > 10:1

Source: Data are from references 2, 6, 7, and 8.

Box 20.3 Daily Energy, Protein, and Fluid Needs for Clients With Pressure Ulcers (Calculated on actual body weight)

Energy needs: minimum of 30 to 35 kcal/kg body weight

Protein needs: 1.2 to 1.5 g of protein/kg body weight. Note: 1.5 g/kg may not promote protein synthesis and may cause dehydration in the elderly or those with impaired renal function (16).

Fluid needs: minimum of 1,500 mL (unless medically contraindicated) or 30 mL/kg body weight (or an amount equal to kilocalorie requirements). 10 to 15 mL for air-fluidized beds; 150 cc for every degree of elevated temperature.

---

for Healing (PUSH) (Figure 20.3 [23]). This tool gives a numeric score that indicates change in an ulcer over time and includes length and width, exudate amount, and predominant tissue. Reimbursement is often compromised when pressure ulcers are documented as healing by regression to a Stage I or a Stage II pressure ulcer. Air-fluidized beds and other treatments and therapies required to promote healing are often denied on the basis of the current payment system.

Box 20.4   Selected Nutrient Needs for Clients With Pressure Ulcers

Glutamine

Glutamine stimulates the release of human growth hormone and preserves lean body mass. Enteral formulas designed for wound healing contain added glutamine to compensate for the drop in glutamine levels during stress. Some studies indicate that supplemental glutamine does not have noticeable effects on wound healing (9).

Arginine

Arginine stimulates collagen synthesis, assists in cell growth and replication, and enhances cellular immune mechanisms. A study of older adults with normal renal function who were hydrated concluded that they could tolerate the increased nitrogen loads when they were on enteral formulas supplemented with arginine (10,11).

Micronutrients

Among the micronutrients most essential for skin integrity are vitamin A, the B vitamins, vitamin C, zinc, and copper. Vitamin A is required for inflammatory response, although excessive amounts of this vitamin may exacerbate the inflammatory response. Vitamin B is required for cross-linking of collagen fibers in rebuilding tissue. Vitamin C may increase the activation of leukocytes and macrophages to the wound site. Copper is required for cross-linking of collagen fibers in rebuilding tissue. Zinc is an essential cofactor for formation of collagen, protein synthesis, DNA, and RNA.

Vitamin A. Vitamin A supplements have been effective in promoting healing for corticosteroid-dependent clients (12,13). Because vitamin A stimulates cellular differentiation in fibroblasts and collagen formation and the maintenance of epithelium, a daily dietary source of this vitamin is suggested (12,13).

Vitamin C. Protein and lysine work with vitamin C during collagen synthesis. A deficiency in vitamin C extends the healing time and reduces resistance to infection. Older adults who do not consume a diet adequate in vitamin C or those who have Stage III or IV pressure ulcers may benefit from a daily supplementation of 500 to 1,000 mg of vitamin C daily, if conditions exist, such as acute stress or malnutrition, which increase the requirements (14-17).

The RDA for vitamin C is 75 mg/day for healthy adult females and 90 mg/day for healthy males, plus an additional 35 mg/day for those who smoke (18). Smoking increases the metabolic turnover of vitamin C. The upper tolerable limit (UL) for ascorbic acid is 2,000 mg/day for adults (18); therefore, the dietetics professional should assess the older adult for signs and symptoms of possible vitamin C deficiency before recommending doses higher than the UL.

Zinc. Zinc deficiency can occur from wound drainage, from excessive gastrointestinal fluid loss, or from long-term poor dietary intake. High serum zinc intakes can inhibit healing, impair phagocytosis, and interfere with copper metabolism (19-22).

Zinc supplementation of 50 mg/day (ie, twice-daily supplements of 220 mg of zinc sulfate) is often recommended for older adults with poor intake or weight loss, who have a stage III or stage IV pressure ulcer. Long-term supplementation is discouraged (8).

Guideline 5

Documentation in the medical record is sufficient to track implementation and outcomes of care.

Documentation in the medical record is consistent with care that is actually provided. The dietetics professional documents in the medical record on a routine basis (ie, energy, hydration, vitamin/mineral needs, weight status, and progress toward goals.)

Many techniques used to promote weight gain are also used for older adults requiring additional protein and energy for healing pressure ulcers. All aspects of nutrition care are documented and reviewed on a routine basis at least monthly until the wounds are healed. The dietetics professional needs to be a member of the wound care team. This team concept improves the quality of care for older adults and ultimately the quality of life (24).

The following skin ulcers should not be confused with pressure ulcers:

- *Venous insufficiency (stasis):* defined as a disturbance in the forward flow of blood in the lower extremities, which may progress to increased hydrostatic pressure, venous hypertension, and ultimately dermal ulceration. Risk factors for venous disease include obesity, deep-vein thrombosis, family history of venous disease, inactivity, and trauma.

Figure 20.2.

Nutrition assessment and support. Reprinted from Bergstrom N, Bennett MA, Carlson CE, et al. *Clinical Practice Guideline Number 15: Treatment of Pressure Ulcers.* Rockville, Md: US Dept of Health and Human Services, Agency for Health Care Policy and Research; 1994:12-13. AHCPR publication 95-0652.

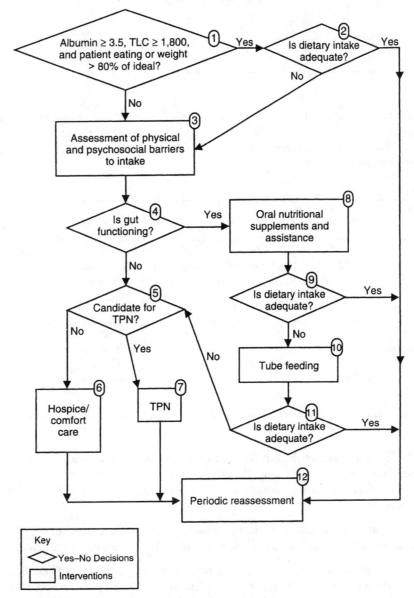

Note: TLC = total lymphocyte count; TPN = total parenteral nutrition.

- *Arterial insufficiency:* defined as insufficient arterial perfusion to an extremity or a location such as the ankle, the heel, or the toe. Risk factors for peripheral vascular disease include history of cardiac disease, hypertension, smoking (a client smoking two packs per day for 20 years has a 40 pack-year smoking history), and diabetes.

- *Peripheral neuropathy:* defined as altered nerve function in the lower extremities—may involve diminished or absent sensation to touch, pain, or temperature; absence of sweating; foot deformities; and altered gait (weight bearing) (25).

Figure 20.3.

Pressure Ulcer Scale for Healing (PUSH Tool 3.0). Reprinted with permission from National Pressure Ulcer Advisory Panel. Copyright © NPUAP, 1997.

PUSH Tool 3.0

Patient Name: _____   Patient ID#: _____

Ulcer Location: _____   Date: _____

DIRECTIONS:

Observe and measure the pressure ulcer. Categorize the ulcer with respect to surface area, exudate, and type of wound tissue. Record a sub-score for each of these ulcer characteristics. Add the sub-scores to obtain the total score. A comparison of total scores measured over time provides an indication of the improvement or deterioration in pressure ulcer healing.

Length	0 0 cm²	1 < 0.3 cm²	2 0.3-0.6 cm²	3 0.7-1.0 cm²	4 1.1-2.0 cm²	5 2.1-3.0 cm²	
X Width		6 3.1-4.0 cm²	7 4.1-8.0 cm²	8 8.1-12.0 cm²	9 12.1-24.0 cm²	10 > 24.0 cm²	Sub-score
Exudate Amount	0 None	1 Light	2 Moderate	3 Heavy			Sub-score
Tissue Type	0 Closed	1 Epithelial Tissue	2 Granulation Tissue	3 Slough	4 Necrotic Tissue		Sub-score
							Total Score

Length × Width: Measure the greatest length (head to toe) and the greatest width (side to side) using a centimeter ruler. Multiply these two measurements (length × width) to obtain an estimate of surface area in square centimeters (cm²). Caveat: Do not guess! Always use a centimeter ruler and always use the same method each time the ulcer is measured.

Exudate Amount: Estimate the amount of exudate (drainage) present after removal of the dressing and before applying any topical agent to the ulcer. Estimate the exudate (drainage) as none, light, moderate, or heavy.

Tissue Type: This refers to the types of tissue that are present in the wound (ulcer) bed. Score as a "4" if there is any necrotic tissue present. Score as a "3" if there is any amount of slough present and necrotic tissue is absent. Score as a "2" if the wound is clean and contains granulation tissue. A superficial wound that is reepithelializing is scored as a "1." When the wound is closed, score as a "0."

4 – **Necrotic Tissue (Eschar):** black, brown, or tan tissue that adheres firmly to the wound bed or ulcer edges and may be either firmer or softer than surrounding skin.

3 – **Slough:** yellow or white tissue that adheres to the ulcer bed in strings or thick clumps, or is mucinous.

2 – **Granulation Tissue:** pink or beefy red tissue with a shiny, moist, granular appearance.

1 – **Epithelial Tissue:** for superficial ulcers, new pink or shiny tissue (skin) that grows in from the edges or as islands on the ulcer surface.

0 – **Closed/Resurfaced:** the wound is completely covered with epithelium (new skin).

continued

PRESSURE ULCER HEALING CHART
(To Monitor Trends in PUSH Scores Over Time)
(use a separate page for each pressure ulcer)

Patient Name: _____   Patient ID#: _____

Ulcer Location: _____   Date: _____

DIRECTIONS: Observe and measure pressure ulcers at regular intervals using the PUSH Tool. Date and record PUSH Sub-scale and Total Scores on the Pressure Ulcer Healing Record below.

PRESSURE ULCER HEALING RECORD														
DATE														
Length × Width														
Exudate Amount														
Tissue Type														
Total Score														

Graph the PUSH Total Score on the Pressure Ulcer Healing Graph below.

PUSH Total Score	PRESSURE ULCER HEALING RECORD													
17														
16														
15														
14														
13														
12														
11														
10														
9														
8														
7														
6														
5														
4														
3														
2														
1														
Healed 0														
DATE														

continued

Figure 20.3.   (*continued*)

Instructions for Using the PUSH Tool

To use the PUSH Tool, the pressure ulcer is assessed and scored on the three elements in the tool:

• Length × Width --> scored from 0 to 10

• Exudate Amount ---> scored from 0 (none) to 3 (heavy)

• Tissue Type ---> scored from 0 (closed) to 4 (necrotic tissue)

In order to ensure consistency in applying the tool to monitor wound healing, definitions for each element are supplied at the bottom of the tool.

Step 1: Using the definition for length × width, a centimeter ruler measurement is made of the greatest head to toe diameter. A second measurement is made of the greatest width (left to right). Multiply these two measurements to get square centimeters and then select the corresponding category for size on the scale and record the score.

Step 2: Estimate the amount of exudate after removal of the dressing and before applying any topical agents. Select the corresponding category for amount & record the score.

Step 3: Identify the type of tissue. *Note:* if there is ANY necrotic tissue, it is scored a 4. Or, if there is ANY slough, it is scored a 3, even though most of the wound is covered with granulation tissue.

Step 4: Sum the scores on the three elements of the tool to derive a total PUSH Score.

Step 5: Transfer the total score to the **Pressure Ulcer Healing Graph.** Changes in the score over time provide an indication of the changing status of the ulcer. If the score goes down, the wound is healing. If it gets larger, the wound is deteriorating.

• *Diabetic wounds:* Clients with diabetes often have vascular disease, placing them at high risk for vascular ulcers. Half the amputations yearly are for diabetic older adults (21). The lack of blood flow to the site interferes with the delivery of leukocytes. The growth of destructive anaerobes is promoted because of the decrease in oxygen to the wound site. A high percentage of diabetic ulcers results in osteomyelitis, which causes extensive tissue damage and is associated with a high mortality rate. Controlling blood sugar levels is critical for the diabetic with wounds.

SUMMARY

A nutrition assessment of the older adult should include a physical assessment of the condition of the skin. The older adult is at risk for the development of pressure ulcers based on multiple risk factors, including physical limitations, disease conditions, and medical treatments. In addition to pressure ulcers, other skin conditions, such as wounds and circulating skin problems, must be visually evaluated by the dietetics professional. The dietetics professional should be an active participant on the wound care team that monitors healing

and recommends protocol changes to advance the healing process. Frequent and detailed documentation in the medical record should support nutrition interventions recommended. Nutrition interventions are developed based on careful assessment of the skin.

Documentation should be:
Factual
Accurate
Complete
Timely

REFERENCES

1. Makelbust J, Sieggreen M. *Pressure Ulcers: Guidelines for Prevention and Nursing Management.* 3rd ed. Springhouse, Pa: Springhouse Corp; 2001:356.
2. Bergstrom N, Allman RM, Alvarez OM, Bennett MA, Carlson CE, Frantz RA, Garber SL, Jackson BS, Kaminski MV, Kemp MG, Krouskop TA, Lewis VL, Maklebust J, Margolis DJ, Marvel EM, Reger SI, Rodeheaver GT, Salcido R, Xakellis GC, Yarkony GM. *Clinical Practice Guideline, Number 15: Treatment of Pressure Ulcers.* Rockville, Md: Agency for Health Care Policy and Research, Public Health Service, US Department of Health and Human Services; 1994. AHCPR Publication No. 95-0652.

3. Braden BJ, Bergstrom N. Predictive validity of the Braden Scale for pressure sore risk in a nursing home population. *Res Nurs Health.* 1994;17:459-470.

4. National Pressure Ulcer Advisory Panel Web site. Available at: http://www.NPUAP.org. Accessed June 24, 2003.

5. F tag 314; Procedures: 483.25(c). 56 *Federal Register* 187 (1991).

6. Reilly J, Hull SF, Alert N, Waller A, Bringardener S. Economic impact of malnutrition: a model system for hospitalized patients. *JPEN J Parenter Enteral Nutr.* 1988;88:371-376.

7. Breslow R. Nutritional status and dietary intake of patients with pressure ulcers. *Decubitus.* 1991;4:16-21.

8. Litchford MD. *Practical Applications in Laboratory Assessment of Nutritional Status.* Greensboro, NC: CASE Software; 2001.

9. McCauley R, Platell C, Hall J, McCulloch R. Effects of glutamine infusion on colonic anastomotic strength in the rat. *JPEN J Parenter Enteral Nutr.* 1991;15:437-439.

10. Barbul A, Lazarou SA, Efron DT, Wasserkrug HL, Efron G. Arginine enhances wound healing and lymphocyte immune responses in humans. *Surgery.* 1990;108:331-337.

11. Kirk SJ, Hurson M, Regan MC, Holt DR, Wasserkrug HL, Barbul A. Arginine stimulates wound healing and immune function in elderly human beings. *Surgery.* 1993;114:155-159.

12. Levenson SM, Demetriou AA. Metabolic factors. In: Cohen IK, Diegelmann RF, Lindbald WJ, eds. *Wound Healing: Biochemical and Clinical Aspects.* Philadelphia, Pa: WB Saunders Co; 1992:248-273.

13. Wound Healing. In: Gottschlich MM, Matarese LE, Shronts EP, eds. *Nutrition Support Dietetics Core Curriculum.* 2nd ed. Silver Spring, Md: ASPEN Publications; 1993:403.

14. *Pressure Ulcer Prevention and Intervention: A Role for Nutrition.* Columbus, Ohio: Ross Products Division, Abbott Laboratories; May 1994.

15. Riet G, Kessels AG, Knipschild PG. Randomized clinical trial of ascorbic acid in the treatment of pressure ulcers. *J Clin Epidemiol.* 1995;48:1453-1460.

16. Levenson SM, Demetriou AA. Metabolic factors. In: Cohen IK, Diegelmann RF, Lindbald WJ, eds. *Wound Healing: Biochemical and Clinical Aspects.* Philadelphia, Pa: WB Saunders Co; 1992:248-273.

17. Institute of Medicine. *Dietary Reference Intakes for Vitamin C, Vitamin E, Selenium, and Carotenoids.* Washington DC: National Academy Press; 2000.

18. Andrews M, Gallagher-Allred C. The role of zinc in wound healing. *Adv Wound Care.* 1999;12:137-138.

19. Haggard J, Houston MS, Williford JH, Meserve LA, Shewokis P. Retrospective study of the effects of zinc supplementation in an elderly institutionalized population with decubitus ulcers [abstract]. *J Am Diet Assoc.* 1999;99(suppl):A11.

20. Fosmire GJ. Zinc toxicity. *Am J Clin Nutr.* 1990;51:225-227.

21. Thomas DR. The role of nutrition in prevention and healing of pressure ulcers. *Clin Geriatr Med.* 1997;13:497-511.

22. Omnibus Budget Reconciliation Act of 1987. Nursing Home Reform Legislation, 1987. Interpretive Guidelines: Transmittal #274. *State Operations Manual.* June 1995.

23. Pressure Ulcer Scale for Healing (PUSH Tool 3.0). National Pressure Ulcer Advisory Panel. 1997. Available at: http://www.npuap.org/push3-0.htm. Accessed March 11, 2004.

24. Feinsod FM, Levenson SA. The importance of differentiating pressure sores from other skin ulcers. *Nursing Home Med.* 1997;5:216-219.

25. Reiber GE. Diabetic foot care. *Diabetes Care.* 1992;15:29-31.

ADDITIONAL RESOURCES

Long CL, Nelson KM, Akin JM Jr, Geiger JW, Merrick HW, Blakemore WZ. A physiologic basis for the provision of fuel mixtures in normal and stressed patients. *J Trauma.* 1990;30:1077-1085.

Panel for the Prediction and Prevention of Pressure Ulcers in Adults. *Clinical Practice Guideline Number 3: Pressure Ulcers in Adults: Prediction and Prevention.* Rockville, Md: US Dept of Health and Human Services, Agency for Health Care Policy and Research; 1994;18. AHCPR publication 92-0047.

Pressure Ulcer Treatment Clinical Practice Guidelines. (Quick Reference No. 15). Rockville, Md: US Dept of Health and Human Services, Agency for Health Care Policy and Research; 1994. AHCPR publication 95-0650.

CHAPTER 21

Hydration

The importance of maintaining fluid homeostasis for older adults is well known. Because dehydration is such a persistent problem for institutionalized older adults, in 1999 the Healthcare Financing Administration (HCFA; now known as the Centers for Medicare & Medicaid Services [CMS]) identified hydration as one of four quality indicators (QI) to be especially scrutinized during surveys of nursing facilities (1). Additionally, CMS identified dehydration as a sentinel event—a QI that represents a significant problem, even if it affects only one or a few residents. Because of the negative outcomes associated with dehydration, dietetics professionals and other health care professionals must carefully assess hydration status, estimate fluid needs, and ensure that clients get adequate and appropriate fluids.

NORMAL HYDRATION STATUS AND DEHYDRATION

Normal hydration status refers to the state in which the body has sufficient water in the right locations and contains the right ratios and amounts of electrolytes (eg, sodium and potassium) (2). Box 21.1 lists organs and body systems that may influence the balance of fluids and electrolytes.

Dehydration is an umbrella term used to describe three fluid-electrolyte-volume-deficit disorders. *Hypertonic dehydration,* also called "water deficit," "volume depletion," or "hypernatremic dehydration," occurs when water losses are greater than sodium losses (3).

Hypertonic dehydration can occur whenever clients lose body water, as with fever; elevated environmental temperature; therapies such as air-fluidized beds and dry oxygen; and medications such as diuretics, laxatives, and cardiac glycosides. Inadequate staffing (4), infirmity, functional dependence, demen-

---

Box 21.1   Organs and Body Systems That May Influence Fluid/Electrolyte Balance

- Central and autonomic nervous system
- Heart and circulation
- Urinary system (including kidneys, ureter and bladder)
- Digestive system (including intestines and liver)
- Skin (including sweat glands)
- Lungs and respiratory system
- Endocrine system (including pituitary, thyroid and adrenal glands)

Source: Reprinted from American Medical Directors Association. *Dehydration and Fluid Maintenance. Clinical Practice Guideline.* Columbia, MD: American Medical Directors Association; 2001:3, with permission from American Medical Directors Association. Copyright © 2001, American Medical Directors Association. All rights reserved.

---

tia, and reduced consciousness can also contribute to hypertonic dehydration, because these conditions can inhibit clients' water intake.

The other two types of dehydration occur when there are aberrations in water and electrolyte balance. *Isotonic dehydration* results when equal amounts of body water and sodium are lost. Gastrointestinal (GI) fluid losses, through diarrhea, vomiting, or excessive GI ostomy output, put people at risk for isotonic dehydration. This risk is due to the fact that loss of GI fluids results in loss of water and electrolytes.

Hypotonic dehydration, also called "water and electrolyte deficit," "hyponatremic dehydration," or "volume and electrolyte depletion," occurs when sodium loss exceeds water loss. In older adults, hypotonic dehydration can occur when diuretics are used along with a low-sodium diet. Other causes include glucocorticoid deficiency, hypothyroidism, and syndrome of inappropriate antidiuretic hormone secretion (5). It is very important to determine the type of dehydration, because treatment depends on correct identification (6).

THE MAGNITUDE OF THE DEHYDRATION PROBLEM AMONG OLDER ADULTS

An early report cited dehydration as the most common fluid and electrolyte disorder among older nursing home residents, giving the incidence at nearly 35% (7). Another early report claimed that more than half of patients hospitalized with a diagnosis of dehydration came from nursing homes (8). Data from 1981 showed that outcome for those hospitalized with dehydration and infection was grim; the mortality rate for these patients was nearly 50% (9). There are few data available about the prevalence of dehydration today. Implementation of the Resident Assessment Instrument in 1993 was associated with a significant decline in prevalence, compared with prevalence in 1990 (10). Still, the problem of dehydration persists. In 1991, dehydration was listed as one of the five reported diagnoses in 731,695 Medicare hospitalizations (11). The 2000 National Hospital Discharge Survey showed that 261,000 people aged 65 years and older were discharged in 2000 with a *primary* diagnosis of volume depletion (12).

Studies demonstrate that older residents routinely do not consume enough fluid (4,13,14). In one study, researchers found that only 1 in 40 older residents consumed an adequate amount of liquids (4).

DEHYDRATION RISK FACTORS

The majority of total body weight is from water: 50% in women and 60% in men. Two thirds of the body's water is intracellular; the remaining third is extracellular, distributed between the intravascular (4% of total body weight) and interstitial (16% of total body weight) spaces. Extracellular fluid travels easily between the two spaces, regulated by blood pressure and colloid osmotic pressure. Sodium, the major extracellular ion, is the primary osmotic parti-

cle maintaining total body water volume and the ratio between extracellular and intracellular fluid volume. In response to sodium concentration, water can rapidly cross cell membranes to maintain equal osmolality between the intracellular and extracellular spaces. When sodium concentration increases, so does extracellular fluid volume. When sodium concentration decreases, extracellular fluid volume contracts (15).

Normally, daily water intake equals daily water output. Daily fluid intake can come from food, beverages, liquids, medical nutritional products, intravenous fluids, and water produced when nutrients are metabolized. Daily fluid output is made up of insensible losses from perspiration and pulmonary evaporative losses (920 to 1,000 mL), stool (80 to 100 mL), and urine (500 to 1,400 mL) (16).

When fluid intake is insufficient, normally the kidneys reduce urine output to as little as 500 mL daily, but the lungs and skin continue to lose up to 1,000 mL of water. When a negative fluid balance occurs, blood osmolality rises (16).

Because maintaining normal blood osmolality (280 mOsm/kg H_2O) is vital, the body has a number of mechanisms for ensuring water balance. A change in blood osmolality as small as 1% to 2% causes the hypothalamus to secrete vasopressin. Vasopressin stimulates thirst and a powerful urge to drink. At the same time, the pituitary gland secretes antidiuretic hormone (ADH), which causes the kidney to concentrate urine and minimize urine volume (15). Because of the relationship between sodium and fluid volume, body sodium content is an important factor in controlling body water. A number of mechanisms regulate body sodium. The kidneys filter about 25,000 mEq of sodium daily. Most of this sodium is reabsorbed. In the face of extracellular fluid depletion, the adrenal cortex secretes aldosterone, causing the kidneys to reabsorb even more sodium. Conversely, extracellular fluid expansion stimulates secretion of atrial natriuretic factor (ANF), which increases glomerular filtration rate and reduces sodium reabsorption by the kidneys (15). Box 21.2 (1) lists risk factors for dehydration and fluid/electrolyte imbalance.

THE EFFECTS OF AGING

Older adults are less resistant than younger adults to negative fluid balance. Physiological, medical, environmental, and situational factors increase older adults' vulnerability to dehydration.

Box 21.2   Conditions and Factors That May Increase Risk for Dehydration or Fluid/Electrolyte Imbalance

Critical Conditions

- Dementia or cognitive impairment
- Fever (including low-grade fever)
- Diarrhea
- Vomiting
- Dependence on staff for eating and drinking
- Use of medications that can cause dehydration (eg, diuretics, phenytoin, lithium, laxatives)
- Draining wounds or pressure ulcers
- Excessive sweating
- Rapid breathing
- Gastrointestinal bleeding
- Previous episodes of dehydration
- Difficult or painful swallowing
- Depression
- Small amount of dark or concentrated urine

- Excessive urination
- Nothing-by-mouth or fluid-restriction orders
- Chronic comorbidities (eg, stroke, diabetes, congestive heart failure)
- Infection
- Dizziness

Environmental Factors

- Tube feeding
- Use of specialty beds
- Lack of social or family support
- Inadequate staffing
- Language barriers
- Isolation
- Restraints
- Facility-specific factors that may expose patients to excessive heat (eg, malfunctioning air conditioners)

Source: Reprinted from American Medical Directors Association. *Dehydration and Fluid Maintenance. Clinical Practice Guideline.* Columbia, MD: American Medical Directors Association; 2001:11, with permission from American Medical Directors Association. Copyright © 2001, American Medical Directors Association. All rights reserved.

Physiological Factors

Aging is associated with reduced thirst perception. Older adults do not feel as thirsty, and they do not drink as much in response to volume depletion as do younger people. Consequently, they do not respond to fluid deprivation and blood hyperosmolality by voluntarily increasing fluid intake (17). Kidney function declines with aging. Aged kidneys are less able to concentrate urine (18). Also, ill older adults are less able to respond to vasopressin (19).

Total body water also declines with aging. Age is associated with decreased total body water, which increases risk of cellular dehydration (20).

Medical Factors

A number of medical conditions and therapies interfere with fluid homeostasis. One study (21) identified the following factors associated with volume depletion:

- Febrile illness
- Infirmity

- Surgery
- High-protein diets
- High-solute intravenous fluids
- Diabetes
- Diarrhea
- GI bleeding
- Diuretics
- Renal dialysis

Older adults are especially prone to infections (22). Infections account for up to 25% of acute hospitalizations or emergency room visits for this group (23). Fevers associated with infections increase insensible losses through perspiration, respiration, and increased metabolism. Water losses increase by 100 to 150 mL/day for each degree of temperature above 37°C (98.6°F) (24).

Polypharmacy has been associated with dehydration in older people. Some medications, such as diuretics and cardiovascular agents, contribute directly to the risk of dehydration. The antiseizure medication phenytoin interferes with the action of vasopressin (25). Other classes of medications indirectly contribute to dehydration risk. Sedative and ethanol use in older adults, as well as conditions that depress the level of consciousness, can interfere with adequate intake of fluids.

GI fluid losses due to vomiting, bleeding, nasogastric and fistula draining, laxative abuse, and diarrhea increase risk of dehydration. Unless additional fluid is given, high-solute IVs and high-protein intakes can cause dehydration, because they increase renal solute load, which increases fluid needed for urinary excretion of solute. Urine volume must parallel renal solute load. In adults, each gram of protein theoretically contributes 5.7 mOsm to renal solute load (26).

Environmental Factors

Older adults are very sensitive to heat-related fluid losses, especially in conditions of elevated ambient temperature or low humidity (27). Other causes of evaporative fluid losses that may not be well recognized include use of dry oxygen and air-fluidized beds (28).

Situational Factors

Older adults often depend on others to meet their needs for fluid. When staffing is inadequate, older nursing-facility clients often do not get enough fluid (4).

ASSESSING HYDRATION STATUS

Because dehydration is associated with significant morbidity and mortality in older adults, CMS launched a Nutrition/Hydration Awareness Campaign, to call attention to early warning signs of unintended weight loss and dehydration among residents of long-term-care facilities (29). See Box 21.3 for a list of indicators of dehydration.

In 2001, the American Medical Directors Association (AMDA) published dehydration and fluid maintenance clinical practice guidelines (1). These guidelines state that, for a clinical diagnosis of dehydration to be made, the following minimal criteria must be present:

- Suspicion of increased output and/or decreased intake
- At least two physiologic or functional signs or symptoms suggesting dehydration (eg, dizziness, dry mucous membrane, functional decline)

Box 21.3 Indicators of Risk or Presence of Dehydration

- Has one or more of the following:
  - Change in mental status
  - Cracked lips
  - Diarrhea
  - Dry mouth
  - Fever
  - Postural hypotension
  - Pulse >100 beats per minute and/or systolic blood pressure < 100 mmHg
  - Recent, rapid weight loss
  - Small amounts of dark urine
  - Sunken eyes
  - Urinary tract infection
  - Vomiting
- Needs help drinking from a cup or glass
- Drinks less than 6 cups of liquids daily
- Trouble swallowing liquids
- Easily confused/tired
- Lethargic/weak
- Falls frequently
- Increased combativeness/confusion
- Change in abilities to perform activities of daily living (ADL)

- A BUN:creatinine ratio of > 25:1 *or* orthostasis (defined as a drop in systolic blood pressure ≥ 20 mmHg with a change in position) *or* a pulse of > 100 beats/minute *or* a pulse change of 10 to 20 beats/minute above baseline with a change in position

The dilemma with using either the CMS criteria or the AMDA guidelines is that, by the time these nonspecific signs and symptoms appear, an older person is already dehydrated. Because older adults develop dehydration readily and are slow to respond to therapy, it is vital to not wait for signs and symptoms to appear but to act as soon as conditions associated with increased fluid need or loss are recognized.

PREVENTING AND TREATING DEHYDRATION

Preventing dehydration is preferable to treating it. The first step is to estimate fluid needs. A number of equations for estimating fluid needs are available (13), but the simplest method is to estimate a baseline of 30 mL of water per kilogram of body weight, (making sure to provide a minimum of 1,500 to 2,000 mL), and adjust per individual need (30). (See Box 21.4 [31].)

The dietetics professional should make sure that the appropriate type of fluid is provided. In cases of evaporative fluid loss, water from beverages, food, medical nutritional supplements, tube feedings, or IVs is the appropriate replacement fluid. When GI fluid is lost, however, water and electrolytes must be replaced, because both water and electrolytes have been lost. An oral rehydration solution (32) or an appropriate IV solution can be used.

Overhydration leading to congestive heart failure is rare, especially when the oral/enteral route is used. However, cardiac and pulmonary monitoring should be done to detect fluid overload in clients with a history of cardiac problems.

Box 21.4   Adult Fluid Requirements

Hydration status as a part of nutritional status is often overlooked. This can affect interpretation of biochemical measurements, anthropometry and the physical exam. Assessment of hydration is quick and easy and should include assessment of fluid intake.

Method I: Wt (kg) x 30 mL = Daily Fluid Requirement
Fluid requirements may differ for those clients with cardiac problems, renal failure, dehydration or for those requiring fluid restrictions.

Method II: 100 mL/kg for 1st ten kg body weight
+ 50 mL/kg for 2nd ten kg body weight
+ 15 mL/kg for remaining kg body weight

Shortcut Method II:
[(kg body weight – 20) x 15] + 1500 = mL fluid requirement

Source: Reprinted from Chidester JC, Spangler AA. Fluid intake in the institutionalized elderly. *J Am Diet Assoc.* 1997;97:23-28, with permission from American Dietetic Association.

SUMMARY

Because of factors associated with aging, older adults are at special risk for developing dehydration. Preventing dehydration is key to good outcomes. Dietetics professionals and other health care professionals can help improve the quality of their older clients' lives by responding to risk factors and intervening before the development of overt signs and symptoms of dehydration.

REFERENCES

1. Advocate of Nonprofit Services for Older Ohioans. HCFA changes to survey process. Available at: http://www.aopha.org/pubpolicy/som10sum.htm. Accessed March 20, 2004.
2. American Medical Directors Association. *Dehydration and Fluid Maintenance: Clinical Practice Guideline.* Columbia, Md: American Medical Directors Association; 2001.
3. Reese J. Fluid volume deficit: 1 and 2. In: Maas M, Buckwalter KC, Hardy MA, eds. *Nursing Diagnoses and Interventions for the Elderly.* Redwood City, Calif: Addison-Wesley Nursing; 1991:131-142.
4. Kayser-Jones J, Schell ES, Porter C, Barbaccia JC, Shaw H. Factors contributing to dehydration in nursing homes: inadequate staffing and lack of professional supervision. *J Am Geriatr Soc.* 1999;47:1269-1270.
5. Krugler JP. Hyponatremia and hypernatremia in the elderly. *Am Fam Physician.* 2000;61:3623-3630.
6. Mange K, Matsuura D, Cizman B, Soto H, Ziyadeh FN, Goldfarb S, Neilson EG. Language guiding therapy: the case of dehydration versus volume depletion. *Ann Intern Med.* 1997;127:848-853.
7. Lavizzo-Mourey R, Johnson J, Stolley P. Risk factors for dehydration among elderly nursing home residents. *J Am Geriatr Soc.* 1988;36:213-218.
8. Himmelstein DU, Jones AA, Woolhandler S. Hypernatremic dehydration in nursing home patients: an indicator of neglect. *J Am Geriatr Soc.* 1983;31:466-471.
9. Mahowald JM, Himmelstein DU. Hypernatremia in the elderly: relation to infection and mortality. *J Am Geriatr Soc.* 1981;29:177-180.
10. Fries BE, Hawes C, Morris JN, Phillips CD, Mor V, Park PS. Effect of the National Resident Assessment Instrument on selected health conditions and problems. *J Am Geriatr Soc.* 1997;45:994-1001.
11. Warren JL, Bacon WE, Harris T, McBean AM, Foley DJ, Phillips C. The burden and outcomes associated with dehydration among US elderly, 1991. *Am J Public Health.* 1994;84:1265-1269.
12. Hall MJ, Owings MF. 2000 National Hospital Discharge Survey. *Adv Data.* 2002;329:1-18.
13. Kleiner SM. Water: an essential but overlooked nutrient. *J Am Diet Assoc.* 1999;99:200-206.
14. Holben DH, Hassell JT, Williams JL, Helle B. Fluid intake compared with established standards and symptoms of dehydration among elderly residents of a long-term care facility. *J Am Diet Assoc.* 1999;99:1447-1450.

15. Rose BD, Post TW. *Clinical Physiology of Acid-Base and Electrolyte Disorders*. 5th ed. New York, NY: McGraw-Hill Inc; 2001.

16. Water and Sodium Metabolism. Available at: http://www.merck.com/mrkshared/mamanual/section2/chapter12/12b.jsp. Accessed November 11, 2003.

17. Kenney WL, Chiu P. Influence of age on thirst and fluid intake. *Med Sci Sports Exerc*. 2001;33:1524-1532.

18. Rowe JW, Shock NW, Defronzo RA. The influence of age on the renal deprivation in man. *Nephron*. 1976;17:270-278.

19. Sonnenblick M, Algur N. Hypernatremia in the acutely ill elderly patients: role of impaired arginine-vasopressin secretion. *Miner Electrolyte Metab*. 1993;19:32-35.

20. Ritz P. Investigators of the Source Study and of the Human Nutrition Centre-Auvergne. Chronic cellular dehydration in the aged patient. *J Gerontol*. 2001;56:M349-M352.

21. Snyder NA, Feigal DW, Arieff AI. Hypernatremia in elderly patients: a heterogeneous, morbid, and iatrogenic entity. *Ann Intern Med*. 1987;107:309-319.

22. Louria DB, Sen P, Sherer CB, Farrer WE. Infections in older patients: a systematic clinical approach. *Geriatrics*. 1993;48:28-34.

23. Warshaw G, Mehdizadeh S, Applebaum RA. Infections in nursing homes: assessing quality of care. *J Gerontol A Biol Sci Med Sci*. 2001;56:M120-M123.

24. O'Shea MH. Fluid and electrolyte management. In: Woodley M, Whelan A, eds. *Manual of Medical Therapeutics*. Boston, Mass: Little, Brown and Co; 1992:42-61.

25. Davis KM, Minaker KL. Disorders of fluid and electrolyte balance. In: Hazzard WR, Andres R, Bierman EEL, Blass JP, eds. *Principles of Geriatric Medicine and Gerontology*. New York, NY: McGraw-Hill; 1990:1079-1083.

26. Foman SJ, Ziegler EE. Water and renal solute load. In: Foman SJ (ed). *Nutrition of Normal Infants*. St Louis, Mo: Mosby; 1993:91-102.

27. Worfolk JB. Heat waves: their impact on the health of elders. *Geriatr Nurs*. 2001;21:70-77.

28. Breslow RA. Nutrition and air-fluidized beds: a literature review. *Adv Wound Care*. 1994;7:57-58,60,62.

29. Nursing Homes, Nursing Home Awareness Campaigns. Nutrition and hydration awareness: nutrition care alerts. Medicare Web site. Available at: http://www.medicare.gov/Nursing/Campaigns/NutriCareAlerts.asp. Accessed March 11, 2004.

30. Chernoff R. Meeting the nutritional needs of the elderly in the institutionalized setting. *Nutr Rev*. 1994;52:132-136.

31. Chidester JC, Spangler AA. Fluid intake in the institutionalized elderly. *J Am Diet Assoc*. 1997;97:23-28.

32. Bennett RG. Oral rehydration therapy for older adults. *Diet Currents*. 1992;19:1-4.

CHAPTER 22

Involuntary Weight Loss

Involuntary weight loss (IWL) that continues unchecked week after week is clearly detrimental to the health and welfare of the older adult, particularly one who resides in a nursing facility (1). Typically, a resident of a nursing facility with IWL also loses critical lean body mass (2) and is more prone to falls, nonhealing wounds, dehydration, decreased immune system response, and failure to thrive (3). Also, the health care facility is more prone to inspection citations and litigation for malnutrition and dehydration (4). The problems of IWL and protein-energy malnutrition (PEM) are often underappreciated in the United States, because more attention is generally focused on the treatment of obesity. IWL, however, adversely affects a significant portion of ill and infirm older adults across the continuum of care. Box 22.1 outlines conditions often associated with anorexia or weight loss (5).

DEFINING INVOLUNTARY WEIGHT LOSS

Involuntary weight loss is defined as any unplanned weight loss from the usual adult body weight. This weight loss may occur slowly over time or have a rapid onset. The Centers for Medicare & Medicaid Services (CMS; formerly Health Care Finance Administration [HCFA]) Minimum Data Set, version 2.0 (MDS 2.0), which oversees long-term-care facilities, defines clinically significant weight loss as a loss of 5% of usual body weight in a period of 30 days or a 10% weight loss in 180 days (6). To determine the percentage of weight loss, the following formula is used:

$$\frac{\text{Usual Wt} - \text{Current Wt}}{\text{Usual Weight}} \times 100 = \% \text{ Wt Loss}$$

For example, if a person usually weighs 110 pounds and currently weighs 103 pounds, this person has lost

Box 22.1 Conditions Often Associated With Anorexia or Weight Loss

- Dementia/delirium
- Depression
- Chronic pain
- Constipation
- Use of multiple medications
- Chronic infections
- End-stage major organ system disease
- Terminal illness

Source: Reprinted from American Medical Directors Association. *Altered Nutritional Status: Clinical Practice Guideline.* Columbia, Md: American Medical Directors Association; 2001:3, with permission from American Medical Directors Association. Copyright © 1998 American Medical Directors Association. All rights reserved.

6.4% of his or her body weight. If this occurred over a 1-month period, it would be considered a clinically significant weight loss that requires appropriate intervention and documentation.

Downward weight trends should be considered significant, even if they do not precisely meet the CMS criterion. A person's weight will often fluctuate week to week due to fluid retention, the time of day the weight was obtained, or other temporary factors. After several weeks, the true trend should be apparent, and if the client has demonstrated a slow and steady decline, prompt nutrition intervention is warranted. Table 22.1 traces a downward weight trend. In this example, the client has not

TABLE 22.1. Example of a Downward Weight Trend

Date	Weight (lb)
July 1	135
August 1	132 (30 days = 2.2% loss)
September 1	129
October 1	127
November 1	125
December 1	123 (180 days = 8.9% loss)

TABLE 22.2. General Guidelines for Calculation of Nutritional Requirements

Calories	*kcal/kg/day*
Normal	25-30
PEM*	30-35
Critically ill or injured*	35-40
Protein	*g/kg/day*
RDA	0.8
PEM*	1.5
Critically ill or injured*	1.5-2.0
Fat	< 30% kcal
Water	1 L/1000 kcal

Abbreviations: PEM, protein-energy malnutrition; RDA, recommended dietary allowance.

*Nutrient supplementation required.

Source: Reprinted with permission from Collins N. Involuntary weight loss in the long-term care setting: a suggested nutritional intervention treatment algorithm. *Wounds.* 2001;13(4 Suppl D):32D-37D.

met the CMS criterion for a 10% weight loss in 180 days but has clearly entered a downward spiral that requires nutrition intervention.

THE STRESS RESPONSE

When the body is under stress, either physical or psychological, there is an amplification of the fright-flight response. For example, the stressor may be a disease, such as human immunodeficiency virus (HIV), cancer, a burn or other wound, or any chronic illness. The initial insult leads to local and generalized inflammation and an increase in the level of the stress hormones, particularly catecholamines and cortisol (1). Concurrently, there is a decrease in levels of anabolic hormones, such as human growth hormone and testosterone. This imbalance in the hormonal milieu leads to a catabolic and hypermetabolic state.

A catabolic state is one in which the body breaks down components in order to release energy to meet increased energy demands. Imagine the body working much harder and faster than usual to fight off the stressor and regain homeostasis or balance. Working harder and faster means an increase in the metabolic rate (hypermetabolic) and an increase in body temperature. To keep up this pace, the body needs an increased supply of glucose, which may come from gluconeogenesis or by rapidly breaking down lean body mass as a means to get more energy. If this cycle continues for an extended period of time, the person will lose weight and, more importantly, lean body mass. The loss of lean body mass leads to many complications, including increased susceptibility to infection, decreased healing, and pneumonia. As the catabolism of lean body mass progresses, the medical complications escalate. If a 40% loss of lean body mass is reached, death will result, usually from pneumonia (2).

GOALS OF NUTRITION INTERVENTION

The goals of nutrition intervention for IWL are to maintain or replete lean body mass and to meet the daily energy and protein needs of the older adult. It is important to distinguish between lean body mass and fat mass. Lean body mass is the metabolically active component of the body and contains all the skeletal and smooth muscles, collagen, enzymes, and viscera (7). Fat mass is the metabolically inactive energy reserve. Obese clients who lose weight due to a stress response typically lose lean body mass and retain their fat reserves (8). It is imperative to recognize that the energy and protein needs of stressed older adults are higher than those of healthy individuals. Table 22.2 summarizes the guidelines for calculating energy, protein, and fluid needs for different populations (8-10).

NUTRITION PROTOCOLS

Every health care facility should have a nutrition protocol in place to treat IWL. Protocols have also been called maps, pathways, treatment algorithms, and policies.

Although the names may be slightly different, the goal remains the same—to have a well-defined plan in place to treat IWL promptly and efficiently. Often IWL is treated haphazardly, with no systematic course of treatment defined. This can lead to negative client outcomes, and it leaves the facility open for liability. It is much more effective to have a prescribed course of treatment that outlines a progressive and orderly implementation of nutrition interventions.

A protocol should be administratively manageable, cost effective, legally defensible, and current with the scientific developments in the field of nutrition. An administratively manageable protocol is one that is clear and easily understood by all personnel. It is cost effective because it does not use excessive amounts of time for documentation. A properly designed plan begins with the least costly, least invasive nutrition interventions first and advances to the more costly and more invasive interventions only as needed. Close monitoring is designed into the protocol, to achieve the best possible outcome with the least cost. The protocol is legally defensible by being based on the latest scientific evidence and compliant with all current regulations. It should be instituted in a timely manner for all and should allow for individualization depending on a specific resident's needs. Finally, the protocol must take into account the new developments and products available to treat IWL. Each month, new breakthroughs and clinical trial results are available that impact the standard of care. Thus, the protocol should be reviewed at periodic intervals, to make certain that it reflects the most current treatment methods.

INCREASING INTAKE WITH FOOD

Once IWL has been identified, action is needed immediately. All interventions must be documented in the medical record in a clear and concise manner. Each step of the plan of care must be communicated to the care plan team, the physician, the resident, and the resident's family.

After IWL is identified, the first step is to determine whether the gastrointestinal system is functional. If the gut is nonfunctional, parenteral nutrition should be used, if consistent with advance directives. In most cases, however, this is not the cause of IWL, and other factors must be examined. In the first level of intervention, the dining situation and meal environment should be examined, in an effort to increase meal consumption. Adequate nutritional substrate must be consumed in order to meet energy and protein needs. In long-term care, all residents should be encouraged to dine in the dining room rather than in their room. Isolation can occur in the room, and supervision is far more difficult if residents are eating in several locations.

Often, residents are asked to state their dining preference immediately upon admission to a facility. At this time, many older adults are ill at ease or depressed and state that they will stay in their room for meals. After adjusting to their new surroundings, many residents will then change their decision and venture out to the dining room. Staff must check back with residents once the adjustment to the facility has been made.

The dining room should be a pleasant and enjoyable place to dine, without the distraction of loud televisions or other noises. Each resident should be seated at a table of appropriate height to promote self-feeding and with appropriate tablemates to encourage socialization. Assistance should be offered as needed. Many residents require "tray set-up," which includes opening the food packages and arranging the tray on the table, making sure that everything is within reach of the resident. It is important to encourage the use of the smaller tray items, such as butter pats, creamers, and condiments. These items add extra energy and should be added to foods liberally.

Some older adults require total assistance at meals. Assisting these individuals at mealtime is a time-consuming process that cannot be rushed. Residents should be allowed adequate time to chew and swallow. Verbal cues and praise should be used to foster better meal consumption.

At times, inadequate meal intake is the result of unfamiliar foods and unacceptable meal times. Each resident must be asked to list favorite and comfort foods, as well as foods that they wish to avoid. Many parts of the United States have a culturally diverse population with very specific food preferences. Effort should be made to serve foods that meet the cultural needs of older adults. Meals should be served at the standard time usually found in the local community and in accordance with the usual pattern the older adult followed at home. Some people are early risers, and others prefer brunch rather than breakfast. The evening meal is often too early for many when it is served at 5:00 p.m. Policies and procedures must be flexible enough to accommodate the individual preferences of older adults.

TABLE 22.3. Sample Snack and Supplement Rotation Schedule

Day	10:00 AM	2:00 PM	7:00 PM
Monday	High-calorie shake	High-protein cookies	Fortified pudding
Tuesday	Yogurt	Energy bar	High-calorie shake
Wednesday	Fortified pudding	Ice cream	High-protein cookies
Thursday	Energy bar	Yogurt	High-calorie custard
Friday	High-calorie shake	Fortified pudding	Ice cream
Saturday	High-calorie custard	High-calorie shake	Energy bar
Sunday	High-protein cookies	Ice cream	Yogurt

Weekly Number of Servings
Shakes: 4
Cookies: 3
Pudding: 3
Yogurt: 3
Energy bar: 3
Custard: 2
Ice cream: 3

Reprinted with permission from Collins N. Involuntary weight loss in the long-term care setting: a suggested nutritional intervention treatment algorithm. *Wounds.* 2001;13(4 Suppl D):32D-37D.

Snacks are served between meals to provide extra energy and protein. However, if the snacks are served too close to mealtime, the meal intake may be reduced. Care should be taken to space out snacks and meals throughout the day. House supplements are typically liquid beverages or shakes. Most older adults tire quite quickly from the same supplement day after day and would prefer a variety of flavors and textures. A sample supplement schedule is shown in Table 22.3 (10). This demonstrates the use of a variety of products to avoid food and flavor fatigue.

If snacks interfere with meal consumption, a high-energy/high-protein supplement can be served with medications. Instead of using water to swallow pills, 2 ounces of a liquid supplement may be served. If a product containing 2 kcal/mL is used, a 2-ounce serving will provide 120 kcal. If medicines are given three or four times per day, the total energy intake with medications will be 360 or 480 additional kcal (5).

Additional protein can be provided in many ways. Hard-boiled eggs are a cost-effective and easy snack that provides additional energy and protein. Adding an extra ounce of the entree at each meal is another way to encourage higher protein intake. Protein powder may be added to prepared food and is usually well accepted. There are many commercially available protein powders that provide high-quality protein in a ready-to-use form.

A hidden cause of poor intake may be food-drug interactions or the timing of medication administration. It is important to review and evaluate the older adult's medication list and determine whether this may be interfering with proper oral intake (11). Box 22.2 lists several common drugs that are associated with IWL and anorexia (12).

PHARMACEUTICAL INTERVENTIONS

If meal intake has not improved and IWL continues even after all environmental and food factors have been corrected, it is time to advance the interventions along the continuum of care. In order to ensure that 100% of the RDAs are met each day, a daily multivitamin and mineral supplement should be considered (5).

APPETITE STIMULANTS

As the name suggests, an appetite stimulant helps improve or regain the older adult's desire to eat. People with many different conditions may benefit from an appetite stimulant. Older adults with altered mental status, significant weight loss, or a

Box 22.2   Drugs Associated With Involuntary Weight Loss and Anorexia

- Amlodipine
- Ciprofloxacin
- Conjugated estrogens
- Corticosteroids
- Digoxin
- Enalapril maleate
- Esomeprazole magnesium
- Famotidine
- Fentanyl transdermal system
- Furosemide
- Ipratropium bromide
- Levothyroxine sodium
- Narcotic analgesic
- Nifedipine
- Nizatidine
- Omeprazole
- Paroxetine HCl
- Phenytoin
- Potassium replacement
- Propoxyphene
- Ranitidine HCl
- Risperidone
- Sertraline HCl
- Warfarin

Adapted with permission from Council for Nutrition Clinical Strategies in LTC Web site. Available at: http://www.ltcnutrition.org/anorexia/treatable.cfm. Accessed April 7, 2003.

developed dislike for eating due to an illness or certain medications are often given an appetite stimulant to maintain or gain body weight and to prevent the immune system from deteriorating.

Many products are used as appetite stimulants. Table 22.4 outlines the products commonly used (13). Dronabinol (Marinol, Unimed Pharmaceuticals, Inc., Marietta, GA 30062) is a synthetic delta-9-tetrahydrocannabinol (delta-9-THC). Delta-9-THC is also a naturally occurring component and is found in marijuana. The indication for dronabinol is anorexia associated with weight loss in patients with AIDS and for the nausea and vomiting associated with cancer chemotherapy in those clients who have failed to respond to conventional antiemetic treatments. Dronabinol is an oral drug that can be prescribed in dosages that range from 2.5 to 20 mg per day (14). The lowest effective dose should be used. It is recommended to begin with 2.5 mg twice per day and to measure the therapeutic effect of the drug before increasing to a higher dose.

Megestrol acetate, marketed as Megace Oral Suspension (Bristol-Myers Squibb Company, Princeton, NJ 08543), contains a synthetic derivative of the naturally occurring steroid hormone progesterone. Each mL of the oral suspension contains 40 mg of micronized megestrol acetate. Megace is indicated for the treatment of anorexia, cachexia, or unexplained, significant weight loss in patients with a diagnosis of AIDS. It is also used to treat metastatic endometrial and breast cancer and has been shown to improve appetite and weight (15). It is important to prescribe Megace at the recommended dose of 20 mL (800 mg) once per day. Some residents may see an improvement in appetite in a short period of time, but the drug should be administered for 8 to 12 weeks to fully evaluate weight change and appetite improvement (16).

Cyproheptadine, formerly marketed under the brand name Periactin (Zenith Goldline Pharmaceuticals, Miami, FL 33137) but now available in generic form, is an antihistamine. Cyproheptadine blocks the effects of the naturally occurring chemical histamine in the body and is prescribed for the treatment of perennial and seasonal allergic rhinitis, hay fever, and other allergies (17). The therapeutic range is 4 to 20 mg a day, with most of those receiving the drug requiring 12 to 16 mg a day. Periactin is available in both tablet and syrup form. The syrup is used mainly in pediatrics and for those who cannot swallow pills. Although not approved by the Food and Drug Administration (FDA) for appetite stimulation, Periactin is commonly used for this purpose. It has been observed that Periactin increases appetite, but no mechanism of action has yet been determined (18,19).

Eldertonic (Merz Pharmaceuticals, Greensboro, NC 27419) is an over-the-counter, sherry-based beverage that is recommended for older adults experiencing malaise, lack of energy or appetite, weight loss, or other signs of reduced vitality due to surgery, illness, stress, or use of multiple medications (20). It contains a mixture of many vitamins and minerals, including thiamin, riboflavin, B-6, B-12, and zinc.

TABLE 22.4. Common Appetite Stimulants*

Drug*	Components	Form	Dosage	Side Effects
Marinol *Dronabinol*	Delta-9-THC; active ingredient of marijuana	Capsules	2.5-20 mg/day	Euphoria, sleepiness, thinking abnormalities, paranoid reactions, depression, nightmares, flushing, vision difficulties
Megace *Megestrol acetate*	Female hormone derivative; progesterone	Oral suspension	800 mg/day (20 mL/day)	Hyperglycemia, glucose intolerance, nausea, vomiting, mood changes, lethargy, sweating, rash, water retention, bloating
Periactin *Cyproheptadine*	Calcium phosphate, lactose, magnesium stearate, and starch	Tablet or syrup	4-20 mg/day, most patients require 12-16 mg/day	Drowsiness, dizziness, dry mouth, throat, and nose, thickening of mucus in nose or throat
Eldertonic	B vitamins and minerals	Liquid	One tablespoon (15 mL) 3 times daily	None listed
Remeron *Mirtazapine*	Hydroxypropyl cellulose, magnesium stearate, lactose	Tablet	15-mg single dose, usually before bedtime; maximum dose is 45 mg/day	Drowsiness, decreased alertness, weight gain, increased appetite, dizziness, dry mouth, constipation, edema, urinary frequency

Note: Appetite stimulation is not noted on the product labeling. Although off-label usage is common, the clinician should be fully aware of the product labeling and the research supporting additional usages.

*Marinol is a registered trademark of Unimed Pharmaceuticals, Inc., Marietta, GA 30062. Megace is a registered trademark of Bristol-Myers Squibb Co., Princeton, NJ 08543. Periactin is a registered trademark of Zenith Goldine, Miami, FL 33109. Eldertonic is a registered trademark of Merz Pharmaceuticals, Greensboro, NC 27419. Remeron is a registered trademark of Organon Inc., USA, West Orange, NJ 07052.

Source: Adapted with permission from Collins N, Schafer P. Appetite stimulants: an overview. *Ext Care Prod News.* January/February 2002:1,16-17.

The usual dose for Eldertonic is one tablespoon (15 mL) three times daily, with or before meals (21).

Mirtazapine tablets, known as Remeron (Organon, Inc., West Orange, NJ 07052), is a commonly prescribed antidepressant, usually used with "major depression," a continuously depressed mood that interferes with everyday life. Remeron is thought to correct the chemical imbalance found in depression by increasing the release of both norepinephrine and serotonin from nerve cells in the brain. It is often taken as a 15-mg tablet in a single dose before bedtime. The maximum dose is 45 mg. The most common side effects are drowsiness, decreased alertness, and an increased appetite and weight gain (22).

CONCERNS WITH APPETITE STIMULANTS

Since the goal of an appetite stimulant is for the older adult to eat more food, careful attention should be paid to individuals with diabetes. An increase in food intake means an increase in blood sugar. If the dosage of insulin is not adjusted, the older adult will most likely develop high blood sugar and the accompanying side effects. Physicians and other health care team members should monitor the blood sugar levels of diabetics regularly, especially if treatment with an appetite stimulant is prescribed. Proper adjustment of the diabetic regimen should be made to account for the increased food consumption (15).

Many products commonly prescribed for appetite stimulation have very specific product indications and are often used beyond the approved product labeling. Although this practice of off-label use is very common, the prescriber should be fully aware of the product labeling and the research supporting additional uses. Frequently, the research is anecdotal and, sometimes, off-label uses are not reimbursed.

ANABOLIC AGENTS

Unfortunately, some older adults continue to lose weight despite optimal nutrition interventions. This may be due to changes in the way nutrients are used during the catabolic state. In the presence of the stress response, the normal nutrient partitioning process may be disrupted, particularly for protein. It is theorized that a percentage of the amino acids are diverted from the normal protein partition into the energy partition. There is also a greater net amino acid excretion due to inefficient anabolism (23). In these cases, it may be best to combine the nutrition approach with an anabolic agent.

Anabolic agents work to reverse the catabolic state and return nutrient partitioning to normal. This can allow older adults in a negative nitrogen balance to stop losing nitrogen and to retain it. Anabolic agents are derivatives of testosterone and attenuate the catabolic state by decreasing protein breakdown and increasing protein synthesis. They also improve intracellular reutilization of amino acids, so that nitrogen is retained in the body and not excreted. A successful effort has been made to separate the anabolic activity from the androgenic or virilizing activity of testosterone, which means fewer side effects (7). Although there are several different agents available on the market, oxandrolone (Oxandrin, Savient Pharmaceuticals, East Brunswick, NJ 08816) is widely used, because of its high level of anabolic activity and safety. Oxandrolone has 6.3 times greater anabolic activity than methyltestosterone (24). Oxandrolone also has the status of being the only FDA-approved oral anabolic agent for adjunctive treatment to promote weight gain after IWL due to surgery, chronic infections, or severe trauma, or for any resident who fails to gain or to maintain normal weight. It is also approved to offset the protein catabolism associated with prolonged corticosteroid use (25). Oxandrolone is an oral medication that may be crushed if necessary. It is contraindicated for residents with known or suspected cancer of the prostate or male breast, cancer of the breast in females with hypercalcemia, those with nephrosis or hypercalemia, and during pregnancy. Oxandrolone has not been extensively studied in the long-term-care population.

Anabolic agents such as oxandrolone must have some nutritional substrate on which to exert their mechanism of action. If inadequate nutritional substrate is consumed, an appetite stimulant may be used to encourage a greater oral intake. An alternate means of providing nutritional substrate is via a feeding tube. Feeding-tube placement requires a great deal of thought and consideration on the part of the older adult and the family. Often this topic is avoided until the person has lost considerable weight and must consider this as an immediate option. It would be far more beneficial to educate the older adult and family members on tube feeding procedures at an earlier point in the continuum of care. It is important to explain the progression of interventions in a clear and thorough manner and allow time for questions and discussion. These education sessions must be documented in detail in the medical record, so that the entire care plan team is aware of the plan.

ETHICAL CONSIDERATIONS

If an older adult is in the end stages of a terminal disease, including dementia, the more invasive and more advanced interventions may not be appropriate. At times, it may be that IWL cannot be halted and is an expected part of the disease progression. In these cases, the interventions may only include providing favorite and comfort foods and allowing the resident to enjoy whatever he or she likes. Explaining the effects of continued lean body mass loss and possible dehydration to the resident and family members will help them to understand what may transpire in the future. All discussions of this nature must be documented in the medical record, so that all caregivers can be aware of the wishes and directives of the resident.

SUMMARY

The treatment of IWL is imperative to ensure optimal resident outcomes. IWL is a debilitating illness that must be halted in the early stages. Nutrition interventions should be offered in a logical and well-planned order. It is best to begin with the least costly, least invasive interventions and advance to the newer and cutting-edge technologies only as needed. Dining should be a pleasant and social time, with eye-appealing meals. Food is the first-line intervention, and creative techniques to serve the most nutrient-dense meals should be used. Creativity in snack and supplement programs will also help to maintain resident interest in food. If IWL persists despite optimal intervention or if the older adult is in a severely stressed or catabolic state, an anabolic agent can be used to promote lean body mass synthesis. Feeding tubes are necessary in some instances and should be offered as an option when appropriate. Every health care discipline has a role on the IWL treatment team. It is only through early and aggressive nutrition intervention that the war against IWL can be won.

REFERENCES

1. Himes D. Protein-calorie malnutrition and involuntary weight loss: the role of aggressive nutritional intervention in wound healing. *Ostomy Wound Manage.* 1999;45:46-55.
2. Demling RH, Stasjk L, Zagoren AJ. Protein-energy malnutrition and wounds: nutritional intervention. In: *Treatment of Chronic Wounds Number 10.* Hauppauge, NY: Curative Health Services; 2000:1-10.
3. Morley JE. Nutrition in the elderly. *Curr Opin Gastroenterol.* 2002;18:240-245.
4. US General Accounting Office. *Nursing Homes: Additional Steps Needed to Strengthen Enforcement of Federal Quality Standards.* Washington, DC: US General Accounting Office 1999. Available at: http://www.access.gpo.gov/su_docs/aces/aces160.shtml. Accessed April 7, 2003.
5. American Medical Directors Association. *Altered Nutritional Status: Clinical Practice Guideline.* Columbia, Md: American Medical Directors Association; 2001.
6. *Minimum Data Set. Resident Assessment Instrument for Long Term Care Facilities* [database]. Version 2.0.R-20. Baltimore, Md: Health Care Financing Administration; 1994.
7. Demling RH, DeSanti L. The stress response to injury and infection: role of nutritional support. *Wounds.* 2000;12:3-14.
8. Chang, DW, DeSanti L, Demling RH. Anticatabolic and anabolic strategies in critical illness: a review of current treatment modalities. *Shock.* 1998;10:155-160.
9. DeBiasse MA, Wilmore DW. What is optimal nutrition support? *New Horizons.* 1994;2:122-130.
10. Collins N. Involuntary weight loss in the long-term care setting: a suggested nutritional intervention treatment algorithm. *Wounds.* 2001;13(4 Suppl D):32D-37D.
11. Cicero LA. The nature and management of involuntary weight loss in the elderly. *Consult Pharm.* 2001;16(suppl):1.1-1.6.
12. Council for Nutrition Clinical Strategies in LTC Web site. Available at: http://www.ltcnutrition.org/anorexia/treatable.cfm. Accessed April 7, 2003.
13. Collins N, Schafer P. Appetite stimulants: an overview. *Ext Care Prod News.* January/February 2002:1,16-17.
14. Marinol [package insert]. Marietta, Ga: Unimed Pharmaceuticals, Inc; 2001.
15. Megace [package insert]. Princeton, NJ: Bristol-Myers Squibb Co; 2001.
16. *Megace Oral Suspension: Focus on the Treatment of Age-Related Anorexia and Cachexia: An Interview With Morris Green.* Princeton, NJ: Bristol-Myers Squibb Co; 1998. Current and Future Directions for Elderly Patients in Long-term Care Facilities series.
17. Periactin product literature. Available at: http://www.zenithgoldline.com. Accessed April 7, 2003.
18. William B, Waters D, Parker K. Evaluation and treatment of weight loss on adults with HIV disease. American Academy of Family Physicians 1999. Available at: http://www.aafp.org/afp/990901ap/843.html. Accessed March 20, 2004.
19. Cyproheptadine hydrochloride [package insert]. Spring Valley, NY: Par Pharmaceuticals; 2002. Available at: http://www.parpharm.com/downloads/cyproheptadine_po.pdf. Accessed March 20, 2004.
20. Eldertonic product literature. Available at: http://www.eldertonic.com. Accessed April 7, 2003.
21. Eldertonic dosing schedule. Available at: http://www.eldertonic.com/eldertonic.htm#Eldertonic%20Dosing%20Schedule. Accessed March 10, 2004.
22. Remeron product literature. Available at: http://www.remeronsoltab.com. Accessed April 7, 2003.
23. The Problem of Burn-Induced Catabolism. Available at: http://www.burnsurgery.org/Modules/anabolic/page_02.htm. Accessed February 20, 2002.
24. Fox M, Minot AS, Liddle GW. Oxandrolone: a potent anabolic steroid of novel chemical configuration. *J Clin Endocrinol Metab.* 1962;22:921-924.
25. Oxandrin [package insert]. East Brunswick, NJ: Savient Pharmaceuticals; 2001.

CHAPTER 23

Rehabilitating the Eating-Disabled Client

A key clinical indicator for unintentional weight loss is a reduced functional ability (1). Providing clients with interventions and strategies that promote their independence and ability to self-feed and maintain the highest practicable level of functioning is critical (2,3). In addition to the physical task of eating, the social aspects of dining may be significant to the older adult.

This chapter provides an overview of considerations and information to assist older adults with eating disabilities in achieving optimal nutritional status, recognizing that food and dining have a psychosocial as well as physiological importance.

DINING EXPERIENCE

One of the first steps in promoting eating independence and maximizing intake for older adults is to evaluate the eating environment. Lifestyle and family changes may affect the client living at home. If eating alone, there is less incentive and greater difficulty in preparing foods for one person. For older adults who have become residents in a nursing facility or assisted-living facility, the dining experience may be very different from what they were accustomed to at home. This represents another major lifestyle change to which the client must become accustomed.

ATMOSPHERE AND ENVIRONMENT

Food and the atmosphere in which the food is served have an impact on quality of life (4-6). Dining atmosphere is one of the most crucial aspects of creating a pleasurable dining experience. A pleasant atmosphere consists of attractive physical surroundings and, more importantly, a climate of friendship and respect. Because of the social significance of mealtime, every effort should be taken to make each meal a positive experience (3,7-10).

Evaluation of the dining atmosphere includes the following considerations:

- Comfortable sound levels
- Atmosphere free from distractions (ie, loud conversations, television, and radio)
- Attractive setting
- Adequate lighting
- Comfortable temperature and adequate ventilation
- Absence of odors

DINING ROOM AND MEAL SERVICE ORGANIZATION

Organization of the delivery of meals and food in a congregate dining setting is critical to all but especially to the eating-disabled client. The goal is to provide a calm atmosphere and prevent client frustration.

Well-planned meal delivery and distribution contributes to the positive atmosphere in a dining room and enables staff who are assisting to maximize time spent with clients. This helps to prevent the client from becoming discouraged, which may result in diminished appetite (10-14).

The following considerations may affect dining room and meal service delivery:

- Table placement and table height are correct for mealtime. If dining rooms serve as multi-purpose rooms, the dining room should be checked before meals, to ensure that tables and chairs are correctly arranged and at the proper height, if adjustable tables are available.
- Established seating assignments should honor clients' seating preferences.
- All clients seated at a table are served meals at the same time. Meals should be delivered

from the kitchen to the dining room in order, so that facility staff can serve clients in the order in which they are seated.

- Independent diners are served first. Staff can then proceed to serving and assisting more dependent diners who require greater staff time.
- The dining area is not crowded, and staff and clients can maneuver among tables.
- Staff who provide one-to-one assistance are seated during the meal.
- Before the meal is served, an activity is conducted while clients wait for their food.
- Meals are provided on time.
- Adequate staff is specifically assigned to each dining room.
- Alternates or substitutes for meal items are readily available.

PHYSICAL PLANT AND EQUIPMENT

The physical structure and equipment in the dining room affect all clients, but the eating-disabled person is especially impacted (3,15).

The following are considerations to review in evaluating the physical plant:

- Lighting is indirect with no glare.
- There is sufficient space for clients and staff to maneuver.
- There are sufficient furnishings—tables, chairs, and storage units.
- Table heights accommodate wheelchairs. The distance from the plate to the mouth should be within 12 to 18 inches or individualized as needed.
- Dining room chairs have armrests and a sturdy base to allow for correct positioning.
- Chairs are available for staff to use while providing assistance.
- Space for storage of needed supplies is available.
- Staff wash or sanitize their hands before and while assisting each client to eat.
- There is space to allow for carts, steam tables, or other equipment needed to deliver and serve meals.
- The dining room is neat and without clutter.
- The dishware contrasts with the tablecloth or placemat, to overcome vision deficits.

PERSONAL CONSIDERATIONS

Consideration of basic personal needs before meal service provides for comfort and basic infection control measures (3).

- The client's hands and face are washed before the meal.
- Personal assistive devices, such as proper dentures, eyeglasses, and hearing aids, are in place.
- Assistive devices and adaptive eating equipment, as identified in the client's plan of care, are available.
- Clients are appropriately dressed, with hair combed.
- Incontinence care and toileting are provided before meals.
- Clients are properly positioned in chairs and wheelchairs.
- Clients are positioned at an appropriate distance from the table.

CONDITIONS AND DISORDERS AFFECTING EATING ABILITIES

Dysphagia

Eating and swallowing disorders may be neurologic, mechanical, or functional in their etiology. For older adults, any combination of illness or acute injury may affect swallowing abilities. As the body ages, changes in mobility, flexibility, and ability to compensate for daily occurrences of aspiration are experienced.

Dysphagia is impairment in any or all stages of swallowing, resulting in the reduced ability to obtain adequate nutrition by mouth and/or reduced safety during oral feeding. Difficulty for the older adult may depend on the consistency of the food or liquid, the time of day, and medical status. Box 23.1 lists signs and symptoms of dysphagia (16-19).

Serious complications of dysphagia include choking and aspiration. Aspiration occurs when food or liquid enters the lungs rather than the stomach. Aspirated food or liquid irritates the lung tissue and may cause an infection or pneumonia.

The *National Dysphagia Diet,* published in 2002, introduced textural property considerations of foods for dysphagia and recommended three solid-food texture levels and three altered liquid consistencies (16). The food textures are

- Level 1: Dysphagia Pureed
- Level 2: Dysphagia Mechanically Altered
- Level 3: Dysphagia Advanced

Box 23.1. Signs and Symptoms of Dysphagia

- Excessive mouth movement during chewing and swallowing
- The need to swallow two and three times with each bolus
- Food remaining on the tongue after swallowing
- Coughing or choking before, during, or after swallowing food, liquids, or medication
- Nasal regurgitation, excessive drooling
- "Wet" vocal quality; hoarse, breathy voice or gargly breathing
- Frequent throat clearing
- Feeling of something caught or sticking in throat
- Pocketing of food in mouth
- Repetitive rocking of tongue from front to back
- Weight loss
- Dehydration
- Fever

The liquid consistencies are

- Nectar-like
- Honey-like
- Spoon-thick

Direct and Indirect Treatment Techniques

Based on the problems identified in a clinical bedside evaluation, the rehabilitation professional will develop an individualized exercise and treatment program written specifically for the client to follow. Treatment goals may include the following:

- Increasing the strength of the lips, tongue, and pharyngeal muscles
- Increasing the range of motion of the lips, tongue, and palate
- Improving the sensation of the swallowing mechanism
- Improving laryngeal closure and airway protection during swallowing

Retraining strategies and techniques to improve the client's ability to swallow include the following:

- Direct and indirect techniques to improve oral-motor functioning

- Manipulation of the food bolus
- Positioning to enhance the function of the swallowing mechanism
- Staff and family training

Box 23.2 outlines tips for caring for a client with swallowing difficulties.

Interventions

Altering the texture of the food may allow the client to form a bolus more effectively, chew more completely, or initiate a swallow in a more timely manner. Finger foods or enhanced foods may also be indicated based on the nature of the disorder. See Box 23.3 (20).

Treatment efficacy of thickened liquids is currently being confirmed by research protocols. From a subjective standpoint, thickened liquids may be easier for the client to manage in the mouth when there is disordered strength or sensation of swallowing. Thickened fluids tend to be more cohesive than thinner liquids and may therefore help the client with bolus formation and airway protection during swallowing.

Dementia

The cognitive losses associated with dementia have significant ramifications on eating abilities. Clients with dementia may forget whether or not they have eaten, how to feed themselves, or how to chew and swallow.

Clients with dementia have impaired depth perception and spatial orientation. Impairments in depth perception may be manifested by the person placing a cup on the plate instead of next to the plate. Consider the color contrast of the table setting when providing meals for clients; a white plate against a white tablecloth or placemat while serving chicken, mashed potatoes, and corn may result in the client's limited ability to find the food on the plate. In addition, meal presentation may be visually confusing or overwhelming for the client (3).

Motor Control

Eating abilities may be affected by progressive or acute neurologic changes. Gross motor and fine motor movements may be impaired, resulting in difficulty bringing food from the plate to the mouth. Grasp strength, proximal and distal control, and regulation of speed of movement are required for a smooth movement to occur. Trunk stability is also necessary for effective arm movement.

Box 23.2 Caring for a Client With Swallowing Difficulties

DO

- Check tray for proper diet.
- Help client to eat slowly.
- Sit on the client's weaker side.
- Present small bites of food. Each bite should be approximately one teaspoon or less, as directed by the therapist.
- Allow sufficient time for the client to swallow.
- Encourage the client to "double swallow"; that is, first swallow food, then dry swallow once.
- Check that the client's mouth is empty before continuing.
- Encourage the client to use tongue movements.
- Make sure that the client's head is tilted slightly forward.
- Create an environment free of distractions.
- Guarantee that the client's dentures are in place and fit well.
- Ensure adequate lighting, but not glaring light.
- Check that food is within 12 inches of reach, if the client is self-feeding.
- Present foods, drinks, and medications from the midline position.
- Alternate food and liquids.
- Serve food at appropriate temperatures.
- Provide adequate time for the client to eat or to be assisted (up to 45 minutes).
- Ensure safety by having suctioning equipment readily available.
- Be certain that the client sits upright for 30 minutes after the meal.
- Perform complete oral hygiene after all meals.
- Report any choking or coughing to the nursing supervisor and/or rehabilitation professional.

DO NOT

- Stand to assist clients, because that causes them to lift their heads and extend their necks.
- Assist the client if the client is lying down or reclining.
- Rush the client or assist with meals too rapidly.
- Assist the client when head is tilted backwards ("bird feeding").
- Provide medicine during choking or coughing.
- Change the client's program without consulting the therapist or supervisor.

Box 23.3 Finger Food Diet

Objective: To provide food that is of a consistency that can be easily eaten by hand.
Indications: For residents who are unable or will not use silverware to feed themselves.
General Information

1. All foods can be eaten without the aid of utensils.

2. The sodium and sugar content of this diet may make it difficult to combine with all types of therapeutic diets.

3. This texture modification cannot be combined with any other texture modifications (ie, pureed or mechanical soft).

Nutritional Adequacy: This diet can be planned to meet the Recommended Dietary Allowances.

Specifics of the Diet

Food Group	Foods Allowed	Foods to Avoid
Beverages	All	None
Breads and cereals	Any breads or rolls that can be picked up to eat by hand	Hot cereals
	Cold cereals that are formed in large pieces, served without milk	

continued

Box 23.3 Finger Food Diet (continued)

Specifics of the Diet

Food Group	Foods Allowed	Foods to Avoid
Desserts	Cookies, cake cut into pieces prior to meal service, ice cream bars, pudding pops, gelatin cubes, bar cookies, tarts, eclairs, donuts, ice cream cones, popsicles, turnovers	Pies, pudding, gelatin-based desserts, crisps, cobblers
Eggs	Scrambled, poached, fried, omelets cut into small pieces, hard-boiled	None
Fats	All	None
Fruits	Canned fruits cut into bite-sized pieces or slices Any fresh fruit cut into pieces or served whole if able to bite off pieces	Canned halves of fruit, applesauce or other pureed fruits
Meat, fish, poultry, cheese, legumes	Meats sliced and placed between bread to serve as a sandwich cut into fourths prior to meal service Meat patties cut into bite-sized pieces Chicken legs, thighs, wings, and breasts if not in a sauce Sliced chunks of cheese Peanut butter on crackers Any chicken or fish nuggets, fish sticks	Cottage cheese, meats covered with gravy or thick sauces, large pieces of meat, casseroles
Potatoes or substitutes	Tater tots, boiled or baked potatoes cut into pieces	Rice; mashed, creamed, scalloped, or au gratin potatoes; pasta, spaghetti; macaroni and cheese, tuna noodle, and other casseroles; stuffing and dressing
Soups	All if served in a mug	None if served in a mug Avoid adding too many crackers or it will be necessary to use a spoon to eat.
Vegetables	Raw vegetable pieces, any vegetables cooked to crisp-tender, corn on the cob, large slices of vegetables, corn nuggets, butter-dipped vegetables, vegetable juices	Vegetable casseroles, spinach, very soft vegetables, corn, peas, mixtures of small vegetable pieces may be very tiresome to eat. Vegetable salads with sauces
Sugar, sweets	All	Any that are gooey or need to be eaten by spoon
Miscellaneous	Popcorn, pickles, olives, nuts, salt, pepper	Relish only if on a food, cream sauces, gravies

Source: Diet developed by Mary Auch, MS, RD. May be copied for use. For more information, contact CD-HCF at cdhcf@cdhcf.org. Reprinted with permission from Finger food diet. In: Niedert KC, ed. *Pocket Resource for Nutrition Assessment.* Chicago, Ill: Consultant Dietitians in Health Care Facilities; 2001:260-262.

Apraxia is defined as the inability to plan and execute a skilled movement in the absence of sensory and motor deficits. The client with apraxia is not able to demonstrate a movement on verbal request (21).

Vision

Vision changes associated with aging also affect eating abilities. An older person requires more light than a younger person. Many older adults have difficulty focusing between distant and near objects. It may be difficult for them to look at food close up and try watch the events taking place in the dining room.

Poor acuity or low vision problems, resulting from conditions such as cataracts, glaucoma, macular degeneration, or diabetic retinopathy, are also commonplace in older adults (4).

ADAPTATIONS FOR INDEPENDENCE

Maintaining independence with self-feeding is one of the most important goals for the eating-disabled client. Adaptive equipment may assist the client to increase independence with self-feeding and swallowing. See Box 23.4.

Positioning

Positioning provides the key for maximizing eating independence and the framework on which other interventions may be added, to promote independence in eating and to make the client more comfortable during mealtimes.

The ideal eating position begins with the use of a standard dining room chair with armrests for support. While in the chair, the client can get close to the table by sliding the chair arms under the table. Being close to the table is a key element in being independent with eating. The ideal position places the client's mouth approximately 12 inches from the plate. Body alignment should be maintained so that weight is evenly distributed. Pillows, trunk supports, lap boards, or chair arms may be useful to assist in maintaining posture, so the person can concentrate on chewing and swallowing. See Figure 23.1 for correct positioning. Box 23.5 lists positioning tips.

Wheelchair-Bound Clients

The use of regular dining room chairs, rather than wheelchairs, should be encouraged, to facilitate the best mealtime positioning. Clients who generally use wheelchairs need to be encouraged to use dining

---

Box 23.4 Examples of Adaptive Equipment

- *Cutout cup/nosey cup:* prevents head tilting back when drinking.
- *Straws:* may be helpful when range of motion (ROM) is limited or tremor is present, may control amount of liquid intake. Straws may be dangerous for those clients with dysphagia.
- *Dycem/nonslip materials:* Holds utensils and dishes in place.
- *Weighted utensils/wrist weights:* May decrease tremors and provide distal stability.
- *Universal cuff:* Reduces the amount of movement required to bring food from plate to mouth for eating. Compensates for reduced grip strength.
- *Built-up flatware:* May compensate for decreased grasp. Provides distal stability.
- *Plate guard/divided dish/scoop dish/inner lip plate:* Allows the client to load the utensils for self-feeding. **Note:** Do not use these devices simply because a client is on a mechanically altered diet.

Figure 23.1
Correct position.

Box 23.5 Positioning Tips

- In most cases, the person should be positioned with the head slightly flexed.
- Head should be at a 90° angle with chin just slightly tucked.
- Shoulders should be slightly forward.
- Trunk should be leaning slightly forward.
- Hips should be flexed at slightly more than 90°.
- Knees should be flexed at 90°.
- Feet should be flat on the floor.
- The upper extremities should be placed so that elbows can be used to increase stability if needed.

Figure 23.2
Incorrect position.

room chairs at mealtime. Transferring from a wheel-chair to a dining room chair allows the additional benefit of position change. For clients who are unable or unwilling to transfer from a wheelchair to a dining room chair for meals, proper positioning in the wheelchair is very important and should comply with the following parameters (4):

- The table may need to be elevated, to allow the wheelchair to roll under the edge.
- The client must be within 12 inches of the plate.
- The wheelchair must be locked into position, with the client's abdomen close to the table and the hips at a 90° angle.
- The client needs solid support from the wheelchair seat and back, and foot support with foot rests or feet directly on the floor, to help maintain the hips at a 90° angle.
- If the client cannot be positioned at the table, a lap tray attached to the wheelchair should be provided.
- Position the client to promote normal dining room conversation.
- Note that, in nursing facilities, the lap tray may be considered a restraint, even when used for positioning.

Poor Sitting Balance and Poor Neck Control

If a client has a tendency to fall forward from the waist, with his or her head on the table, while seated at the table in a regular dining room chair, several techniques are available to help maintain an upright position. First, the chair must be secure, so that the client does not slide away from the table (see Figure 23.2). If the client's hips are sliding forward in the seat of the chair, the client's head tends to lean back, and the distance from plate to mouth increases. With this increased distance, independence in eating becomes more difficult. The best position begins with the client's hips at a 90° angle at the back of the chair. A nonslip netting or other non-slip material on the seat of the chair helps prevent the client from sliding forward. Avoid multiple layers of cushions on the chair seat, because this can result in the hips sliding forward (4).

If these interventions are unsuccessful, then a seat belt may be considered for use on the chair during mealtime. A seat belt would be used for positioning but would still be considered a restraint. Placement of the seat belt should allow the belt to come from under the chair and pass over the client's hips, not waist, to help keep the hips at the 90° angle at the back of the chair (4).

Bed-Bound Client

Occupational and/or physical therapists can be a great resource in evaluating the bed-bound client for positioning interventions. If clients cannot sit in a chair, the following positioning tips can be used (4):

- Raise the head of the bed to the fullest upright position.
- Position a pillow behind the client's shoulder blades and neck so that the neck is slightly forward and the chin is tucked under.

- Keep the head in a midline position.
- Maintain the head in an upright position, to reduce the chances of aspiration.
- Position the knees at a 90° flexion, by adjusting the bed or by supporting the knees with pillows. (Additional pillows may be needed to maintain this position.)
- Reposition the resident frequently to prevent pressure ulcers.

Remember to raise the bedside table, and position it close to the client. The table should be between waist and breast level, to reduce the distance from plate to mouth. Positioning is improved and a positive mealtime experience is promoted by close attention to the following (4):

- Clearing and cleaning the bedside table before serving the meal
- Placing all necessary items within reach
- Avoiding unpleasant smells
- Limiting distractions, eg, from visitors and loud televisions
- Providing periodic supervision and assistance as needed

Verbal and Hand-Over-Hand Cueing

Independent eating skills might include being able to hold a glass, direct the glass to the mouth, and drink independently. Caregivers may need to use verbal prompts to remind the client to pick up the glass and drink, or they may need to support the client's hand to help hold the glass and direct the glass to the mouth. This hand-over-hand assistance allows the client to continue to go through the motions of picking up the glass and directing the glass to the mouth, which fosters less chance of losing this ability (4).

Hand-over-hand assistance can also be used to help the client eat with utensils. As the client becomes stronger or more independent, the caregiver needs to withdraw assistance gradually. For instance, instead of hand-over-hand assistance, the client may benefit from the assistance or support of the caregiver's hand under the forearm or at the elbow. Once the client has food on the eating utensil, the caregiver can help direct the filled utensil to the mouth by providing assistance at the client's elbow to lift and direct the arm. It is important not to provide more assistance than the client needs. To increase independence, gradually reduce the amount

of physical assistance while using only verbal prompts to provide the required direction (4).

Cognitively impaired clients capable of moving their hands to their mouths need to be involved in independent eating. These individuals may need only verbal prompting, or they may need prompting at every step of the eating process. The prompt might follow this sequence:

> "(Client's name), pick up your spoon."
> "Scoop some potatoes onto your spoon."
> "Put the potatoes in your mouth."
> "Swallow the potatoes."

When verbal prompting is unsuccessful, the caregiver should try hand-over-hand assistance (4).

Repetition is an essential element of rehabilitation. The same is true for maintaining or regaining independent eating skills. Repetition and consistent approaches are necessary and may take several weeks to achieve progress. Encouraging the client to use repetitive motions, such as tooth brushing, face washing, hair combing, and shaving, is helpful in the rehabilitation process, because similar muscles are used for eating (4).

SUMMARY

Quality of life improves when nutritious meals that meet individual food preferences are served in a pleasant, friendly atmosphere that promotes socialization. With older adults, these approaches may be more beneficial than restricted therapeutic diets. Older adults benefit from an environment in which they are encouraged to function at their highest physical and mental levels. Appropriate mealtime positioning promotes independence in eating. Monitoring for problems at mealtime and providing interventions can maximize the rehabilitation of eating-disabled clients.

REFERENCES

1. Gilmore S, Robinson G, Posthauer M, Raymond J. Clinical indicators associated with unintentional weight loss and pressure ulcers in elderly residents of nursing facilities. *J Am Diet Assoc.* 1995;95:984-992.
2. Centers for Medicare & Medicaid Services. Survey Protocol for Long-term Care Facilities: Investigative Protocol Dining and Food Service. 1999 (pp 47-50). Available at: http://www.cms.hhs.gov/manuals/pub07pdf/AP-P-PP.pdf. Accessed March 10, 2004.
3. Robinson G, Leif B, eds. *Nutrition Management and Restorative Dining for Older Adults: Practical Interventions For Caregivers.* Chicago, Ill: American Dietetic Association; 2001.

4. Russell C, ed. *Dining Skills: Practical Interventions for the Caregiver of Eating-Disabled Older Adults.* Chicago, Ill: Consultant Dietitians in Health Care Facilities; 2001.

5. Dwyer JT. *Screening Older Americans' Nutritional Health: Current Practices and Future Possibilities.* Washington, DC: Nutrition Screening Initiative; 1991.

6. Langer EJ, Rodin J. The effects of choice and enhanced personal responsibility for the aged: a field experiment in an institutional setting. *J Personality Soc Psychol.* 1976;34:191-198.

7. Evans B, Crogan N. Quality improvement practices: enhancing quality of life during mealtimes. *J Nurses Staff Dev.* 2001;17:131-136.

8. Mathey M, Vanneste V, de Graaf C, de Groot L, van Staveren W. Health effect of improved meal ambiance in a Dutch nursing home: a 1-year intervention study. *Prev Med.* 2001;32:416-423.

9. Hotaling D. Adapting the mealtime environment: setting the stage for eating. *Dysphagia.* 1990;5:77-83.

10. American Medical Directors Association. *Altered Nutritional Status: Clinical Practice Guideline.* Columbia, Md: American Medical Directors Association; 2001:18-20.

11. Miceli B. Nursing unit management maintenance program: continuation of safe-swallowing and feeding beyond skilled therapeutic intervention. *J Gerontol Nurs.* 1999;25(8):22-36.

12. Bower M. The resident dining room: a CQI project. *J Nutr Elder.* 1996;15:46-54.

13. Porter C, Schell ES, Kayser-Jones J, Paul SM. Dynamics of nutrition care among nursing home residents who are eating poorly. *J Am Diet Assoc.* 1999;99:1444-1446.

14. Simmons S, Babineau S, Garcia E, Schnelle J. Quality assessment in nursing homes by systematic direct observation: feeding assistance. *J Gerontol A Biol Sci Med Sci.* 2002;57:M665-M671.

15. McDaniel J, Hunt A, Hackes B, Pope J. Impact of dining room environment on nutritional intake of Alzheimer's residents: a case study. *Am J Alzheimer's Dis.* 2001;16:297-302.

16. National Dysphagia Diet Task Force. *National Dysphagia Diet: Standardization for Optimal Care.* Chicago, Ill: American Dietetic Association; 2002.

17. Zenner P. The clinical examination for dysphagia. In: Mills R, ed. *Evaluation of Dysphagia in Adults: Expanding the Diagnostic Options.* Austin, Texas: Pro-Ed; 2000: 27-63.

18. Miller RM. Clinical examination for dysphagia. In: Groher M, ed. *Dysphagia Diagnosis and Management.* 3rd ed. Newton, Mass: Butterworth-Heinemann; 1997: 143-162.

19. Perlman A. Dysphagia: populations at risk and methods of diagnosis. *Nutr Clin Pract.* 1999;14 (suppl):S2-S9.

20. Finger food diet. In: Niedert KC, ed. *Pocket Resource for Nutrition Assessment.* Chicago, Ill: Consultant Dietitians in Health Care Facilities; 2001:260-262.

21. National Institute of Neurological Disorders and Stroke. Apraxia information page. Available at: http://www.ninds.nih.gov/health_and_medical/disorders/apraxia.htm. Accessed March 10, 2004.

CHAPTER 24

Enteral and Parenteral Nutrition Support

Enteral and parenteral nutrition therapies provide nutrients for maintenance or restoration of nutritional status for persons who are unable or unwilling to consume an adequate diet. Technological advances and the proliferation of home care providers have made nutrition support more available to individuals outside the traditional acute-care hospital setting. Nutrition support is common for institutionalized older adults and is used to counteract decreased oral intake and decreased assimilation of nutrients resulting from malnutrition and chronic diseases in this population.

The basic indications for and principles of nutrition support are the same in older adults as in their younger counterparts. However, there are physiologic and sociological factors unique to older adults that must be evaluated, because they can affect the timing and route of nutrition support, the type and amount of substrates administered, and the type and degree of monitoring. Changes in body composition and function that occur with aging leave older adults with diminished reserves and impaired compensatory mechanisms (1). It may be difficult, at times, to distinguish between these age-related physiologic changes and abnormalities due to malnutrition. Older adults are more likely to take multiple medications that can affect the absorption, metabolism, or excretion of nutrients (2). Ethical issues, such as those related to quality of life, are more commonplace among older adults and must be considered (3).

The role of the registered dietitian includes assessing nutritional status, identifying appropriate candidates for nutrition support, determining the route and timing of administration, monitoring tolerance and efficacy of therapy and making the appropriate adjustments, and documenting the nutrition care plan.

NUTRITION ASSESSMENT

Establishing nutrition support goals for older adults begins with a comprehensive nutrition assessment and history. Many age-related factors affecting the nutritional state of older adults need to be considered in designing and implementing the nutrition support care plan.

BODY COMPOSITION AND ORGAN SYSTEM CHANGES

Body composition changes associated with senescence (growing old) include decreased lean body mass (LBM), increased body fat, and loss of height. Lean body mass, including skeletal muscle, smooth muscle, and body organs, decreases from about 45% of total body weight at age 30 years to 27% at age 70 years. There is a proportional increase in total body fat to approximately 30% of total body weight at age 70 years from 14% at age 30 years. Total body water parallels the loss of LBM and decreases to 53% of total body weight at age 70 years (3).

Type 2, or senile, osteoporosis causes a loss of height with aging, and occurs at a rate of 1 cm per decade after the age of 20 years. In addition, women may experience postmenopausal osteoporosis (type 1), which further decreases bone density significantly (4).

The aging process affects multiple organ systems. The following list summarizes some age-related effects on organs (1):

- Skin: dryness, wrinkling, loss of elasticity
- Gastrointestinal tract: decreased absorption and peristalsis
- Cardiovascular: thickening, decreased heart size
- Pulmonary: decreased vital and breathing capacity

- Renal: decreased blood flow, glomerular filtration rate, creatinine excretion, and renal concentrating ability
- Endocrine: altered circulating hormones, decreased insulin sensitivity
- Nervous: decreased cognition, memory, and muscle response to stimuli

The aging process, as well as common chronic diseases, can negatively affect nutritional status in older adults. Chronic diseases, such as cardiac, renal, and pulmonary diseases, can lead to altered nutrient absorption and metabolism. Multiple medications frequently prescribed for older adults may further contribute to altered nutrient absorption, metabolism, and decreased appetite (2).

Other risk factors associated with malnutrition in older adults include dementia, depression, alcohol or substance abuse, and adverse social conditions, such as isolation and poverty. Altered physical and cognitive ability contribute to difficulties with food shopping and preparation (1).

NUTRITION SCREENING

Nutrition assessment of older adults incorporates the use of anthropometric, clinical, biochemical, dietary, and psychosocial data. The Nutrition Screening Initiative, a collaborative effort between the American Dietetic Association, the American Academy of Family Physicians, and the National Council on the Aging, developed tools for nutrition screening and evaluation of nutritional status of older persons. These screening tools are used to query individuals about dietary habits, functional status, social environment, and biochemical and anthropometric data (5).

Serum albumin is a marker of visceral protein status and has been associated with poor outcome in hospitalized clients. In the hospital setting, hypoalbuminemia in older adults is associated with increased length of stay, complications, readmissions, and mortality (6,7). In community-dwelling older persons, some studies have suggested that low albumin levels are associated with functional limitations, sarcopenia, increased health care use, and mortality (8-10).

Subjective global assessment (SGA) is another useful screening tool, which incorporates elements of the client's history and physical findings. From these data, clients are categorized as well nourished, moderately malnourished, or severely malnourished. SGA has demonstrated predictive value for nutrition-related complications and mortality in older adult residents of a nursing facility superior to that of hypoalbuminemia (11).

Malnutrition is more common in older clients of nursing facilities and other long-term-care facilities than in community-dwelling individuals. The incidence of malnutrition in nursing facilities is reported between 37% and 85%: it is approximately 40% in hospitalized older adult clients (2). These rates of malnutrition, along with the many confounding factors that affect the nutritional status of older adults, suggest that aggressive nutrition intervention is indicated. This may include early nutrition support with enteral or parenteral feeding.

NUTRITIONAL REQUIREMENTS

Energy

Energy needs of adults decrease with age, because of a decreased basal metabolic rate associated with diminished LBM. The decrease in energy expenditure is approximately 1% to 2% per decade for adults aged 20 to 75 years (2). The recommended dietary allowance (RDA) (1989) of energy for adults > 51 years is 30 kcal/kg of body weight (12). However, the dietary reference intakes (DRIs) (2002) for estimating energy requirements are based on age, gender, weight, height, and level of activity (sedentary, low active, active, or very active) (13). The DRIs provide an equation for predicting total energy expenditure using these variables. When determining energy needs of older adults, it is also important to consider the disease state or whether acute or chronic illness is present. As with any client receiving nutrition support, energy levels should be adjusted as needed to meet the established goal weight.

Protein

The protein DRI for adults 51 to 70 years and for those older than 70 years is 0.8 g/kg body weight (13). It is important to consider the level of activity and the disease state when determining protein requirements. Acute illness or conditions of metabolic stress or infection warrant increased provision of protein. Older adults who are bedridden or immobile need increased protein because of the negative nitrogen balance associated with inactivity. Inadequate provision of protein may contribute to loss of LBM. Conditions that require decreased protein intake include hepatic failure or age-related diminished renal function (3).

Carbohydrate

The DRI for adults for carbohydrate (CHO) is 45% to 65% of energy, with a minimum of 130 g/day (13). Aging adversely affects CHO metabolism, and older adults are more likely to experience hyperglycemia than younger adults (2). Enteral and parenteral formulas with a high CHO content may not be well tolerated. Selecting lower CHO or diabetic enteral formulas or three-in-one admixtures of parenteral nutrition formulas may be necessary to help control hyperglycemia. The addition of insulin to parenteral nutrition may be necessary.

The trace element chromium has a role in CHO metabolism, and clients experiencing hyperglycemia may be chromium deficient. Serum chromium may be checked, and the parenteral nutrition supplemented with additional chromium if the serum level is below normal limits (14).

Fat

Fat provides a source of energy and essential fatty acids, and it is necessary for absorption of fat-soluble vitamins. The DRI for fat for the adult is 20% to 35% of total energy needs (13). Standard 1-kcal/mL enteral products provide approximately 30% of the energy as fat. Clients receiving parenteral nutrition should receive at least 10% of their energy from intravenous fat emulsion, to meet their essential fatty acid requirement (15).

Vitamins and Minerals

The intake of vitamins and minerals in older adults parallels their decreased energy intake. Because of age-related decreased absorption in the gastrointestinal (GI) tract, deficiencies may develop, especially during an acute illness secondary to decreased body stores. DRIs include the age categories of 51 to 70 years and > 70 years (16-19). Enteral formulas contain vitamins and minerals providing 100% or more of the RDAs in 1,000 mL to 1,500 mL of formula. Intravenous injections of multivitamin and mineral preparations are added to parenteral nutrition formulas (20).

Fluid

Older adults have fewer compensatory mechanisms than younger adults for restoring and maintaining homeostatic norms due to age-related declines in renal and cardiac function, which have a negative effect on the ability to maintain adequate hydration. Dehydration is the most common fluid and electrolyte disturbance in older clients (1). Fluid recommendations include 1 mL fluid/kcal or 30 mL/kg of body weight (1,2). Older clients should be closely monitored for adequate fluid balance.

ETHICAL CONSIDERATIONS

The decision to initiate nutrition support in older clients is based on the same medical indications and principles used for younger adults. However, ethical considerations are more likely to play a factor in the decision to initiate nutrition support in older adults. These include the client's desires, estimated duration of nutrition support, expected benefits, prognosis, and effect on quality and quantity of life. Older adults with advance directives or who have made their wishes known to family members may help outline the decisions for implementing or discontinuing nutrition support, especially if it is expected to be long-term or will require institutionalization for administration (21).

HOME ENTERAL AND PARENTERAL NUTRITION

The older adult may be a candidate for enteral or parenteral home nutrition support. As is the case whenever home nutrition support is being considered, it is necessary to thoroughly assess the client's medical condition, the client or caregiver's level of independence and ability to learn home nutrition support procedures, psychological and social life aspects, and medical insurance coverage. The evaluation process is best accomplished by a multidisciplinary team of experts, including the physician, nurse, registered dietitian, psychiatrist, social worker, and case manager/discharge planner (22). Home nutrition support has an impact on the client's and the caregiver's lifestyle. Sleep, travel, and social life have been found to be significantly affected by home nutrition support therapies (23). One of the most important aspects for successful home nutrition support is the availability, commitment, and support of the client's family or caregiver.

In many situations, the older adult may not be a good candidate for home nutrition support but may be a candidate for nutrition support in a rehabilitation or nursing facility. Nutrition support in a nursing facility may be permanent or temporary while a client undergoes rehabilitation, wound management, or training of home parenteral nutrition procedures before discharge to home. Lack of evidence of potential benefit of home nutrition support, including improved nutritional state or disease state, may preclude the older adult as a home nutrition support candidate.

ENTERAL NUTRITION SUPPORT

Older adults who are unable to meet their nutritional requirements orally may be candidates for enteral nutrition. Enteral nutrition is appropriate when the GI tract is functional and safely accessible. Enteral nutrition can be used to provide full nutrition needs or as a supplement to oral intake or parenteral nutrition. Box 24.1 lists indications for tube feeding in older persons (1) .

The decision to proceed with enteral nutrition should involve the client, support person(s), the physician, and the health care team. The client's medical status, comorbidities, quality of life, and prognosis should be taken into consideration. Older adults should be frequently screened for nutritional risk factors, because their nutritional status tends to decline more rapidly than that of younger adults and because they respond more slowly to nutrition therapy (3). Enteral nutrition may be needed beyond the hospital stay and may be continued in the nursing facility or home setting.

For certain subgroups of older adults, particularly those who have dementia, the risks may outweigh the benefits of enteral nutrition. Older clients with swallowing disorders receiving home enteral nutrition tend to have poorer outcomes than younger adults (24). Among older adults with dementia, there is evidence of increased mortality with advancing age and postgastrostomy, particularly in those with existing poor nutritional status and hypoalbuminemia (25,26). Data may be insufficient to demonstrate that enteral nutrition helps to reduce aspiration or to improve functional status and wound healing among older adults with dementia (25). Box 24.2 lists contraindications to enteral nutrition support (21).

Enteral Feeding Access

Once enteral nutrition is decided upon, selecting the most appropriate enteral access is the next step. Determining the optimal access route for enteral nutrition depends on the anticipated duration of therapy, gastric function, lower esophageal sphincter competence, and the risk of aspiration. Figure 24.1 outlines how to determine the optimal feeding model (27). Box 24.3 lists conditions that may preclude intragastric feeding (28).

Nasogastric/Enteric Feeding-Tube Placement

Clients who require enteral nutrition support for fewer than 4 to 6 weeks may benefit from a feeding tube placed through the nose into the stomach, duodenum, or proximal jejunum (29).

Box 24.1 Indications for Tube Feeding in Older Persons

Oncologic disease
  Neoplasm
  Chemotherapy
  Radiation therapy
Inability to swallow
  Cerebrovascular accident
  Dysphagia
  Head trauma or comatose state
  Advanced dementia
Degenerative or debilitating disease
  Huntington's chorea
  Advanced Parkinson's disease
  Demyelinating disease
**Hypermetabolism or inadequate
  oral intake > 5 days**
  Sepsis
  Surgery
  Severe malnutrition
  Burns
  Organ failure
Other
  Depression
  Failure to thrive

Source: Reprinted with permission from McGee M, Binkley J, Jensen GL. Geriatric nutrition. In: Gottschlich MM, ed. *The Science and Practice of Nutrition Support, A Case-Based Core Curriculum.* Dubuque, Iowa: Kendall/Hunt Publishing Co; 2001:382.

Box 24.2 Contraindications to Enteral Nutrition Support

Malnourished individuals expected to eat
  within 5-7 days
Severe acute pancreatitis
High output proximal fistula
Inability to gain enteral access
Intractable vomiting or diarrhea
Aggressive therapy not warranted
Expected need less than 5-7 days if malnourished
  or 7-9 days if normally nourished

Source: Reprinted with permission from Charney P. Enteral nutrition: indications, options, and formulations. In: Gottschlich MM, ed. *The Science and Practice of Nutrition Support, A Case-Based Core Curriculum.* Dubuque, Iowa: Kendall/Hunt Publishing Co; 2001:141-166.

Figure 24.1.

Determining the optimal feeding model. Reprinted with permission from Ideno KT. Enteral nutrition. In: Gottschlich MM, Matarese LE, Shronts EP, eds. *Nutrition Support Dietetics: Core Curriculum.* 2nd ed. Silver Spring, Md: American Society for Parenteral and Enteral Nutrition: 1993:83.

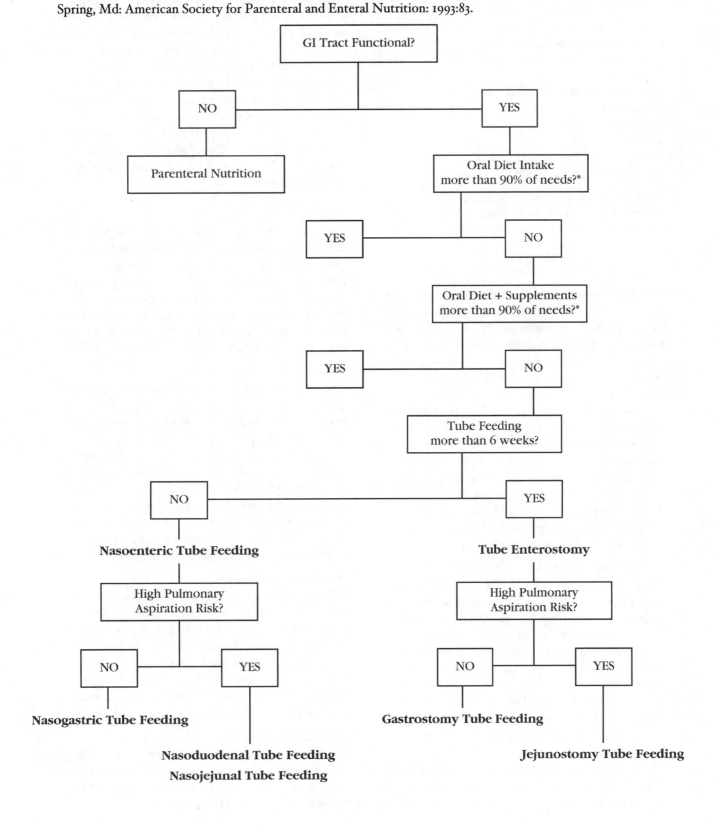

* Demonstrated by daily calorie counts.

Box 24.3   Conditions That May Preclude Intragastric Feeding

Gastroparesis/gastric ileus
Recent abdominal surgery
Sepsis
Significant gastroesophageal reflux
Pancreatitis
Aspiration
Ileus

Source: Reprinted with permission from Minard G, Lysen LK. Enteral access devices. In: Gottschlich MM, ed. *The Science and Practice of Nutrition Support: A Case-Based Core Curriculum.* Dubuque, Iowa: Kendall/Hunt Publishing Co; 2001:167-189.

Nasogastric/enteric tubes are generally made of soft, biocompatible materials, such as polyurethane or silicone. These tubes range in length from 90 cm (nasogastric) to 150 cm (intestinal). Clients with gastroparesis or diseases involving the stomach, or those at risk for pulmonary aspiration may require a tube placed beyond the pylorus into the small bowel.

Nasoduodenal and nasojejunal feeding tubes may be placed by a variety of methods, including (*a*) spontaneous passage, in which the tube migrates to the small bowel by peristalsis or with the help of prokinetic agents (eg, metoclopramide, cisapride, erythromycin): (*b*) active bedside placement, such as the Zaloga technique (30): or (*c*) by fluoroscopic and endoscopic methods. The method used depends on the training of the clinician and availability of equipment.

Enterostomy Feeding-Tube Placement

Clients who require access to the GI tract for more than 4 to 6 weeks may have a gastrostomy or jejunostomy tube placed surgically, endoscopically, or radiologically. A surgical gastrostomy is performed under general anesthesia in the operating room, whereas a percutaneous endoscopic gastrostomy (PEG) may be performed at the bedside or in an endoscopic suite with local anesthesia. Gastrostomy tubes are indicated when gastric emptying is normal, a gag reflex is present, and there is no esophageal reflux.

Jejunostomy feeding tubes are generally placed at the time of a surgical procedure or may be placed endoscopically (percutaneous endoscopic jejunostomy [PEJ]). Another method of jejunal feeding-tube placement is by advancing a small-bore feeding tube, called a *jejunal extension tube* (JET) through a PEG into the jejunum. This procedure is referred to as a JET-PEG. Due to the technical difficulty of this method and the high rate of tube complications, the JET-PEG is not commonly used. Indications for jejunal feeding tubes include severe esophageal reflux, obstruction, stricture, fistula(s) or ileus of the upper GI tract, or risk for pulmonary aspiration.

An esophagostomy or cervical pharyngostomy may be performed in clients with head and neck cancer, but these are generally not common sites for enteral feeding access.

Formula Selection

There are a multitude of formulas available for enteral nutrition support. These formulas can be grouped into three main categories: polymeric, hydrolyzed, and modular. Selection of an appropriate formula is based on several factors, including digestive and absorptive capacity, volume status, and overall disease state. See Table 24.1 for specific guidelines regarding the selection of enteral formulas (31).

Polymeric Formulas

These formulas are nutritionally complete, predominantly lactose-free, and casein- or soy protein isolate–based. Normal digestion and absorption are required, because nutrients are in an intact molecular form. Polymeric formulas supply all necessary nutrients for complete nutrition, generally in 2 liters or less. The following varieties of polymeric formulas are available: standard, high nitrogen, fiber supplemented, concentrated, and disease specific (ie, renal, hepatic, glucose intolerance, pulmonary, stress/trauma, and immune-enhancing).

Hydrolyzed Formulas

Minimal digestion is required for the absorption of hydrolyzed formulas. The carbohydrate source is typically glucose oligosaccharides, and protein is provided as short-chain peptides and/or free amino acids. These formulas are usually low in fat and provide a portion of fat in the form of medium-chain triglycerides. Due to hydrolyzation, these formulas tend to have a higher osmolality (32).

Modular Formulas

Modular components of single macronutrients (ie, carbohydrate, protein, and fat) may be used to alter the energy or protein content of a base formula or to create a new tube-feeding formula (31).

TABLE 24.1. Selection of Tube-Feeding Formulas

Type	Description	Indications for Use	Advantages	Disadvantages
Standard	• Nutritionally complete • Lactose-free • Isotonic • 1.0 kcal/mL • 80%-85% water	• General tube-feeding needs • Supplement inadequate oral intake	• Inexpensive • Readily available	• Requires normal digestion and absorption
Fiber-supplemented	• Nutritionally complete • Lactose-free • Fiber source mainly soy polysaccharide • Contains 5-14 g fiber/1000 mL	• Normalize bowel function • Long-term feeding	• Fiber addition well tolerated	• Adequate water needed to minimize gastrointestinal side effects
High-nitrogen	• Nutritionally complete • Lactose-free • Low-residue • Protein > 15% total kcal	• Increased protein requirements	• Increased protein content without increased caloric level	Increased renal solute load may increase water requirements
Concentrated	• Nutritionally complete • Lactose-free • Low-residue • Osmolality of 450–600 mOsm/kg of water • 70%-80% water	• Fluid restrictions • Limited formula volume tolerance	• Allows provision of energy and nutrient needs in a limited volume of formula • Well tolerated in most patients	• Hypertonic • Lower percentage of water may increase risk of dehydration
Disease-specific	• Specific organ dysfunction and/or hypercatabolism	• Renal failure • Diabetes • Respiratory failure • Stress/trauma • Hepatic failure • AIDS	• Alteration of macro- and micro-nutrients for clients with specific diseases	• Higher cost • Controversial efficacy
Predigested	• Nutritionally complete • Low residue • Peptide- and/or amino acid–based • Very low fat content (1%-15% of kcal) • Osmolality of 450-700 mOsm/kg of water • Low in fat or fat mainly in form of MCT	• Malabsorption • Maldigestion • Transition from total parenteral nutrition to enteral nutrition	• Easily digested and absorbed	• Higher cost • Less palatable • Hypertonic

Special Considerations for Older Adults

A standard, 1-kcal/mL polymeric formula can meet the needs of many older clients. However, some older adults may need a specialized formula. Constipation is common among older adults and may be alleviated by a fiber-containing formula and sufficient free-water flushes. A high-nitrogen, 1-kcal/mL polymeric formula, which provides increased protein without increased energy, may be appropriate for older adults with increased protein needs, because their energy needs tend to be lower than those of younger adults. Older adults with medical diagnoses requiring volume restriction, such as those with congestive heart failure, chronic obstructive pulmonary disease, or renal or hepatic failure, may benefit from a concentrated formula (31).

Older adults experience hyperglycemia more frequently than their younger counterparts, and the hyperglycemia may be exacerbated with initiation of enteral nutrition (33). In addition to medical management and avoiding overfeeding, use of a lower-carbohydrate formula or one designed for glucose intolerance may be beneficial for improved glycemic control (33).

Administration Techniques

The method of administration used to provide enteral nutrition support depends on the location of the feeding tube, client tolerance to the feeding regimen, and overall nutrition goals. The two methods of tube feeding are continuous and intermittent/bolus.

Continuous feedings may be given by gravity drip or infusion pump and are provided 24 hours per day. Continuous feedings are generally the best tolerated and are ideal for immobile, comatose, or critically ill clients. When the feeding tube is in the small bowel, continuous feedings are required because of the lack of gastric holding capacity. Alternatively, tube feeding may be administered cyclically by infusion pump over a 10- to 18-hour period (typically during the night). Nocturnal feeding is beneficial when attempting to wean the tube feeding, because it allows the client to eat during the day. Nocturnal feedings also allow clients to engage more easily in activities of daily living and in physical activity.

Intermittent feedings can be given with a syringe as a bolus or via gravity drip or infusion pump for 20 to 30 minutes several times per day (usually 5 to 6 times per day).

Bolus feedings are characterized by the rapid delivery (10 minutes or less) of 300 mL to 400 mL of formula several times per day. Feedings are infused via syringe through the feeding tube into the stomach. This method is frequently used in home and nursing facilities, because it is a more physiologic method of providing nutrition. However, bolus feedings are more likely to result in nausea, diarrhea, vomiting, distention, cramps, or aspiration than are other administration methods (34,35).

Tube feedings, including hypertonic formulas, can generally be initiated at full strength. Isotonic feedings have an osmolality range of 280 mOsm/kg water to 320 mOsm/kg water: whereas hypertonic feedings exceed this range. If intolerance develops with initiation of a hypertonic feeding, it may be changed to half-strength, continuing with the same feeding schedule until the desired rate is achieved, then switching to full strength. Altering the rate and strength at the same time should be avoided. Continuous feedings can be initiated at 20 mL to 50 mL/hour. Advancement may range from 10 mL to 25 mL/hour every 4 to 24 hours until the goal rate is achieved. Intermittent feedings may be initiated at 120 mL every 4 hours and increased by an additional 60 mL every 8 to 12 hours to goal (27). Table 24.2 is an example of initiation and progression of tube feeding (27).

TABLE 24.2. Example of Initiation and Progression of Tube Feeding

Delivery Method	Rate	Time
Continuous tube feeding	50 mL/h	1st 8 h
	75 mL/h	2nd 8 h
	100 mL/h	3rd 8 h
		Goal: 24 h
Intermittent/bolus tube feeding	120 mL every 4 h	1st 8 h
	180 mL every 4 h	2nd 8 h
	240 mL every 4 h	3rd 8 h
		Goal: 24 h

Medication Administration

The administration of medications through enteral feeding tubes should be avoided if possible, because of the risk of tube occlusion and incompatibility of medications with tube-feeding formulas (36). Alternative routes for medication administration, such as oral, intravenous, or intramuscular, should be used. When medications must be administered through the enteral feeding tube, the following guidelines are suggested (37):

1. Flush the feeding tube with 15 mL to 30 mL of warm tap water before and after administering any single medication.

2. If a medication is to be given on an empty stomach, check gastric residuals before administration.

3. Use only water to flush feeding tubes.

4. When ordering medications for enteral feeding-tube administration, provide this information to the dispensing pharmacist, so that the most appropriate solution or suspension can be used.

5. Administer medications as liquid, crushed tablets, or opened capsules diluted in 10 mL to 15 mL of room-temperature tap water.

6. Administer each medication separately.

7. Dilute hypertonic medications with water.

8. Administer medications known to cause GI irritation when formula remains in the GI tract

9. Avoid potential food-drug interactions by using alternative administration routes, by alternating formulas or medications, by altering feeding or medication schedules as indicated, and with multidisciplinary team input.

Monitoring

Appropriate monitoring may prevent or reduce complications associated with tube feeding. Monitoring is more critical in older adults because of diminished compensatory mechanisms. Tube-fed clients should have the following parameters monitored daily: body weight, presence of edema/ascites, fluid intake/output, bowel function, vital signs, and medications. Clients with diabetes or glucose intolerance may need to have blood glucose levels monitored several times daily.

Laboratory studies, including electrolytes (ie, sodium, potassium, and chloride), blood urea nitrogen, creatinine, phosphorous, calcium, liver function tests, magnesium, albumin, and transferrin, should be checked on initiation of enteral nutrition and as needed for medically unstable clients (38). Laboratory studies may only need to be monitored every 1 to 6 months for stable, long-term, tube-fed clients. Table 24.3 provides guidelines to help prevent complications of tube feedings.

Complications

Although generally considered to be safe, tube feeding is not without complications. Problems related to the delivery of tube feeding may be classified as mechanical, infectious, gastrointestinal, or metabolic.

Mechanical Issues

Feeding-tube displacement and migration is a serious mechanical complication of enteral nutrition and may result in aspiration, diarrhea, or peritonitis (with gastrostomy or jejunostomy tubes). Verification of tube placement by x-ray is necessary before feedings are started or when tube malposition is suspected (39).

Formula coagulation, obstruction by pill fragments, tube kinking, and precipitation of incompatible medications may lead to feeding-tube obstruction. It is preferable to dislodge the obstruction rather than to replace the tube (40). See Medication Administration section of this chapter for guidelines regarding the delivery of medications via feeding tubes.

Nasogastric and nasoenteric tubes are associated with pressure necrosis. This may also lead to sinusitis, mucosal ulceration, abscess formation, and perforation. The risk of pressure necrosis can be minimized by use of a soft, small-bore feeding tube or by replacing nasally inserted tubes with gastrostomy/jejunostomy tubes for long-term nutrition (41).

Leakage of feeding-tube contents can be secondary to several different problems. Although rare, leakage around the exit site of a feeding tube may be due to infection or trauma from the tube itself. To prevent or treat infection around the exit site, antibiotic therapy, debridement, and/or feeding tube removal may be indicated (42).

Infections

Gastroesophageal reflux can occur as a result of diminished gastric emptying. Pulmonary aspiration, which may result from reflux, is one of the most serious complications of enteral nutrition and can

TABLE 24.3. Tube-Feeding (TF) Monitoring

Monitoring Parameter	Frequency for Continuous TF	Frequency for Intermittent TF (Includes Cyclic and Bolus)
Maintain head of bed at 30° minimum	Continuously and for 30 min after TF discontinuation	During TF administration and for 30 min after TF discontinued
Check gastric residuals (gastric feedings only)	Every 4-8 h	Before administering TF (every 4-8 h if feeding longer than 8 h)
Flush feeding tube with 20-30 mL of water	After TF discontinued or interrupted Before and after any medication infused via feeding tube Every 4-8 h	After TF discontinued or interrupted Before and after any medication infused via feeding tube Before and after each period of TF administration
Change TF delivery container and tubing (excluding feeding tube)	Daily	Daily
Flush TF administration container and tubing with water	Every 4-8 h Before adding fresh formula to empty TF container	After each TF administration period
Refill TF administration container with fresh formula—open system	Every 4-8 h Limit formula hang time to no more than 8 h per feeding period	Beginning each feeding period Limit formula hang time to no more than 8 h per feeding period
Hang new TF administration container—closed system	Limit formula hang time to no more than 24 h or according to manufacturer's directions	Limit formula hang time to no more than 24 h or according to manufacturer's directions

lead to pneumonia and death in a debilitated, older adult (39). Elevating the head of the bed, the use of aggressive oral hygiene, regular assessment of feeding-tube tip location, minimal use of narcotics, and the use of continuous feeding regimens are recommended measures to prevent aspiration during tube feeding (43). Additional measures to prevent aspiration include regularly checking gastric residuals, using small-bore feeding tubes, and placing the feeding tube beyond the pyloric sphincter (36).

Contamination of any tube-feeding system may originate from nonsterile ingredients, unsanitary equipment, and failure to maintain a clean technique in the preparation of the feeding by the client or caretaker. The risk of contamination may be minimized by proper hand washing, clean preparation methods, use of ready-to-hang/closed system

formulas, and adherence to the tube-feeding monitoring techniques listed in Table 24.3 (36).

Gastrointestinal Complications

GI complications may result from the administration of tube feeding. One of the most common complications associated with tube feeding is diarrhea, which occurs in up to 30% of all tube-fed clients (22). Causes such as antibiotic therapy, osmotically active medications, infection (eg, *Clostridium difficile*), hypoalbuminemia, and microbial contamination of the tube-feeding formula should be ruled out before the tube-feeding formula is considered as the source of diarrhea (41). If the formula is the suspected cause, changing from a hypertonic to an isotonic formula or changing a standard formula to one containing fiber may help to alleviate diarrhea (38). Clients may also demonstrate less diarrhea with tube feeding provided by continuous infusion vs intermittent or bolus schedules (38). Finally, use of antidiarrheal agents or added fiber (eg, banana flakes or psyllium) may be of benefit (38).

Additional GI complications include nausea, vomiting, abdominal distention, and pain. Often the client's medical status and medications are the primary cause of such symptoms. When GI dysmotility is an underlying cause, provision of tube feeding at a slow, continuous infusion or use of prokinetic agents may ease symptoms. Antiemetic medications may also relieve nausea and vomiting (44).

Metabolic Complications

Dehydration, electrolyte disturbances, and azotemia (retention of excessive amounts of nitrogenous compounds in the blood) may occur in an unconscious or debilitated older adult who is unable to communicate or to alleviate thirst. These complications may be reduced by the delivery of adequate amounts of free water, especially to clients who have an elevated temperature or who have additional fluid losses from ostomies, fistulas, and/or drains (41). Overhydration may also occur if a client is receiving excessive amounts of fluid. Accurate daily assessment of fluid intake/output and frequent monitoring of weights and laboratory values are needed to help minimize these complications and to ensure that the client is receiving the prescribed amount of tube feeding (41).

Refeeding syndrome is a potential complication of tube-feeding delivery in the severely malnourished client. This occurs when carbohydrate is reintroduced as the major source of energy, and insulin release is stimulated. As a result, potassium, magnesium, and phosphorous move intracellularly. Electrolyte abnormalities created by refeeding may result in cardiac dysfunction, excess sodium and water retention, and death from respiratory or cardiac failure. The risk of refeeding can be minimized by taking several days to reach nutrition goals in severely malnourished clients. Electrolytes can be repleted by providing supplementation orally or via tube feeding or parenterally (38).

PARENTERAL NUTRITION SUPPORT

Parenteral nutrition is the provision of macronutrients, vitamins, minerals, and electrolytes via a central or peripheral vein. The route of administration depends on the length of the anticipated therapy, nutritional requirements, available intravenous (IV)

Box 24.4 Indications for Parenteral Nutrition Support

- Nonfunctioning GI tract
  - Severe malabsorption
  - Short bowel syndrome
  - Obstruction
  - Intractable diarrhea or vomiting
  - GI bleeding
  - Radiation enteritis
  - Bowel ischemia
  - High output fistula (> 200 mL)
- Bowel rest (eg, severe pancreatitis)
- GI tract not accessible or unsafe for enteral nutrition support

---

access, and fluid status. The indications for nutrition support are the same for older adults as for their younger counterparts. Age alone should not be a contraindication to nutrition support. The threshold for initiating parenteral nutrition, however, may be lower in older adults than in the young, because age-related decreases in muscle mass and organ function leave this population with diminished reserves and impaired compensatory mechanisms (1). Furthermore, older adults may not be able to respond as efficiently to nutritional repletion as younger adults (45). Box 24.4 shows indications for parenteral nutrition support.

Intravenous Access

There are a variety of IV access devices that can be used to administer parenteral nutrition. Choosing the most appropriate type of catheter can be a complex decision, but factors that should be considered include the clinical and nutritional status of the client and the anticipated length of therapy. Age should not be a factor.

IV access devices are generally categorized as either peripheral or central and either temporary or permanent. Peripheral catheters can be used to administer peripheral parenteral nutrition (PPN) in an acute-care setting. The advantages of a peripheral catheter are that (*a*) it can be placed at bedside by a nurse, and (*b*) it has a low rate of serious complications. The disadvantages of a peripheral catheter are that (*a*) a PPN solution may not be able to provide adequate calories and protein to meet the client's requirements, because of concerns with osmolarity: and (2) the catheter needs to be changed every few days, making it impractical for long-term use (46).

Central catheters used to administer total parenteral nutrition (TPN) include temporary central catheters, which do not require surgery, may be inserted at the bedside by a physician, and are generally used in the hospital only; tunneled catheters (ie, Hickman, Broviac, Groshong), which are inserted surgically or radiologically, are tunneled subcutaneously, and have an exit site on the chest wall; and implantable devices (eg, MediPort, Port-a-cath), which are also inserted surgically, are completely under the skin, and are accessed using a special needle. A peripherally inserted central catheter (PICC) is another type of long-term IV access device. A PICC can be inserted radiologically or at the bedside by a specially trained nurse and is typically used to administer IV antibiotics but can also be used for TPN. Permanent catheters (ie, tunneled catheters, implanted devices, or PICCs) are usually required for administration of TPN in nursing facilities or at home (47).

Regular and meticulous care of central catheters is imperative to prevent catheter-related problems such as infection or sepsis. Catheter sepsis is the most common therapy-related reason for readmission of clients receiving home parenteral nutrition (48). Catheter care protocols must be in place in any insti-

tution or home parenteral therapy program where catheters are used for nutrition support (49).

Components of Parenteral Nutrition Solutions

Macronutrients

The macronutrients used in parenteral nutrition solutions are dextrose, amino acids, and lipids (see Table 24.4). Requirements are based on the clinical and nutritional status of the client. Dextrose is the primary source of calories, because it is relatively inexpensive and generally well tolerated. Dextrose provides 3.4 kcal/g and is available in concentrations ranging from 5% to 70%. Amino acids provide 4.0 kcal/g and are available in concentrations ranging from 3% to 15% as standard solutions or disease-specific formulas for clients with renal or liver failure. The disease-specific formulas are generally designed for short-term use in an acute-care setting and are rarely indicated in long-term parenteral nutrition. Lipids provide 9.0 kcal/g and are available in 10%, 20%, or 30% concentrations. Lipids provide essential fatty acids (EFAs) in addition to being a source of energy. Requirements for EFAs can be met by admixing lipids in the parenteral nutrition solution or by infusing 500 mL of 20% fat emulsion once per week or 250 mL of 20% fat emulsion three times per week separately. Table 24.4 gives macronutrients in parenteral nutrition solutions.

TABLE 24.4. Macronutrients in Parenteral Nutrition Solutions

Macronutrient	Concentration	g/L	kcal/L
Dextrose	5%	50	170
	10%	100	340
	20%	200	680
	50%	500	1700
	70%	700	2380
Amino acids	3%	30	120
	7%	70	280
	8.5%	85	340
	10%	100	400
	15%	150	600
Lipids	10%	122	1100
	20%	222	2000
	30%	333	3000

The macronutrient composition of parenteral nutrition solutions administered to older adults may need to be adjusted to compensate for age-related changes in body composition, nutrient metabolism, and organ function (1). Energy expenditure is generally lower because of decreased muscle mass (1). Glucose and protein intolerance is more common because of impaired carbohydrate metabolism and renal function with age (1). These physiological changes may favor a lipid-based parenteral nutrition solution with a modest protein content for the older adult. Insulin may need to be added to the solution, even in clients without diabetes (1).

Fluid

Parenteral nutrition solutions must meet fluid requirements for individuals who are unable to maintain hydration enterally. Fluid intake must be adequate to replace normal losses via urine, feces, sweat, and respiration, along with abnormal losses such as output from ostomies, fistulas, wounds, or a chest tube. Maintaining fluid homeostasis is more difficult in older adults, because of age-related alterations in thirst perception and decreases in cardiovascular and renal function (1). Careful monitoring and documentation of fluid input/output, weight, labs, and vital signs is necessary for managing fluid status in clients receiving parenteral nutrition.

Micronutrients

Electrolytes, minerals, vitamins, and trace elements are essential for normal cellular function and need to be added daily to the parenteral nutrition solution. Requirements vary among individuals based on clinical status, nutritional status, renal function, and medications (see Tables 24.5 and 24.6) (39). There are no established standards for IV requirements for micronutrients specifically for older adults. Electrolytes are commercially available as single or multiple additives and can be added as needed to the parenteral nutrition solution, except in the case of calcium and phosphorus. Excessive concentrations of calcium and phosphorus can result in the formation of a precipitate, which can be life threatening if the solution is infused (50). A pharmacist should be consulted for guidelines.

TABLE 24.5. Average Daily Electrolyte Requirements During Total Parenteral Nutrition

Electrolyte	Daily Requirement
Sodium	1-2 mEq/kg
Potassium	1-2 mEq/kg
Chloride	As needed to maintain acid-base balance
Acetate	As needed to maintain acid-base balance
Calcium	11-15 mEq
Magnesium	8-20 mEq
Phosphorus	20-40 mmol

Source: Adapted with permission from ASPEN Board of Directors and Clinical Guidelines Task Force. Guidelines for the use of parenteral and enteral nutrition in adult and pediatric clients. *JPEN J Parenter Enteral Nutr.* 2002;26:22SA.

TABLE 24.6. Parenteral Vitamin and Trace Element Requirements for Adults

Nutrient	Requirement
Vitamins	
A	1 mg
D	5 µg
E	10 mg
K	150 µg
Ascorbic acid	200 mg
Folic acid	600 µg
Niacin	40 mg
Riboflavin	3.6 mg
Thiamin	6.0 mg
B-6	6.0 mg
B-12	5.0 µg
Pantothenic acid	15 mg
Biotin	60 µg
Trace elements	
Chromium	10-15 µg
Copper	0.3-0.5 mg
Manganese	60-100 µg
Zinc	2.5-5.0 mg
Selenium	20-60 µg

Source: Reprinted with permission from ASPEN Board of Directors and Clinical Guidelines Task Force. Guidelines for the use of parenteral and enteral nutrition in adult and pediatric clients. *JPEN J Parenter Enteral Nutr.* 2002;26:23SA.

It is important to be aware of the content of commercially available multivitamin and trace element preparations. Multivitamin preparations may contain vitamin K, which may interfere with anticoagulation therapy. Multiple trace element preparations contain anywhere from four to six components. Some vitamins and trace elements can be ordered as single additives if needed.

Medications

It is important to be aware of all medications prescribed to clients who are receiving parenteral nutrition because of potential drug-nutrient interactions. Older adults are at higher risk for drug-nutrient interactions, because they are more likely to be on multiple medications (2).

The use of parenteral nutrition as a method for administering medications is generally not recommended, because of potential incompatibility between the drug and other components of the solution, the inability to adjust or discontinue the dosage without discontinuing the solution, and the necessity to infuse medications continuously rather than intermittently. Potential advantages of using parenteral nutrition solutions to deliver medications include cost savings due to decreased use of materials and labor, fluid savings due to a decrease in the number of IVs, and a lower risk of contamination due to less manipulation of the IV lines. Medications routinely added to parenteral nutrition solutions include heparin to prevent catheter occlusion, insulin to control blood sugars, and H2 blockers (eg, famotidine) to prevent gastric ulcer formation. Other medications that have been added to parenteral nutrition include antibiotics, aminophylline, metoclopramide, octreotide, and steroids. A pharmacist should be consulted before adding any medication to a parenteral nutrition solution.

Administering Parenteral Nutrition

Formula selection

Parenteral nutrition solutions are usually categorized as either central or peripheral and either two-in-one (ie, dextrose + protein) or three-in-one (ie, dextrose + protein + lipids). The type of formula is determined by the clinical and nutritional status of the client, as well as the type of IV access. PPN requires a formula that is modest in osmolarity, to prevent thrombophlebitis (inflammation of a vein). Lipids are the primary source of calories in PPN, because dextrose, amino acids, and electrolytes con-

tribute to osmolarity. Solutions with a final dextrose concentration of less than 10% and an osmolarity below 900 mOsm/kg are generally well tolerated by peripheral veins (51).

TPN is not limited by osmolarity, because it is infused through a larger vein and therefore can be concentrated as either a two-in-one or a three-in-one solution. Dextrose-based solutions are preferred in clients who can tolerate the high-carbohydrate concentration, because of concerns with compatibility and immunosuppression associated with IV lipids (52). With dextrose-based TPN, lipids can be infused one to three times per week, to prevent fatty acid deficiency, usually by "piggybacking" into the IV line using a "Y" set. Lipid-based solutions are indicated when minimizing carbohydrate intake is desired. Older adults, who are more likely to have some degree of glucose intolerance than are the young, may tolerate lipid-based solutions better than the young, because of less reliance on dextrose as a source of energy (1).

The stability of three-in-one solutions can be disrupted by improper admixing or inappropriate levels of macronutrients causing a separation of the aqueous and lipid portions of the solution, referred to as creaming or cracking. If this occurs, the parenteral nutrition solution should not be infused, and a pharmacist should be consulted to adjust the levels of macronutrients (53).

Standard parenteral nutrition solutions are available in many institutions and may be appropriate for clients who are medically stable. However, it is important to be able to make appropriate adjustments in the parenteral nutrition formula when necessary, including determining the dextrose, amino acid, and lipid content of solutions (see Boxes 24.5 and 24.6) (53).

Administration Techniques

Parenteral nutrition is usually administered continuously in the hospital, because it requires minimal effort and manipulation of the IV lines and facilitates management of fluid and electrolytes. For clients in nursing facilities or at home, parenteral nutrition is usually cycled over 8 to 16 hours, to allow time away from the IV pump. See Box 24.7 (22). Cycling parenteral nutrition may be more difficult in older adults, because it requires increasing the infusion rate of fluid and dextrose in the face of age-related declines in renal and cardiovascular function and carbohydrate metabolism.

Box 24.5 Determining Parenteral Nutrition Prescription

A. Calculate energy and protein content given final concentrations and volume.

   Example: D_{25} $AA_{4.25}$ $L_{3.0}$ @ 2,400 mL/day

   1. Calculate grams of dextrose, amino acids, and lipids using the formula:

   (Concentration x Volume of Solution in Liters) x 10

   Examples: (25% dextrose $\times$ 2.4 L) $\times$ 10 = 600 g dextrose
   (4.25% amino acids $\times$ 2.4 L) $\times$ 10 = 102 g amino acids
   (3.0% lipids $\times$ 2.4 L) $\times$ 10 = 72 g lipids

   2. Calculate energy for dextrose, amino acids, and lipids by multiplying grams by kilocalories per gram.

   Examples: 600 g dextrose $\times$ 3.4 kcal/g = 2040 kcal
   102 g amino acids $\times$ 4 kcal/g = 408 kcal
   72 g lipid $\times$ 9 kcal/g = 648 kcal

   3. Add kilocalories from dextrose, amino acids, and lipids to determine total energy.

   Example: 2040 + 408 + 648 = 3096 kcal

B. Calculate energy and protein content given volume of base solutions.

   Example: 357 mL D_{70}, 1200 mL AA_{10}, 250 mL L_{20}

   1. Convert volume of base solutions into liters.

   Examples: 357 mL D_{70} = 0.357 L
   1200 mL AA_{10} = 1.2 L
   250 mL L_{20} = 0.250 L

   2. Multiply volume (L) by number of kilocalories per liter for base solutions.

   Examples: 0.357 L D_{70} $\times$ 2380 kcal/L = 850 kcal
   1.2 L AA_{10} $\times$ 400 kcal/L = 480 kcal
   0.250 L L_{20} $\times$ 2000 kcal/L = 500 kcal

   3. Add kilocalories from base solutions to determine total energy.

   Example: 850 + 480 + 500 = 1830 kcal

   4. Multiply volume of amino acid solution (L) by grams per liter to determine protein content.

   Example: 1.2 L AA_{10} $\times$ 100 g/L = 120 g amino acids

---

Tapering (ie, gradually increasing or decreasing the infusion rate at the beginning or end of a cycle) is used to prevent severe changes in blood glucose due to the abrupt infusion or discontinuation of carbohydrate. Clients receiving cyclic parenteral nutrition usually need to be tapered down at the end of the cycle to prevent rebound hypoglycemia. It may also be necessary to taper the parenteral nutrition up for 1 or 2 hours, to avoid hyperglycemia at the start of infusion.

If the parenteral nutrition needs to be stopped unexpectedly, it should be replaced by D_{10} for 1 hour, to prevent rebound hypoglycemia. If time allows, parenteral nutrition should be decreased to half-rate for at least 1 hour before discontinuing.

Box 24.6 Worksheet for Determining Parenteral Nutrition Prescription*

A. Calculate energy and protein content given final concentrations and volume

Example: D_{25} $AA_{4.25}$ $L_{3.0}$ @ 2400 mL/day

1. Record concentration of dextrose, amino acids, and lipids in solution (below).

2. Calculate grams of dextrose, amino acids, and lipids by multiplying concentration by volume of solution in liters ($\times$ 10).

_____% dextrose	$\times$	_____ L $\times$ 10	=	_____ g dextrose
_____% amino acids	$\times$	_____ L $\times$ 10	=	_____ g amino acids
_____% lipids	$\times$	_____ L $\times$ 10	=	_____ g lipids

3. Calculate energy from dextrose, amino acids, and lipids by multiplying grams by kilocalories per gram.

_____ g dextrose	$\times$	3.4 kcal/g	=	_____ kcal
_____ g amino acids	$\times$	4.0 kcal/g	=	_____ kcal
_____ g lipids	$\times$	9.0 kcal/g	=	_____ kcal

4. Add kilocalories from dextrose, amino acids, and lipids (from #3) to determine total energy.

_____total kcal

B. Calculate energy and protein content given volume of base solution.

Example: 357 mL D_{70}, 1200 mL AA_{10}, 250 mL L_{20}

1. Convert volume of dextrose, amino acids, and lipids to liters by dividing volume in milliliters by 1000.

_____ mL dextrose/1000	=	_____ L
_____ mL amino acids/1000	=	_____ L
_____ mL lipids/1000	=	_____ L

2. Multiply volume (L) by kilocalories per liter for base solutions.

_____ L dextrose	$\times$	_____ kcal/L	=	_____ kcal
_____ L amino acids	$\times$	_____ kcal/L	=	_____ kcal
_____ L lipids	$\times$	_____ kcal/L	=	_____ kcal

3. Add kilocalories from dextrose, amino acids, and lipids (from #2) to determine total energy.

_____ total kcal

4. Determine protein content by multiplying volume of amino acids (L) by grams per liter for base solution.

*Omit lipid calculations for dextrose-based solutions.

Monitoring Parenteral Nutrition

Careful monitoring, catheter care, and formula preparation and administration will help to prevent parenteral nutrition-associated complications. Serum levels of electrolytes, blood urea nitrogen, creatinine, visceral proteins, blood or urine sugars, weight, fluid intake and output, vital signs, and current medications should be monitored routinely when parenteral nutrition is administered in a nursing facility or at home. See Table 24.7 (54). Older adults may need to be monitored more closely than would younger adults, because of age-related decreases in compensatory mechanisms. When complications occur, it is important to understand the cause and the treatment. See Table 24.8 (55).

Box 24.7 Calculating Total Parenteral Nutrition Cycling Rates*

1-Hour Taper Down
   Main rate = Total volume/(Cycle hours – 1/2 hour)
   1st-hour taper rate = Main rate/2

2-Hour Taper Down
   Main rate = Total volume/[(Cycle hours –2 hours) + 0.75]
   1st-hour taper rate = Main rate/2
   2nd-hour taper rate = 1st-hour taper rate/2

1-Hour Taper Up, 1-Hour Taper Down
   Main rate = Total volume/(Cycle hours – 1 hour)
   Taper rates = Main rate/2

1-Hour Taper Up, 2-Hour Taper Down
   Main rate = Total volume/[(Cycle hours – 2 hours) + 0.25]
   1st-hour taper up and 1st-hour taper down rates = Main rate/2
   2nd-hour taper down rate = 1st-hour taper rate/2

2-Hour Taper Up, 2-Hour Taper Down
   Main rate = Total volume/ [(Cycle hours – 3 hours) + 0.50]
   2nd-hour taper up rate and 1st-hour taper down rate = Main rate/2
   1st-hour taper up rate and 2nd-hour taper down rate = 2nd-hour taper up rate/2

Rates are expressed in mL/hour.

Source: Reprinted with permission from Matarese LE, ed. *The Cleveland Clinic Foundation Nutrition Support Handbook.* Cleveland, Ohio: Cleveland Clinic Foundation; 1997:102.

TABLE 24.7. Laboratory Monitoring for the Adult Client on Long-term Parenteral Nutrition

Frequency	Laboratory Data
Weekly	Serum glucose, serum electrolytes, BUN, creatinine, serum magnesium, and serum phosphorus until stable. Other laboratory data as clinically indicated.
Monthly for 3 months, then every other month	CBC, serum proteins, serum triglyceride, serum glucose, serum electrolytes, BUN, creatinine, serum magnesium, serum phosphorus, serum calcium. Other laboratory data as clinically indicated.
Quarterly	Serum albumin, AST, alkaline phosphatase, total bilirubin, prothrombin time, INR every 3-6 months. Micronutrients as clinically necessary and/or if deficiency suspected.

Abbreviations: AST, aspertate aminotransferase: BUN, blood urea nitrogen: CBC, complete blood cell count: INR, international normalized ratio.

Source: Reprinted with permission from ASPEN Board of Directors. *Clinical Pathways and Algorithms for Delivery of Parenteral and Enteral Nutrition Support in Adults.* Silver Spring, Md: American Society for Parenteral and Enteral Nutrition; 1998:8-11.

TABLE 24.8 Metabolic Complications of Total Parenteral Nutrition (TPN)

Complication	Possible Causes	Clinical Findings	Prevention	Treatment
Macronutrient substrate complications				
Hyperglycemia	• Diabetes mellitus • Excessive dextrose infusion • Metabolic stress/sepsis • Corticosteroids • Peritoneal dialysis or Continuous arteriovenous hemodialysis • Obesity • Chromium deficiency	• Elevated blood glucose (> 200 mg/dL)	• Limit initial dextrose infusion to approximately 200-250 g/day. • Do not exceed maximum glucose utilization rate (5 mg/kg/min). • Monitor serum glucose.	• Decrease total dextrose (may need to increase fat kcals). • Add regular insulin to TPN or give subcutaneous or IV solution.

Hyperglycemic, hyperosmolar, nonketotic, dehydration/coma	• Sustained, uncontrolled hyperglycemia	• Very high blood glucose levels
		• Elevated serum osmolarity
		• Osmotic diuresis
		• Metabolic acidosis
		• Lethargy and confusion
		• Coma
			• Goal ≤ 200 mg/dL: < 250 mg/dL if at risk for hypoglycemia
			• Monitor:
			  • Blood, urine, glucose closely
			  • Serum OSM
			  • Fluid status (weight, I&Os, skin turgor)
				• Immediate discontinuation of TPN
				• IV hydration, insulin
				• Correction of metabolic acidosis

Hypoglycemia	• Sudden discontinuation of TPN • Exogenous insulin administration not decreased when TPN discontinued	• Sweating • Lethargy and palpitations • Agitation • Faintness • Confusion • Coma	• Taper TPN over 1-2 hours. • Check glucose 1 hour after TPN discontinued in patients with impaired glucose metabolism.	IV dextrose
Hypercapnia (elevated paCO2)	• Excessive dextrose or total caloric intake in patients with obstructive or restrictive lung disease	• Increased paCO2 • Respiratory distress	• Avoid excessive caloric or dextrose infusion. • Obtain indirect calorimetry measurement. • Adjust TPN regimen to meet needs.	• Decrease total caloric intake and/or increase calories as lipid.

TABLE 24.8 *Continued*

Complication	Possible Causes	Clinical Findings	Prevention	Treatment
Macronutrient substrate complications				
Azotemia	• Dehydration • Renal insufficiency • Excessive amino acid infusion • Lean tissue catabolism	• Elevated BUN	• Adequate hydration prior to TPN initiation • Carefully assess protein requirements: avoid excessive amino acid infusion. • Provide adequate nutrition to minimize lean tissue catabolism. • Provide adequate nutrition to minimize lean tissue catabolism. • Monitor BUN.	• Free water administration • Decrease amino acid infusion.
Hypertriglyceridemia	• Excessive lipid infusion • Decreased clearance (stress/sepsis, liver failure) • Sustained hyperglycemia • Preexisting hyperlipidemia	• Lipemia	• Avoid excessive lipid infusion. • Monitor triglycerides weekly.	• Decrease lipid infusion. • If severe, provide only enough lipid to prevent Essential fatty acid deficiency (500 mL 10% fat emulsion 2-3 times/week).
Fluid and electrolyte disturbances/metabolic, acidosis, alkalosis				

Fluid overload	• Excessive fluid administration
	• Renal dysfunction, congestive heart failure, liver disease, trauma
		• Rapid weight gain
		• Fluid intake exceeds output
		• Increased blood pressure
		• Decreased serum sodium and hematocrit
		• Edema
			• Avoid excessive fluid administration.
			• Close monitoring of:
			  • Weights
			  • Intake/output
			  • Laboratory parameters
			  • Physical signs (eg, pitting edema)
				• Concentrate TPN solution: use 20% lipid emulsion.
				• Fluid restriction
				• Sodium restriction, if appropriate
				• Diuretic therapy

Dehydration	• Inadequate fluid intake • Excessive diuresis • Increased GI losses • Fever	• Decreased urine output • Orthostatic blood pressure • Increased serum sodium, BUN, hematocrit • Poor skin turgor • Thirst • Rapid weight loss	• Provide adequate fluid. • Replace insensible and GI losses. • Monitor fluid status.	• Fluid replacement

continued

TABLE 24.8 Metabolic Complications of Total Parenteral Nutrition (TPN) (continued)

Complication	Possible Causes	Clinical Findings	Prevention	Treatment
Hypokalemia	• Inadequate potassium supplementation during anabolism/refeeding • Increased GI losses (vomiting, diarrhea, fistulas) • Medications (eg, Lasix, amphotericin B, cisplatin, etc)	• Metabolic alkalosis • Cardiac arrhythmias • Muscle weakness • Ileus	• Adequate potassium in TPN • Measure and replace losses. • Monitor serum levels daily until stable; biweekly thereafter.	• Increase potassium in TPN if mildly to moderately depleted. • Additional IV supplementation if severely depleted
Hyperkalemia	• Renal insufficiency • Excessive potassium administration • Medications (eg, spironolactone) • Catabolism	• Weakness • Paresthesias • Hyporeflexia • Cardiac arrhythmias	• Avoid excessive potassium administration. • Monitor serum levels daily until stable; biweekly thereafter. • Monitor serum potassium daily in patients with renal insufficiency; restrict as appropriate.	• Decrease potassium in TPN.
Hyponatremia	• Fluid overload • Syndrome of inappropriate antidiuretic hormone • Excessive losses (urinary, GI, or through skin)	• Irritability • Confusion • Lethargy • Seizures	• Adequate sodium in TPN • Avoid excessive fluid administration. • Monitor serum sodium daily until stable; biweekly thereafter.	• Fluid restriction • Increase sodium in TPN if sodium depleted.
Hypernatremia	• Dehydration • Excessive sodium administration • Osmotic diuresis secondary to hyperglycemia • Pituitary tumors	• Thirst (difficult to assess in critically ill patients) • Restlessness • Muscle tremor and rigidity • Hyperactive reflexes • Coma • Convulsions	• Provide adequate fluid. • Avoid excessive sodium administration. • Monitor intake/output, urine, sodium, Osm. • Monitor serum sodium daily until stable; biweekly thereafter.	• Replace fluid if dehydrated. • Decrease sodium in TPN if appropriate.

TABLE 24.8 *Continued*

Complication	Possible Causes	Clinical Findings	Prevention	Treatment
Metabolic acidosis	• Increased intestinal losses of bicarbonate (diarrhea, fistulas) • Renal bicarbonate losses • Ketoacidosis (diabetes, starvation) • Lactic acidosis (shock, cardiac arrest) • Chronic renal failure or renal tubular acidosis • Excessive chloride in TPN (rare)	• Headache • Nausea/vomiting • Diarrhea • Convulsions	• Measure and replace intestinal losses. • Avoid excessive chloride in TPN.	• Increase acetate and decrease chloride in TPN.
Metabolic alkalosis	• Gastric acid losses (increased NG output) • Excess base administration	• Nausea/vomiting • Diarrhea • Sensory changes • Tremoring • Convulsions	• Measure and replace NG output	• Treat underlying cause. • Increase chloride and decrease acetate in TPN. • If severe, may need IV hydrochloric acid.
Mineral imbalances				
Hypocalcemia	• Hypoalbuminemia • Hypomagnesemia • Hyperphosphatemia • Hypoparathyroidism • Malabsorption • Inadequate calcium in TPN	• Muscular/abdominal cramping • Irritability • Confusion • Tetany • Seizures	• Adequate calcium in TPN • Monitor serum calcium biweekly: check ionized calcium if total calcium decreased.	• Correct magnesium deficiency. • Increase calcium in TPN if ionized calcium low.
Hypercalcemia	• Neoplasm • Renal insufficiency • Excessive vitamin D administration • Bone resorption caused by prolonged immobilization/stress	• Confusion • Lethargy • Dehydration • Muscle weakness • Abdominal pain • Nausea and vomiting • Constipation	• Monitor serum levels daily until stable: biweekly thereafter. • Restrict as appropriate.	• Decrease calcium in TPN. • Hydrate with isotonic saline.

continued

TABLE 24.8 Metabolic Complications of Total Parenteral Nutrition (TPN) (continued)

Complication	Possible Causes	Clinical Findings	Prevention	Treatment
Hypo-magnesemia	• Increased GI losses (vomiting, diarrhea, fistula) • Increased urinary losses secondary to drugs (eg, cisplatin, amphotericin B) • Inadequate magnesium supplementation during anabolism/refeeding	• Weakness • Muscle tremors • Ataxia • Tetany • Paresthesias • Dizziness • Disorientation/irritability • Seizures • Cardiac arrhythmias	• Adequate magnesium in TPN • Monitor serum levels daily until stable; biweekly thereafter.	• Increase magnesium in TPN if mildly to moderately depleted. • Additional IV supplementation if severely depleted.
Hypermagne-semia	• Renal insufficiency • Excessive magnesium administration	• Nausea/vomiting • Lethargy/weakness • Cardiac arrhythmias • Hypotension • Respiratory depression	• Monitor serum levels daily until stable; biweekly thereafter. • Monitor serum levels daily in patients with renal insufficiency; restrict as appropriate. • Avoid excessive magnesium administration.	• Decrease magnesium in TPN.
Hypophos-phatemia	• Inadequate phosphorus supplementation during anabolism/refeeding • Exogenous insulin administration • Chronic use of phosphate-binding antacids • Alcoholism • Diabetic ketoacidosis	• Paresthesias • Confusion • Altered speech • Lethargy • Respiratory failure • Decreased red blood cell function • Coma	• Supplement in TPN above standard amounts in patients at risk (diabetes, alcoholism, protein-calorie malnutrition). • Monitor serum levels daily until stable; biweekly thereafter.	• Increase phosphorus in TPN if mildly to moderately depleted. • Additional IV supplementation if severely depleted.

TABLE 24.8 *Continued*

Complication	Possible Causes	Clinical Findings	Prevention	Treatment
Hyperphosphatemia	• Renal insufficiency • Excessive phosphorus administration	• Prolonged elevations may lead to tissue calcification.	• Monitor serum levels daily until stable; biweekly thereafter. • Monitor serum levels daily in patients with renal insufficiency; restrict as appropriate. • Avoid excessive phosphorus administration.	• Decrease phosphorus in TPN.

Other

Complication	Possible Causes	Clinical Findings	Prevention	Treatment
Refeeding syndrome	• Rapid or excessive dextrose infusion (especially in malnourished patients)	• Hyperglycemia • Hypophosphatemia • Hypokalemia • Hypomagnesemia • Edema • Pulmonary edema/CHF	• Identify patients at risk (chronically malnourished, nutritionally depleted patients). • Replete serum electrolyte deficiencies prior to TPN initiation. • Limit initial dextrose infusion to approximately 150-200 g/day. • Supplement phosphorus in TPN. • Advance TPN cautiously. • Routinely administer 3 mg thiamin/day. • Monitor serum glucose, electrolytes, phosphorus, and magnesium daily until stable; biweekly thereafter.	• Decrease infusion rate. • Replete serum electrolyte, phosphorus, magnesium deficiencies; monitor closely. • Limit fluid in presence of edema.
Essential fatty acid deficiency (EFAD)	• Prolonged insufficient lipid infusion	• Dry, scaly skin • Hair loss • Thrombocytopenia • Triene:tetraene > 0.4	• Provide at least 500 mL 10% fat emulsion 2-3 times/week.	• Daily lipid infusion • Cutaneous application of linoleic acid–rich oils if IV lipid contraindicated

continued

TABLE 24.8 Metabolic Complications of Total Parenteral Nutrition (TPN) (continued)

Complication	Possible Causes	Clinical Findings	Prevention	Treatment
Trace mineral deficiencies	• Inadequate supplementation during long-term TPN • Excessive losses via GI tract (diarrhea, fistula output)	• Varies depending upon specific deficiency	• Adequate supplementation	• Supplement deficient nutrient.

Metabolic bone disease	• Etiology unclear/ possibly multifactorial
	• Possible etiologies include:
	  • Altered vitamin D metabolism
	  • Aluminum toxicity
	  • Cyclic versus continuous TPN
	  • Protein-induced calcium loss
		• Bone pain
		• Back pain
		• Pathological fractures
		• Hypercalciuria
			• Moderate nutrient provision
			• Monitor minerals and other TPN solutions for presence of aluminum.
				• Omit vitamin D from TPN for several months; monitor symptoms.
				• Continuous versus cyclic TPN

Source: Reprinted with permission from Green K, Cress MJ. Metabolic complications of parenteral nutrition. *Support Line.* 1993;15:7-9.

SUMMARY

Enteral and parenteral nutrition support, once predominantly confined to acute-care settings, is becoming more commonplace in nursing facilities. Technological advances in nutrition support, the aging of the population, and the changing focus toward health care outside the hospital will ensure the continuation of this trend. Registered dietitians play a vital role in ensuring that nutrition support is provided in a safe and efficacious manner, by assisting in the design and implementation of the nutrition care plan, monitoring and documenting the client's response to therapy, and recommending appropriate adjustments when necessary.

REFERENCES

1. McGee M, Binkley J, Jensen GL. Geriatric nutrition. In: Gottschlich MM, ed. *The Science and Practice of Nutrition Support: A Case-Based Core Curriculum.* Dubuque, Iowa: Kendall/Hunt Publishing Co; 2001:373-389.
2. Watters JM. Parenteral nutrition in the elderly client. In: Rombeau JL, Rolandelli RH, eds. *Clinical Nutrition: Parenteral Nutrition.* 3rd ed. Philadelphia, Pa: WB Saunders Co; 2001:429-443.
3. Johnston RE, Chernoff R. Geriatric nutrition support. In: Matarese LE, Gottschlich MM, eds. *Contemporary Nutrition Support Practice: A Clinical Guide.* Philadelphia, Pa: WB Saunders Co; 1998:365-372.
4. Lipschitz D. Nutrition and aging. In: Evans JG, Williams TF, eds. *Oxford Textbook of Geriatric Medicine.* New York, NY: Oxford University Press; 1992:870.
5. *Nutrition Interventions Manual for Professionals Caring for Older Americans.* Washington, DC: Nutrition Screening Initiative; 1992.
6. D'Erasmo E, Pisani D, Ragno A, Romagnoli S, Spagna G, Acca M. Serum albumin level at admission: mortality and clinical outcomes in geriatric clients. *Am J Med Sci.* 1997;314:17-20.
7. Friedmann JM, Jensen GL, Smiciklas-Wright H, McCamish MA. Predicting early nonelective hospital readmission in nutritionally compromised older adults. *Am J Clin Nutr.* 1997;65:1714-1720.
8. Jensen GL, Kita K, Fish J, Heydt D, Frey C. Nutrition risk screening characteristics of rural older persons: relation to functional limitation and health care charges. *Am J Clin Nutr.* 1997;66:819-828.
9. Corti MC, Guralnik JM, Salive ME, Sorkin JD. Serum albumin level and physical disability as predictors of mortality in older persons. *JAMA.* 1994;272:1035-1042.
10. Baumgartner RN, Koehler KM, Romero L, Garry PJ. Serum albumin is associated with skeletal muscle in elderly men and women. *Am J Clin Nutr.* 1996;64:552-558.

11. Sacks G, Dearman K, Replogle B, Canada T. Evaluation of malnutrition with subjective global assessment in geriatric long-term care facility clients. *JPEN J Parenter Enteral Nutr.* 1998;22:S11.

12. National Research Council. *Recommended Dietary Allowances.* 10th ed. Washington, DC: National Academy Press; 1989.

13. Institute of Medicine. *Dietary Reference Intakes for Energy, Carbohydrate, Fiber: Fat, Fatty Acids, Cholesterol, Protein, and Amino Acids.* Washington, DC: National Academy Press; 2002.

14. Jeejeebhoy KN, Chu RC, Marliss EB, Greenberg GR, Bruce-Robertson A. Chromium deficiency, glucose intolerance, and neuropathy reversed by chromium supplementation, in a patient receiving long-term total parenteral nutrition. *Am J Clin Nutr.* 1997;30:531-538.

15. Skipper A. Principles of parenteral nutrition. In: Matarese LM, Gottschlich MM, eds. *Contemporary Nutrition Support Practice: A Clinical Guide.* Philadelphia, Pa: WB Saunders Co; 1998:233.

16. Institute of Medicine. *Dietary Reference Intakes for Calcium, Phosphorus, Magnesium, Vitamin D, Fluoride.* Washington, DC: National Academy Press; 1997.

17. Institute of Medicine. *Dietary Reference Intakes for Thiamin, Riboflavin, Niacin, Vitamin B6, Folate, Vitamin B12, Pantothenic Acid, Biotin, and Choline.* Washington, DC: National Academy Press; 1999.

18. Institute of Medicine. *Dietary Reference Intakes for Vitamin C, Vitamin E, Selenium, and Carotenoids.* Washington, DC: National Academy Press; 2000.

19. Institute of Medicine. *Dietary Reference Intakes for Vitamin A, Vitamin K, Arsenic, Boron, Chromium, Copper, Iodine, Iron, Manganese, Molybdenum, Nickel, Silicon, Vanadium, and Zinc.* Washington, DC: National Academy Press; 2001.

20. Food and Drug Administration. Parenteral multivitamin products: drugs for human use: drug efficacy study implementation: amendment. *Federal Register.* 2000;65:21200-21201.

21. Charney P. Enteral nutrition: indications, options, and formulations. In: Gottschlich M, ed. *The Science and Practice of Nutrition Support: A Case-Based Core Curriculum.* Dubuque, Iowa: Kendall/Hunt Publishing; 2001:141-166.

22. Home nutrition support. In: Matarese LE, ed. *The Cleveland Clinic Foundation Nutrition Support Handbook.* Cleveland, Ohio: Cleveland Clinic Foundation; 1997:97-105.

23. Hammond KA, Szeszycki E, Pfister D. Transitioning to home and other alternate sites. In: Gottschlich MM, ed. *The Science and Practice of Nutrition Support: A Case-Based Core Curriculum.* Dubuque, Iowa: Kendall/Hunt Publishing Co; 2001:701-729.

24. Howard L, Malone M. Clinical outcome of geriatric clients in the United States receiving home parenteral and enteral nutrition. *Am J Clin Nutr.* 1997;66:1364-1370.

25. Sheiman SL. Tube feeding the demented nursing home resident. *J Am Ger Soc.* 1996;44:1268-1270.

26. Nair S, Hertan H, Pitchumoni CS. Hypoalbuminemia is a poor predictor of survival after percutaneous endoscopic gastrostomy in elderly clients with dementia. *Am J Gastroenterol.* 2000;95:133-136.

27. Ideno KT. Enteral nutrition. In: Gottschlich MM, Matarese LE, Shronts EP, eds. *Nutrition Support Dietetics: Core Curriculum.* 2nd ed. Silver Spring, Md: American Society for Parenteral and Enteral Nutrition; 1993:71-104.

28. Minard G, Lysen LK. Enteral access devices. In: Gottschlich MM, ed. *The Science and Practice of Nutrition Support: A Case-Based Core Curriculum.* Dubuque, Iowa: Kendall/Hunt Publishing Co; 2001:167-189.

29. Vanek VW. Ins and outs of enteral access. Part 1: short-term access. *Nutr Clin Pract.* 2002;17:275-283.

30. Zaloga GP. Bedside method for placing small bowel feeding tubes in critically ill clients: a prospective study. *Chest.* 1991;100:1643-1646.

31. Franzi LR, Seidner DL. Enteral nutrition. In: Parekh NR, DeChicco RS, eds. *The Cleveland Clinic Foundation Nutrition Support Handbook.* Cleveland, Ohio: Cleveland Clinic Foundation; 2004:61-77.

32. Fussell ST. Enteral formulations. In: Matarese LE, Gottschlich MM, eds. *Contemporary Nutrition Support Practice: A Clinical Guide.* Philadelphia, Pa: WB Saunders Co; 2001:188-200.

33. Hurley DL, Neven AK, McMahon MM. Diabetes mellitus. In: Gottschlitch MM, ed. *The Science and Practice of Nutrition Support :A Case-Based Core Curriculum.* Dubuque, Iowa: Kendall/Hunt Publishing Co; 2001:663-675.

34. Rhoney DH, Parker D, Formea CM, Yap C, Coplin WM. Tolerability of bolus versus continuous feeding in brain injured patients. *Neurol Res.* 2002;24:613-620.

35. Coben RM, Weintraub A, DiMarino AJ, Cohen S. Gastroesophageal reflux during gastrostomy feeding. *Gastroenterology.* 1994;106:13-18.

36. Beyer PL. Complications of enteral nutrition. In: Matarese LE, Gottschlich MM, eds. *Contemporary Nutrition Support Practice: A Clinical Guide.* Philadelphia, Pa: WB Saunders Co; 2001:215-226.

37. Thomson CA, Rollins CJ. Nutrient-drug interactions. In: Rombeau JL, Rolandelli RH, eds. *Enteral and Tube Feeding.* 3rd ed. Philadelphia, Pa: WB Saunders Co; 1997:523-539.

38. Russell M, Cromer M, Grant J. Complications of enteral nutrition therapy. In: Gottschlich MM, ed. *The Science and Practice of Nutrition Support: A Case-Based Core Curriculum.* Dubuque, Iowa: Kendall/Hunt Publishing Co; 2001:189-209.

39. ASPEN Board of Directors and Clinical Guidelines Taskforce. Guidelines for the use of parenteral and enteral nutrition in adult and pediatric clients. *JPEN J Parenter Enteral Nutr.* 2002;26(suppl): 1SA-138SA.

40. Kudsk KA. Clinical applications of enteral nutrition. *Nutr Clin Pract.* 1994;9:165-171.

41. Lord L, Trumbore L, Zaloga G. Enteral nutrition implementation and management. In: *The ASPEN Nutrition Support Practice Manual.* Silver Spring, Md: ASPEN; 1998:5-1-5-16.

42. Holmes S. Enteral feeding and percutaneous endoscopic gastrostomy. *Nurs Stand.* 2004;18:41-43.

43. Proceedings of the North American Summit on Aspiration in the Critically Ill Patient. *JPEN J Parenter Enteral Nutr.* 2002;26(Suppl 6):S1-S85.

44. Parish CR. Enteral feeding: the art and science. *Nutr Clin Pract.* 2003;18:76-85.

45. Shizgal HM, Martin MF, Gimmon Z. The effect of age on the caloric requirement of malnourished individuals. *Am J Clin Nutr.* 1992;55:783-789.

46. Orr ME. Vascular access device selection for parenteral nutrition. *Nutr Clin Pract.* 1999;14:172-177.

47. Steiger E. Obtaining and maintaining vascular access in the home parenteral nutrition patient. *JPEN J Parenter Enteral Nutr.* 2002;26(suppl):S17-S20.

48. Howard L, Ament M, Fleming CR, Steiger E. Current use and clinical outcome of home parenteral and enteral nutrition therapies in the United States. *Gastroenterology.* 1995;109:355-365.

49. Grant J. Recognition, prevention, and treatment of home total parenteral nutrition central venous access complications. *JPEN J Parenter Enteral Nutr.* 2002;26(suppl):S21-S28.

50. Lumpkin MM. Safety alert: hazards of precipitation associated with parenteral nutrition. *Am J Hosp Pharm.* 1994;51:1427-1428.

51. Isaacs JW, Millikan WJ, Stackhouse J, Hersh T, Rudman D. Parenteral nutrition of adults with a 900 milliosmolar solution via peripheral veins. *Am J Clin Nutr.* 1977;30:552-559.

52. Seidner DL, Mascioli EA, Istfan NW, Porter KA, Selleck K, Blackburn GL, Bistrian BR. Effects of long-chain triglyceride emulsions on reticulendothelial system function in humans. *JPEN J Parenter Enteral Nutr.* 1989;113:614-619.

53. National Advisory Group on Standards and Practice Guidelines for Parenteral Nutrition. ASPEN Board of Directors. Safe practices for parenteral nutrition formulations. *JPEN J Parenter Enteral Nutr.* 1998;22:49-66.

54. ASPEN Board of Directors. *Clinical Pathways and Algorithms for Delivery of Parenteral and Enteral Nutrition Support in Adults.* Silver Spring, Md: American Society for Parenteral and Enteral Nutrition; 1998.

55. Green K, Cress MJ. Metabolic complications of parenteral nutrition. *Support Line.* 1993;15:7-9

CHAPTER 25

Nutrition Care for Palliative Care Clients

Health care professionals are challenged to provide the highest quality of care and quality of life possible for clients and their families. This becomes especially important for clients who are terminally ill and may be receiving palliative care. Clients, family members, facility health care teams, facility administrators, surveyors, risk managers, corporate legal departments, and plaintiff attorneys are all concerned about nutrition care. Regardless of health care setting (nursing facility, home care, hospice or palliative care units of hospitals, assisted-living facilities, or other settings), the dietetics professional has an extremely important role in achieving quality of life and quality of care for older adults who are receiving palliative care. Additionally, all members of the health care team have the responsibility to address the moral, ethical, legal, and risk-management issues associated with nutrition care (1).

THE MEANING AND VALUE OF FOOD AND NUTRITION

Food and drink are among life's greatest pleasures, and our perception of food and drink varies throughout life. When individuals are healthy and their appetite is good, food and drink are generally enjoyed and often taken for granted, regardless of age. When individuals are ill and their appetite may be poor, food and drink can be a source of conflict and take on greater importance. This is especially true for older adults, especially when diagnosed with a terminal illness (2).

It is important for health care providers to understand the psychological aspects of a diagnosis of terminal illness, such as Alzheimer's disease, dementia, cancer, and end-stage liver, kidney, or heart disease. Such diagnoses elicit powerful emotions, including fear and grief, and can have a shat-tering effect on a client's self-image, particularly one who has had a disfiguring surgery (3).

The emotions that burden clients often manifest themselves in eating disorders. Sometimes such emotions can cause overeating, but more often these emotions dampen the appetite (3). A common emotion among clients diagnosed with a terminal disease is the loss of control of life's events and the anxiety over the perceived incompleteness of their lives. Many clients experience guilt associated with their past or present lifestyle, and many focus on failed or strained relationships and failure to accomplish goals. They also may experience fears, such as fear of abandonment, fear of pain, fear of the dying process, fear of physical and mental disability, or fear of dependence on others (4).

The dying process itself can diminish appetite, as well as alter nutritional needs in ways such as the following (5):

- The anatomical, physiological, and metabolic changes that occur because of various diseases can decrease gastrointestinal absorption and increase nutrient requirements, such as frequently occurs in clients with acquired immune deficiency syndrome (AIDS) who often develop severe diarrhea and malabsorption.

- The dying process itself slows many body functions, including gastric emptying, which results in increased satiety, decreased hunger, and frequent food intolerances.

- Medical interventions, such as chemotherapy, alter metabolic processes and frequently result in increased nutrient requirements. Even palliative medications, such as narcotics, impact nutrient needs when side effects, such as nausea, vomiting, and constipation, occur.

GOALS OF NUTRITION CARE

Although clients with a terminal diagnosis often feel a loss of control, nutrition is one aspect of their care about which they often feel they do have control. Giving clients a feeling that they can help with their own well-being through what they eat and drink is important. Clients usually desire a proactive approach to nutrition care early in the diagnosis of their illness.

O'Sullivan Maillet suggests that the responsibility of health care providers to clients early in the diagnosis of a terminal disease is to encourage a varied food intake, weight maintenance for those who are overweight, and weight maintenance or increased weight if possible for those who are underweight (6). Encouraging intake of a varied diet that is calorie appropriate is a way to put control into clients' hands. Liberalization of diets offered can go a long way in giving residents a sense of control and in encouraging them to eat a varied and calorie-appropriate diet (7).

Families of terminally ill clients frequently feel impotent. Including them in nutrition counseling sessions can bring them into the care of their loved one. Family members can reinforce nutrition principles and encourage eating; however, they should be cautioned that there is a fine line between nagging, which is counterproductive, and encouragement (8).

Goals of nutrition care for clients with a terminal disease, whose choice is for palliative care, are as individual as is the client. Goals may also vary as the illness progresses. For example, the nutrition goals for the client whose life expectancy is several months or longer may be to provide tube feeding to prolong length and quality of life. Nutrition support via percutaneous endoscopic gastrostomy (PEG) tube feeding can achieve this goal for a client with amyotrophic lateral sclerosis (ALS) who has dysphagia and is at risk for suboptimal energy and fluid intake, worsening of muscle atrophy, weakness, and fatigue (9). Similarly, tube feeding is appropriate for clients undergoing aggressive cancer therapies or for clients after stroke when rehabilitation is the primary goal (10).

However, the nutrition goal for a palliative care client, whose life expectancy is short, may be to use food and drink as desired by the client, to maximize enjoyment and to minimize pain (5). When eating and mealtimes can accomplish either of these goals, they should be used to advantage. If eating is not an enjoyable experience, however, its practice should not be overemphasized. It is at this time that dietetics professionals can be strong client advocates and family allies by reassuring both that loving care can be demonstrated in ways other than through feeding (11).

THE DIETETICS PROFESSIONAL'S ROLE IN ACHIEVING NUTRITION GOALS

The role of the nurse . . . is first, to come to terms with personal, psychological, and moral and ethical issues surrounding nutrition and hydration on an individual level; and second, to enter into a partnership with the client and family and guide them through the storm of emotions and questions using a framework based on principles of ethics, crisis intervention, and effective communication.

—CM Maurer Baack (12)

Maurer Baack's admonition to nurses applies to dietetics professionals as well. After self-understanding, the dietetics professional will perform several functions to achieve nutrition care goals, such as the following (5):

- Assess the client's physical and psychological condition for the role that curative and palliative treatments, food, and mealtimes have on causing symptoms; ascertain if dietary modifications can alleviate these symptoms and improve well-being.

- Identify the client and family's nutritional concerns and dietary questions.

- Establish goals of treatment and integrate dietary interventions as appropriate into the overall plan of care.

- Counsel the client and family on specific and practical dietary modifications that can enhance well-being.

- Reevaluate nutrition goals and interventions periodically, and implement changes when appropriate.

ASSESSING THE CLIENT'S CONDITION

Assessment is the first component in the provision of nutrition care; a plan of care is only as good as the completeness and accuracy of the data collected and the assessment of the client's condition and the family's situation.

Box 25.1 is an assessment instrument that includes important nutrition-related questions that the facility or home-care nurse might ask the client and family during an initial visit and during ongoing visits. Answers to these questions will give clues about the nutritional status and eating behavior of the client. In addition, use of this tool may alert the nurse to the need for the services of a dietetics professional. Box 25.2 lists conditions and issues that generally require the services of a dietetics professional.

Box 25.1   Nutrition Assessment Instrument

1. Does the client experience any of the following problems?
   - Nausea and/or vomiting

     If yes, is it associated with any of the following?
     - Taste of specific foods
     - Sight or smell of particular foods
     - Temperature of foods
   - Diarrhea
   - Constipation or gastrointestinal obstruction
   - Mouth sores
   - Difficulty swallowing
   - Dry mouth
   - Poor appetite

     If yes, is it caused by any of the following?
     - Pain or other symptoms
     - Depression or anxiety
     - Early satiety, fatigue, or weakness
     - Pressure ulcers

2. Does the client take any vitamin, mineral, or other food supplements?

3. Does the client have a gastrointestinal or intravenous feeding tube in place?

4. Does the client or family express significant remorse about weight change?
   - If the client has lost much weight, does the weight change make the client more dependent on others?
   - Does the client or family want to try to reverse the weight loss with enteral or parenteral nutrition support?
   - If the client has gained weight, is the weight change acceptable to the client?

5. Does the family exhibit any of the following behaviors?
   - Inappropriate use of food as a crutch for emotional problems
   - Belief that disease is caused by what the client did or did not eat
   - Fear that if the client doesn't eat, he or she will feel hunger pains
   - Fear that if the client becomes dehydrated, he or she will die soon
   - Belief in unorthodox nutrition therapies, such as vitamin C, Laetrile, the macrobiotic diet, enzymes

Box 25.2   Suggested Reasons for Referral to a Dietetics Professional or Nutritionist

Physiological Intake Issues
- Presence of tube feeding or total parenteral nutrition
- Client has concerns about weight loss
- Client has concerns about weight gain
- Difficulty with oral intake due to mouth sores, dysphagia, or poor dentition
- Concerns with continued loss of appetite
- Inadequate fluid intake
- Client or family would like additional nutrition suggestions

Clinical Issues
- Presence of wounds
- Uncontrolled diabetes
- End-stage renal disease
- End-stage liver disease (with or without encephalopathy)

- Symptoms not controlled by medications, such as nausea, vomiting, diarrhea, constipation, dyspepsia, or fluid accumulation
- Intestinal obstruction, when oral intake is not contraindicated
- Chronic bleeding with weakness
- Client taking alternative nutrition therapies, such as herbs or supplements

Psychological/Social Issues
- Conflicts regarding the use of food and drink
- Client or caregiver difficulty giving up past diet restrictions
- Issues concerning initiating, withholding, or withdrawing nutrition support
- Client or caregiver needing clarification on dehydration issue
- Financial difficulties affecting intake
- Living conditions affecting intake

IDENTIFYING CLIENT AND FAMILY CONCERNS

Box 25.1 also includes questions about specific nutrition issues and dietary concerns that clients and families may wish to express. The dietetics professional should pay attention to off-hand remarks that expose hidden fears, such as those given below.

- "If I don't drink anything, will dehydration be painful?"
- "If I give up alcohol, will my liver tumor shrink?"
- "I'd like to eat, but I'm afraid I'll choke and be unable to breathe if I eat too much."
- "If I had eaten 'right,' would I have avoided cancer?"

INTEGRATING NUTRITION INTO THE PLAN OF CARE

After the information from the nutrition assessment tool is collected and assessed, and the client and family concerns have been identified, a nutrition problem list can be delineated. Nutrition goals that are consistent with other medical and nursing goals should then be established. After the delineation of appropriate palliative nutrition therapies, the problems, goals, and therapies are written into the plan of care (5).

The ethnic, cultural, and religious background of the client and family must be taken into consideration when identifying goals and suggesting appropriate therapies. Despite the well-known adage that it is hazardous to apply stereotypes to individual clients, peoples of various backgrounds do have different views and do respond differently to food, symptoms, pain, health-care delivery systems, and dying. Older adults also differ from younger adults in their views of death and dying (13). (See Box 25.3.) The views and responses of others are often greatly different from our own. To be helpful to clients and their families, health care providers must not only recognize that individual differences exist but also be supportive of these differences (14). Many references are available to assist in understanding ethnic considerations in end-of-life care (15-20).

Box 25.3 Views of Death and Dying

Older People

- Spend more time thinking about death.
- Have rehearsed death.
- Have a lifetime of coping mechanisms upon which to call.
- Often state that they are not afraid to die.
- View death more calmly and peacefully than the young.

- Tend to espouse more traditional religious feelings and beliefs.
- Think about the last opportunity to see loved ones, bringing business affairs to completion, and reminiscing about life.
- Are less concerned about cessation of experiences.

- Value the quality of the remaining time more than its quantity, often foregoing therapy in the last few months of life that may make them uncomfortable.
- Fear the process of dying more than the end result.

Younger People

- Have limited thoughts or experiences with death.

- Many middle-aged people state that they are afraid to die.
- The very young often indicate no or little fear of death.
- Often cannot identify what beliefs they hold sacred.
- Tend to deal primarily with the experiences of the present.

- Cessation of experiences is a great sorrow to most young people.
- Often endure almost intolerable therapy and side effects to buy a few more days of life.

- Fear the state of death more than the process of dying.

Source: Data are from reference 13.

COUNSELING ABOUT APPROPRIATE DIETARY MODIFICATIONS

The client is generally highly motivated after the decision to implement therapeutic intervention for a terminal illness. Therefore, after minimizing the client and family's guilt about the illness, O'Sullivan Maillet recommends that health care professionals should focus attention on the current diet—how the client is eating properly and what changes may be appropriately made (6). The value of proper nutrition in promoting overall good health and physical well-being should be emphasized but not overpromised. Teach the client that diet cannot cure the terminal illness and that, regardless of diet, an illness that is in remission can recur (6). Nutrition quackery is tempting to clients at this point. The dietetics professional's responsibility is to provide facts without being judgmental and to advise the client as to whether the contemplated therapy is potentially injurious to health. As with any counseling, however, the client makes the final decision, and the decision should be respected even if the dietetics professional disagrees with it (6).

During the time of therapy, the client and family should be helped to focus their dietary concerns on meeting immediate needs for energy, protein, vitamins, minerals, and fluid. Clients sometimes have trouble understanding why a concentrated-energy diet that may be high in fat, protein, and carbohydrate is different from a "prevention" diet, which they may consider to be low in fat and high in fruits, vegetables, and whole grains.

During active therapy, nutrition is often one of the only areas over which the client feels control. The ability of the client to manipulate intake to consume sufficient calories brings a great sense of accomplishment. Courage and determination to survive are often reflected in the client's efforts to eat well despite symptoms (6). If clients know that they are not eating well and are losing weight, they may wish to discuss aggressive nutrition interventions with health care professionals. Health care team members need to demonstrate awareness that clients may be afraid to verbalize their wish to discuss tube feeding or parenteral feeding by offering in advance to discuss these issues should they become important to the client and family at any time.

When therapy is completed, the emotions of the client and family may range from severe depression to unbridled (but cautious) joy—depending on the outcome of treatment. Relief will be felt by all to some extent (8). When therapy is complete, nutrition in promoting the return of physical strength is important. Weight goals need to be set, possibly with a margin of safety for future therapy. The merits of diet in secondary prevention need to be considered if the client and family desire, but the merits need to be tempered, to avoid reimposing guilt or overpromising a cure or prevention of recurrence (6).

Clients and their families often go through a period of fear of abandonment when treatment has ceased. Cessation of treatment should not mean cessation of care (21). Most clients and families appreciate being told options in straightforward but empathetic terms.

Counseling for the dying client should address issues such as the following (22):

- How the disease process and the process of dying affect the desire for food
- How changes in appetite and ability to eat cause changes in food intake, bodily appearance, and bodily function
- Specific dietary measures for symptom control
- Relief measures that will be available as the client's condition deteriorates
- The availability of community nutrition and food resources
- How to reach the nurse and dietetics professional when questions arise and assistance is needed

REEVALUATING GOALS AND INTERVENTION

Self-evaluation, evaluation of the established plan of care, and evaluation of the ability of the client and family to achieve desired goals are standard procedure during and after visits by members of the health care team. It is only with such evaluation that progress can be noted and the care plan can be modified as necessary. When goals are not achieved, blame should not be imposed on clients, families, or health care team members. Instead, realistic revisions to the plan should be made (5). Two dietary situations that nurses and dietetics professionals frequently encounter are (a) the client who cannot and will not eat; and (b) the client who can and wants to eat but needs assistance in knowing what to eat and how to maximize the quality of mealtimes.

HELPING THE CLIENT WHO CANNOT AND WILL NOT EAT

Anorexia and cachexia are common phenomena that occur with clients who are receiving palliative care (22). Tumors and medications may cause early satiety (especially with lung, stomach, and pancreatic tumors), specific food aversions (with almost all tumors, and particularly to protein-containing foods, such as beef and pork), nausea and vomiting (especially with liver cancer or metastases to the liver and as a result of narcotics and other therapies), and decreased interest in foods (particularly with an external tumor compression or partial obstruction of any part of the gastrointestinal tract) (5,23). Although weight loss is often a worrisome sign, treatment does not necessarily improve the client's well-being or survival (24,25).

Anorexia and cachexia are not always problems to the client and family. When they are problems, generally they are more problematic for the family than for the client (26). Cachexia may be a problem for clients and families because they do not understand what causes it or how it occurs.

When working with an anxious family of a client who cannot or will not eat, attempts should be made to diminish the effects of the no-win situation (see Boxes 25.4 and 25.5 [14]). Treatment is best directed at ameliorating social consequences, such as embarrassment of the client at his or her gaunt appearance and physical complications. Teaching the family about the effects that the disease and dying process have is also important. The family's anxieties can be diminished and the client can be freed from the pressure to eat when attention is shifted from maintaining the client's nutritional status to enhancing client comfort through providing small appetizing meals. Sometimes it is most appropriate to offer no food unless the client requests it. Although this shift may be difficult at first, it brings considerable relief to both client and family in the long run (15).

Box 25.4 Suggestions for Improving Oral Intake

- Feed the client when hungry, changing mealtimes if needed. Note the client's best meals, and make these the largest meals.

- Serve a small serving of the client's favorite foods on a small plate.

- Gently encourage, but do not nag, the client to eat; remove uneaten food without undue comment.

- Cold foods are generally preferred to hot foods.

- Set an attractive table and plate, using a plate garnish or table flower if enjoyed by the client. In an institutional setting, serve the client's food on trays set with embroidered tray cloths and pretty china or stoneware, rather than on traditional paper underliners and dishes. Allow the client's personal china and utensils from home to be used if feasible.

- Make mealtimes sociable (when desired by the client) and enjoyable, vary the place of eating, and remove unnecessary medical equipment (such as bedpans) from the room.

- Suggest the client rest before eating; most people feel more like eating when they are relaxed.

- Encourage high-calorie foods day or night, including eggnog, milkshakes, custard, pudding, peanut butter, cream soups, cheese, fizzy drinks, pie, sherbet, and cheesecake. In an institutional setting, consider serving foods from a hot trolley instead of or in addition to allowing clients to choose their meals in advance. Consider soup and soft sandwiches for midday meals. Try to supply as much variety in food selection as possible, including regional favorites.

- Provide lipped dishes for those clients who have arm and hand weakness; use rubber grips on ordinary cutlery for those with a weak grip.

- In an institutional setting, have a dining room available, with a home-like atmosphere, where clients can eat and clients and families can eat together. Allow the family to eat with the client in the client's room if desired. Have staff available to assist clients who are unable to feed themselves. Do not hurry clients to eat.

- Liberalize diets as much as possible. Rarely are diabetic or low-sodium diets essential, but if they are, consider low simple sugar foods and no regular salt packets instead of more restricted diets.

Adapted from Gallagher-Allred CR. *Nutritional Care of the Terminally Ill.* Rockville, Md: Aspen Publishers, Inc; 1989:221, 269, with permission of Aspen Publishers, Inc.

Box 25.5 Dietary Therapy for Treating Common Symptoms in Palliative Care

Belching

- Allow the client to make the final choice of foods to eat and avoid, but consider testing the client's tolerance to gas-producing foods, such as the following: beer, carbonated beverages, alcohol, dairy products if lactose intolerant, nuts, beans, onions, peas, corn, cucumbers, radishes, cabbage, broccoli, Brussels sprouts, spinach, cauliflower, high-fat foods, yeast, and mushrooms.

- Encourage the client to eat solids at mealtimes and drink liquids between meals instead of with solid foods.

- Advise the client to avoid eating quickly and reclining immediately after eating; encourage the client to relax before, during, and after meals.

- Advise the client to avoid overeating, to avoid sucking through straws, to avoid chewing gum, and to keep the mouth closed when chewing and swallowing.

Constipation

- Encourage the client to eat foods high in fiber (bran; whole grains; fruits, especially pineapple, prunes and raisins; vegetables; nuts; and legumes) if adequate fluid intake can be maintained. Avoid high-fiber foods if dehydration, severe constipation, or obstruction is anticipated.

- Increase fluid intake as tolerated; encourage fruit juices, prune juice, and cider. If liked by the client, a recipe (1 to 2 ounces with the evening meal of a mixture of 2 cups applesauce, 2 cups unprocessed bran, and 1 cup 100% prune juice) is effective and may reduce laxative use.

- Discontinue calcium and iron supplementation if used; limit cheese, rich desserts, and other foods if constipating.

Diarrhea

- Let the client make the final choice of foods to eat or to avoid, but suggest omission of the following foods if they cause diarrhea: milk, ice cream, whole-grain breads and cereals, nuts, beans, peas, greens, fruits with seeds and skins, fresh pineapple, raisins, cider, prune juice, raw vegetables, gas-forming vegetables, alcohol, and caffeine-containing beverages.

- Encourage the client to eat bananas, applesauce, peeled apple, tapioca, rice, peanut butter, refined grains, crackers, pasta, cream of wheat, oatmeal, and cooked vegetables.

- Encourage the client to avoid liquids with a meal and instead to drink liquids an hour after a meal.

- Encourage the client to relax before, during, and after a meal.

- Enteral and/or parenteral nutrition support in the AIDS client may be appropriate if the client has a lengthy life expectancy and the cause of the diarrhea is known and treatable; if tube feedings or oral diet is appropriate, they should be high in energy and protein and low in fiber, lactose, and fat.

- If dehydration is a problem, encourage high-potassium foods.

Hypercalcemia

- Allow the hypercalcemic client to eat foods high in calcium, such as dairy products if desired, but encourage the client to avoid calcium and vitamin D supplementation; restriction of high-calcium foods is rarely helpful.

- Encourage the client to drink lots of fluids, particularly carbonated beverages containing phosphoric acid if the client enjoys them.

Mental Disorders

- Encourage the client to avoid alcohol and caffeine-containing foods, such as coffee, tea, and chocolate, if they contribute to anxiety, sleep deprivation, or depression.

- If the client is drowsy or apathetic, suggest that the family may need to assist the client with meal intake. Encourage them to prepare the client's favorite foods, usually in soft form to be served with a spoon or bite-sized, so the client may self-feed. Help the family protect the client and others from the client by shutting off or removing knobs from stoves, removing matches, and locking doors to cabinets or closets that contain poisons, alcohol, or medications. Put away electrical appliances, such as mixers, food processors, can openers, and waffle irons; unplug microwave ovens.

- If the client is agitated or confused, caution the family about the dangers of hand-feeding the client. Suggest assisting with a spoon and not allowing the client to handle feeding utensils, plates, glass, etc. Encourage the family to tell the client what time of day it is, what meal is served, and what foods are served. Remind the client that the foods served are favorites. Make mealtimes enjoyable by reminiscing about pleasant events in the client's life. Consider the pros and cons of waking the client if asleep at mealtimes.

continued

Box 25.5 Dietary Therapy for Treating Common Symptoms in Palliative Care (continued)

- If the client is stuporous or comatose, counsel the family that semistarvation and dehydration are not painful to the client; explore with them the pros and cons of enteral and parenteral nutrition support if they request information.

Mouth Problems

- If the client says that foods taste bitter, encourage poultry, fish, dairy products, eggs, milk and cheese; bitter-tasting foods usually include red meat, sour juices, coffee, tea, tomatoes, and chocolate. Suggest cooking foods in glass or porcelain instead of in metal containers, and avoid serving foods on metal or with metallic utensils. Encourage sweet fruit drinks, carbonated beverages, flavored ice chips; and seasonings, herbs, and spices to enhance flavors.

- If the client says that foods taste "old," try adding sugar; sour and salty tastes often taste "old."

- If the client says that foods taste too sweet, suggest drinking sour juices; cooking with lemon juice, vinegar, spices, herbs, and mint; adding pickles to appropriate foods.

- If the client says that foods have no taste, suggest marinating appropriate foods, serving highly seasoned foods, adding sugar, and eating foods at room temperature.

- If the client has difficulty swallowing, suggest small frequent meals of soft foods (pureed if needed), advise against foods that might irritate the mouth and esophagus, such as acidic juices or fruits, spicy foods, very hot or cold foods, alcohol, and carbonated beverages.

- If the client has mouth sores, suggest blenderized and cold foods. Gravies, cream soups, eggnog, milkshakes, cream pies, cheesecake, mousses, macaroni and cheese, souffles, and casseroles are well liked. Suggest that the client avoid alcohol, acidic fruit juices, and vegetable juices; spicy, rough, hot, and highly salted foods also may need to be avoided. Antifungal preparations, if necessary, are available.

- If the client has a dry mouth, suggest frequent sips of water, defatted bouillon, juice, ice chips, flavored ice chips, ice cream, fruitades, or slushy frozen baby foods mixed with fruit juice. Sucking on hard sweets and chewing on sugar-free gum may stimulate saliva. Dry alcoholic beverages may also stimulate saliva production. Solid foods should be moist, pureed as needed, with sauces and gravies, and not too tart or too hot or cold if mouth sores are present. Synthetic salivary substitutes (some prefer citrus added, some prefer refrigerated) are often helpful.

Nausea and Vomiting

- Encourage the client to avoid eating if nauseated or if nausea is anticipated.

- Suggest small meals of cool nonodorous foods, such as dry biscuits, cream crackers, soft toast, dry cereals, lean and white meats, milk, yogurt, pudding, and cheese. Many clients find it helpful to avoid fatty, greasy, or fried foods; avoid mixing hot and cold foods at the same meal; avoid high-bulk meals; and avoid nausea-precipitating foods, such as overly sweet foods, alcohol, spicy foods, and tobacco with meals.

- Encourage the client to eat slowly and to avoid overeating. Relaxing before and after meals and avoiding physical activity and lying flat for two hours after eating may also help.

- Suggest that the client not prepare own food.

Obstruction (Gastrointestinal)

- If oral intake is not contraindicated, encourage the client to eat small meals that are low in fiber, low in residue, and blenderized or strained. Many clients will prefer to eat their favorite foods, enjoy large meals, and then vomit frequently. A gastric tube, open to straight or intermittent drain, may alleviate the need for regular vomiting.

- With the "squashed stomach syndrome," encourage the client to eat small frequent meals, avoid nausea-producing foods, odorous foods, gas-producing foods, and high-fat or fried foods. Limit fluid with meals, taking fluids an hour before and after meals.

Note: Not all of the identified treatments may be appropriate for all diseases or conditions.

Adapted from Gallagher-Allred CR. *Nutritional Care of the Terminally Ill.* Rockville, Md: Aspen Publishers, Inc.; 1989:156-195, with permission of Aspen Publishers, Inc.

Helpful phrases that have been used successfully in discouraging the "he must eat or he will die" syndrome include the following (15):

- "The disease controls his appetite; pushing him to eat won't change the course of the disease."

- "He's sick and will be sick even if he eats."

- "Pushing him to eat may only make him uncomfortable."

- "Let him sit with you and eat what he wants."

- "Try not to worry that he eats poorly; it doesn't seem to bother him."

DEHYDRATION

Dehydration is often assumed to be uncomfortable by clients and families. To the contrary, when dehydration occurs close to the time of death, it appears to become a natural anesthesia, by decreasing the client's perception of suffering perhaps by reducing the level of consciousness or increasing production of endorphins and dynorphin (27-30). The concomitant dry-mouth effect associated with dehydration can be relieved through ice chips, lubricants, and other simple remedies (29). If life expectancy is measured in weeks or days, dehydration, as a natural course of events, may be preferred to aggressive nutrition support through tube feedings and/or total parenteral nutrition (TPN), if such feedings cause discomfort. By foregoing aggressive therapy, the following examples of conditions, which can benefit the client, may result (31,32).

- Decreased gastrointestinal and venous distention

- Decreased nausea, vomiting, and potential for aspiration

- Decreased diarrhea

- Decreased pulmonary secretions, resulting in less coughing, less fear of choking and drowning, and less rattling secretions

- Decreased urinary flow and need to void

- Decreased use of restraints

When life expectancy is longer, fluid intake should be encouraged, and creative ways to increase intake should be implemented, such as varying the flavor and temperature of water, providing liquid nutritional supplements, juices, bouillon, and other liquids. Inadequate fluid intake contributes to con-

stipation, a common problem that detracts from quality of life (5,23). There is also a role for low-volume parenteral hydration, to increase comfort for clients who manifest symptoms of opioid toxicity (agitated delirium, myoclonus, seizures), accompanied as appropriate by switching opioids and use of fewer sedating treatments. Hypodermoclysis for rehydration (usually around 1,000 mL/day) is inexpensive, has few complications, and can be administered at home (33).

HELPING THE CLIENT WHO CAN AND WANTS TO EAT

For clients who want to eat and who can be helped to eat better, the importance of improving their appetite and enabling them to eat as normally as possible cannot be overestimated. Medications such as corticosteroids, megestrol acetate, tricyclic antidepressants, dronabinol, and anabolic steroids, as well as alcohol as an aperitif, can be administered to improve appetite and mood (34,35). Improving a poor self-image, with suggestions about clothes that are worn, a hairdresser appointment, or a dental appointment, can also improve a client's appetite.

If anorexia is due to correctable causes and the client has a predicted life expectancy of several months, the correctable causes can be treated aggressively if desired by the client. Likewise, treatment should be aggressive if the client's anorexia appears to be an isolated symptom and the suspected consequence is malnutrition that could compromise both the quality and quantity of the client's remaining days. Suggestions for improving oral intake of terminally ill clients through the use of food have been summarized in Boxes 25.4 and 25.5. Dorner also provides another excellent source of information for dietary management of troublesome symptoms associated with pain (36).

Medical nutritional supplements may be considered for adult clients and children who want a high-energy intake in a small volume and food intake has failed (5,23). Medical nutritional supplements are often appreciated, because the client can drink the highly fortified liquid products with minimal effort, and the family members feel that they are providing "something special" (5). If a client desires enteral tube feedings in addition to oral intake or as the sole source of nutrition, liquid commercial nutritional products can be administered from a small-bore, flexible catheter, which in most clients is passed directly into the stomach through the abdominal wall or through the nose into the stomach or upper small intestine (37). Generally, formulas to be administered should be isotonic solutions (38). Depending on the ability to tolerate the solution, successful feedings can usually be started with a continuous drip at full strength if isotonic solutions are used, or at half strength if hypertonic solutions are used with a beginning rate of 30 mL to 50 mL/hour (up to a final rate of 100 mL to 125 mL/hour) (38), or the concentration can be increased (half to three-quarter to full strength) over several days, depending on client tolerance and nutrition goals. Many clients and families prefer intermittent tube feedings to continuous drip, because the former method seems more like a meal than drip delivery via pump.

In theory, a continuous drip administration of 100 mL to 125 mL/hour of full-strength (1 kcal/mL) solution is the maximum amount needed if weight maintenance is the goal (2,400 kcal to 3,000 kcal/day) for most clients (38). In practice, however, the author has found that only 1,000 kcal to 1,800 kcal/day (continuous drip for 10 to 15 hours) may be needed to achieve satiety and comfort. McCamish and Crocker recommend 25 kcal to 30 kcal/kg body weight for the hospice patient whose goal it is to maintain or improve strength (39). Greater amounts frequently cause complications, including fluid overload, cramps, diarrhea, reflux, and aspiration (40).

A case can be made for limited use of TPN in palliative care. When clients are in the early stages of their disease, they are often able to lead full and active lives. TPN may be appropriate for those who are unable to ingest enough energy orally or via enteral tube feeding to sustain their activity level because of a poorly functioning or nonfunctioning gastrointestinal tract (41). Two examples of such medical conditions are inoperable bowel obstruction and short-bowel syndrome.

On the other hand, this author has found through years of experience in hospice care that TPN is generally not well tolerated by the terminally ill, and rarely does parenteral feeding reduce the distress of anorexia and cachexia when the terminal stage is reached. Instead, TPN may subject the client to new problems that are more distressing and prolong suffering that would not have been faced had parenteral feeding not been initiated. If TPN is desired, it is generally best begun in the hospital setting before returning to the home or long-term-care facility. Home and nursing-facility administration should be closely monitored by a specially trained care team (41). It has been the experience of

this author that palliative care clients with advanced cancer rarely benefit from aggressive nutrition support via tube or parenteral feedings. Those clients who are allowed to eat and drink as desired and who are not pushed to do so if they do not desire or are unable seem to be at an advantage. A previously placed tube for enteral feedings or an intravenous line for TPN may not need to be discontinued, however, unless the client desires. Even though the feeding tube may be in place, there is no moral reason for using the tube for feeding (42).

FOOD SERVICE SUGGESTIONS

Food service in a facility that provides palliative care must reflect the philosophy of maximizing client comfort and enhancing quality of life (43). Menu development should reflect the ethnic, cultural, and regional food preferences of the population. Regardless of meal pattern selected (eg, three or four meals, lighter meals, or heavier meals), there must be flexibility for reheating menu items or preparing a quick meal when a client desires. Allowing clients to select menus as close to serving time as possible may help to allay anorexia. Small portions attractively garnished and plated in a dining atmosphere conducive to client and family socialization also contribute to better client meal acceptance. Family members' assistance with feeding further enhances the dining experience.

Some clients and families may express a desire for additional fiber, others for low-fat foods, still others for meals that reflect personal nutritional beliefs. Specific dietary modifications, such as low-sodium, low-fat, and diabetic requirements, may be needed. In most cases, however, these restrictions are liberalized, to allow maximum pleasure, variety, and choice (7). Fluctuations in mental alertness, level of responsiveness, dental status, and swallowing difficulties may indicate the need for consistency modifications as soft, mechanical soft, pureed, or blenderized foods (43). Simple, easy-to-prepare foods served in smaller portions are often more acceptable to clients than complicated, labor-intensive recipes. Comfort or familiar foods also are enjoyed and may be better tolerated. Some examples of universally selected comfort foods are macaroni and cheese, grilled cheese sandwiches, peanut butter and jelly sandwiches, toast, crackers, soups, fresh fruits, and soft salads. Inpatient palliative care facilities often provide a family kitchen, including personal china, flatware, and crystal storage; refrigerated storage; and a reheating system to handle foods brought from home (43). A family kitchen allows flexibility for meal service and supports family and friends in their caring efforts. Public health rules for labeling and dating food items and safe storage time limits should be enforced. The importance of food sanitation and safety cannot be overemphasized in a setting in which many clients are immune compromised. By serving nutritious, attractively prepared food for visual and physical pleasure, the palliative care facility's food service staff has the opportunity to enrich clients' lives at a time when the smallest pleasure is truly treasured (43).

ETHICAL AND LEGAL CONSIDERATIONS

The ethical and legal considerations in nutrition support of palliative care clients are increasingly being debated, which is due in part to technological advances in nutrition support that enable us to keep people alive longer than meaningful life sometimes can be maintained (1). Ethical and legal issues surrounding whether or not to implement aggressive nutrition support, such as tube or parenteral feedings, is not as simple as asking the questions "What is right?" and "What is wrong?" The answers you receive will depend on whom you ask (1).

Ethical decision making in the nursing facility is difficult, because agendas often take precedence over medical facts and individual considerations of each case. Collins (1) identifies several possible agendas, such as:

- A state survey is due any day and the nursing-facility administrator would prefer not to have any problems with involuntary weight loss and advises the director of nursing to "make sure everyone is eating," which pressures the director of nursing to encourage tube feeding.

- A client is at peace with palliative care and is not feeling pain, hunger, or thirst, yet the resident's daughter is not ready to let her mother go and wants every intervention possible and pushes for tube feeding.

- A facility recently settled a lawsuit for involuntary weight loss in the presence of a non-healing wound, and the legal department believes that tube feeding might have changed the outcome of the case and issues a memo about the financial consequences of litigation.

- A hospice nurse has passionate feelings about compassionate end-of-life care and encourages comfort measures based only on her personal ethical and moral convictions.

Most nursing-facility clients on tube feeding fall into one of two groups (1). The first group includes those who have been diagnosed with dysphagia and may be at high risk for aspiration pneumonia. These clients often have a neuromuscular disorder, such as Parkinson's disease, or have had a stroke. The second group comprises clients who either cannot or will not consume enough nutrition to prevent involuntary weight loss and malnutrition. Many clients in this category have dementia, Alzheimer's disease, or depression, or are in the end stage of a disease. Collins (1) notes that, if the decision about whether to tube feed or not is made strictly based on medical issues, then questions such as "Does tube feeding prevent aspiration?" or "Does tube feeding prevent further malnutrition and the consequences that accompany it such as pressure ulcers, decreased functional status, and death?" should provide a satisfactory answer 100% of the time. Although Finucane et al (44) and others (45-49) advise against tube feeding demented clients based on their observations of these medical issues, Robinson (50) suggests that the absence of proof should not be confused with proof that there is no benefit.

Hand-feeding by staff or family may provide enjoyment from eating and improve social satisfaction. Hand-feeding programs for home or for hospice or long-term care facilities can maintain and increase weight in terminally ill demented patients, but such programs take time and dedication (51). For caregivers, hand-feeding can also be a psychologically important act of caring. After health care professionals or family members have devoted time and effort to hand-feeding, it may be easier for caregivers to accept that when the client gives up eating this may be the right time to allow the client to die. Those who have not been engaged in such care may be troubled by guilt if they had neither instituted feeding by tube nor hand-fed the client. "To feed or not to feed," as with other methods of medical treatment, requires that those involved with palliative care ask the underlying questions, "What good will it accomplish for the client?" and "Do the benefits of nutrition support outweigh the burdens?" (52-54). To answer these questions, it is important to first establish the clinical facts of each situation and effectively communicate these to the client and family. The benefits and burdens the client may experience by the provision of or the withholding/withdrawal of nutrition support should also be delineated for the client and family (54). The benefits and burdens identified in Box 25.6 can help

Box 25.6   Potential Benefits and Burdens of Artificial Nutrition and Hydration

Potential Benefits of Artificial Nutrition and Hydration

- Added energy and other nutrients may prolong life and give the client and family more time to
  - Allow denial to serve as a natural coping mechanism that protects one from fear that death is nearing
  - Provide emotional support by reducing fear of abandonment
  - Get psychosocial and material affairs in order
  - Allow for a significant family event to occur
  - Improve client and family relationships
  - Add confidence that "everything is being done" to prolong life as long as possible
- Prevents perceived suffering due to fear that death from dehydration and/or starvation is a painful way to die.
- Increases ability to recover from effects of other medical therapies.
- Improves client's overall sense of well being and self-esteem.
- Improves nutritional status to decrease risk of infection, pressure ulcers, and aspiration pneumonia.
- Nutrition (food and fluid) is obligatory if it alleviates discomfort from hunger or thirst (32,55).
- Fulfills moral belief that all persons should be fed (32).
- Fulfills moral belief that artificial nutrition and hydration are basic humane care and society's responsibility to "be thy brother's keeper" (32).

Potential Burdens of Artificial Nutrition and Hydration

- Client may experience pain and physical suffering with
  - Tube or line insertion and usage
  - Uncomfortable distention, nausea, vomiting, diarrhea, possible aspiration and pneumonia, and excess stomal leakage and wound dehiscence with tube feedings
  - Fluid overload, ascites, peripheral edema, pulmonary edema, thrombosis, and possible lung puncture and sepsis with total parenteral nutrition
  - Restriction of activities by tethering to an infusion apparatus
  - Use of restraints
  - Increased need for catheterization in clients too weak to void large volumes
  - Increased nasogastric and/or pulmonary secretions, which may require suctioning
  - Increased pharyngeal secretions with increased fluid intake, resulting in death rattle
  - Psychological distress, including possible indignity of being kept alive beyond time life is meaningful, and sadness of imposing hardships on family and friends
  - Social isolation
  - Spiritual and moral conflict
  - Financial hardship

Data are from references 5, 31, 32, 55, and 56.

---

the health care professional discuss this issue with clients and their families (5,31,32,55,56). The client and family's educated perspectives, based on their personal value system, then should be the cornerstone of the decision making process (32,54,57). These questions, rather than questions surrounding litigation, survey census numbers, reimbursement, guilt, anger, and fear of death, much better define the problem, examine the evidence, and contribute to a solution that best serves the client (1).

For some clients, the process of providing artificial nutrition and hydration to avert cachexia and

dehydration is so onerous that the benefits are inconsequential or meaningless. To others, not to intervene is unacceptable and tantamount to murder. The choice lies in doing what is in the client's best interests, after the goals to be accomplished have been considered and the expected benefits and burdens have been analyzed by the client, the family, and competent health care professionals (58). There are many reasons for which clients and their families choose or do not choose to initiate, withhold, or withdraw artificial nutrition and hydration.

Case law rarely provides definitive answers to the question of "whether or not to feed." A position paper of the American Dietetic Association, entitled "Ethical and Legal Issues in Nutrition, Hydration, and Feeding," reviews relevant cases that address ethical, medical, and legal issues (54). The following three legal opinions have been expressed in US courts of law and are practiced in many other countries as well (39,42,54,59,60).

1. Withholding and withdrawing nutrition support have the same ethical significance.

2. Artificial nutrition and hydration is considered medical therapy and can be refused by competent clients and surrogates of incompetent clients under certain circumstances.

3. Client autonomy is a guiding ethical principle.

In circumstances in which the client dies when artificial nutrition and hydration is withdrawn, the cause of death is generally viewed by clinicians to be the underlying disease or condition, not the withdrawal of the nutrition support. In the past, before the availability of nutrition and hydration support technology, clients would have died of their disease. Advances in nutrition and hydration support technology have not changed this; therefore, absence of such support is not the specific cause of death. This concept is very important to emphasize with clients and their families. Families already carry a sufficiently heavy burden without adding to it the burden of guilt due to a decision to withdraw nutrition and hydration. The publication, *Hard Choices for Loving People,* is a helpful ally when discussing "whether or not to feed" with terminally ill clients and families (61).

Within the same context, withholding and withdrawing artificial nutrition and hydration are considered to have the same ethical significance, even though the removal of artificial nutrition and hydration may be psychologically and emotionally much more difficult. This should not, however, lead to withholding this therapy in an attempt to avoid a difficult decision regarding withdrawing support in the future (58,62).

Health care facilities and programs should develop supportive nutrition care programs, to guide providers in caring for clients who choose palliative care (32,63). Dorner's recommendations for developing a nutritional risk protocol for nursing-home residents at risk for involuntary weight loss and dehydration are applicable to developing a supportive nutrition care protocol for palliative care clients (64). Dorner recommends that providers (64)

1. Carefully review the state's advance directive laws.

2. Include best-practice guidelines for maintaining adequate nutritional status.

3. Include guidelines on weight tracking and weight loss interventions.

4. Note the steps the team will take if significant weight loss occurs.

5. Include the client and family in the decision making process.

6. Note what options the team will consider for continued weight loss.

7. Include as many team members as possible in developing and finalizing the protocol.

8. Define the team's protocol for when advance directives will be reviewed and at what point they can legally be followed.

Providers must listen carefully to each individual's wishes about withholding nutrition and hydration, explain all options available, and describe the benefits and burdens of each option. If the resident is unable to make informed choices, a surrogate decision maker who is familiar with the individual's wishes should assist the care team in making decisions that are individualized and resident centered. When the decision is made to provide palliative care without aggressive nutrition support and to allow the resident to eat whatever is desired whenever it is desired, then a supportive nutrition care program, such as that described in Box 25.7 (15,63), is appropriate.

CONCLUSION

Nutrition and hydration issues are common in caring for clients with a terminal illness. The dietetics professional will experience a great deal of satisfaction in individualizing and implementing an appropriate nutrition care plan for the client and family. Nutrition and hydration have a rightful place in the palliative care team's arsenal of therapies, to enhance the quality of a client's living as well as dying. The best answer to the question of whether or not to tube feed is unlikely to be determined at any time soon, because of the volatile atmosphere surrounding end-of-life issues in the United States. Although many dietetics professionals find it uncomfortable and intimidating to discuss issues surrounding death and dying, it is important that they do so. At the same time, they must examine their own feelings and belief systems and see where their own biases lead them. Only then can they be of greatest assistance to clients and families.

Box 25.7   Supportive Nutrition Care Program

Goal
Allow family and caregivers to provide comfort to failing clients through providing emotional and social benefits of continued oral intake of foods and beverages of choice given ad lib, as tolerated.

Clients
Individuals with significant weight loss and persistent inadequate intake of fluids and nutrition, whose poor oral intake and weight loss represent the inevitable progression of the client's condition.

Characteristics
- Base diet choice on client and family goals.
- Offer food and fluids at usual times and in usual location, or at any time in any location.
- Monitor hunger and thirst.
- Provide mouth care.
- Stop weights.
- Offer family food and beverages.

Documentation
- Multidisciplinary evaluation and team recommendation/decision.
- Lack of standard curative intervention efficacy.
- Discussion of options and family choice.
- Certain outcomes may be inevitable due to decline in client's condition (eg, infection, pressure ulcer, dehydration, decline in independence).
- Elements of comfort care, including symptom control, emotional support, spiritual support.

- "Do not do" list (eg, do not resuscitate, hospitalize, give medications unrelated to symptoms, obtain labs, perform vital signs, treat infection).
- "Will do" list (eg, will provide comfort, compassion, respect and dignity; will be vigilant, treat fever, provide skin care, provide nutrition and hydration whenever possible; will control manageable symptoms with aids such as lip lubricants and ice chips to make mouth feel comfortable; will address shortness of breath and nausea with medications).

Role of the Dietetics Professional
- Listen carefully to the client and family.
- Clarify options.
- Provide pros and cons of supportive nutrition care program vs curative nutrition support.
- Support the client-family choice.
- Encourage deliberative palliative care team decisions that are consistent with client and family wishes.
- Develop and assure delivery of plan of care, as determined by client and caregivers.
- Record client outcomes.
- Periodically reevaluate client and family wishes, goals of therapy, actions, and outcomes.

Adapted with permission from Smucker W. Palliative care in a nursing home: policies, procedures, and outcomes. Presented at the American Medical Directors Association 24th Annual Symposium, March 16, 2001, Atlanta Marriott Marquis Hotel, Atlanta, Ga. and from reference 15 (p240).

REFERENCES

1. Collins N. Tube feeding and dementia: to feed or not to feed—that is the question. *Extended Care Products.* November/December 2002:8-9.
2. Gallagher-Allred C. Dietitians are necessary in hospice programs. *Am J Hospice Care.* 1985;2:11-12.
3. Terrill Ross B. Counseling. In: Bloch AS, ed. *Nutrition Management of the Cancer Patient.* Rockville, Md: Aspen Publishers, Inc; 1990:37-40.
4. Newbury A. The care of the patient near the end of life. In: Penson J, Fisher R, eds. *Palliative Care for People with Cancer.* 2nd ed. London, England: Edward Arnold; 1995:178-197.
5. Gallagher-Allred CR. Nutritional care. In: Penson J, Fisher R, eds. *Palliative Care for People with Cancer.* 2nd ed. London, England: Edward Arnold; 1995:91-107.
6. O'Sullivan Maillet J. Ethical and psychological issues relating to the cancer patient. In: Bloch AS, ed. *Nutrition Management of the Cancer Patient.* Rockville, Md: Aspen Publishers, Inc; 1990:355-358.
7. Dorner B, Niedert KC, Welch PK. Position of the American Dietetic Association: liberalized diets for older adults in long-term care. *J Am Diet Assoc.* 2002;102:1316-1323.
8. Gallagher-Allred CR. Current practice in oncology dietetics: special needs of the home care and terminally ill patient. *Oncology Nutr DPG Newsletter.* 1994;2(1):5-7.
9. Gallagher-Allred CR. Managing ethical issues in nutrition support of terminally ill patients. *Nutr Clin Pract.* 1991;6:113-116.
10. Enteral nutrition. In: *Manual of Clinical Dietetics.* 6th ed. Chicago, Ill: American Dietetic Association; 2000:589-608.

11. O'Sullivan Maillet J, King D. Nutritional care of the terminally ill adult. In: Gallagher-Allred C, O'Rawe Amenta M, eds. *Nutrition and Hydration in Hospice Care: Needs, Strategies, Ethics.* Binghamton, NY: The Haworth Press, Inc; 1993:37-54.

12. Maurer Baack CM. Nursing's role in the nutritional care of the terminally ill: weathering the storm. In: Gallagher-Allred C, O'Rawe Amenta M, eds. *Nutrition and Hydration in Hospice Care: Needs, Strategies, Ethics.* Binghamton, NY: The Haworth Press, Inc; 1993:1-13.

13. Bohnet NL. The dying elderly. In: *Nursing Care of the Terminally Ill.* O'Rawe A M, Bohnet NL, eds. Boston, Mass: Little, Brown & Co; 1986:227-233.

14. Gallagher-Allred CR. *Nutritional Care of the Terminally Ill.* Rockville, Md: Aspen Publishers, Inc; 1989.

15. Mouton CP, Lewis RM, Miles TP, Talamantes MA, Espino DV. Ethnic considerations in end-of-life care. *Geriatric Times.* March/April 2001:30-32.

16. Klessig J. Death and culture: the multicultural challenge. *Ann Long-Term Care.* 1998;6:285-290.

17. Manzanec P, Tyler MK. Cultural considerations in end-of-life care. *Am J Nurs.* 2003;103:50-58.

18. Clarfield AM, Gordon M, Markwell H, Alibhai SMH. Ethical issues in end-of-life geriatric care: the approach of three monotheistic religions—Judaism, Catholicism, and Islam. *J Am Geriatr Soc.* 2003;51:1149-1154.

19. Greiner KA, Perera S, Ahluwalia JS. Hospice usage by minorities in the last year of life: results from the national mortality followback survey. *J Am Geriatr Soc.* 2003;51:970-978.

20. Castor JM, Thomas N, Palmer RM, Hujer ME, Messinger-Rapport BJ. Preferences for long-term tube feeding in a geriatric referral population. *Long-Term Care Interface.* October 2003:33-37,40.

21. Cassileth PA. Common medical problems. In: Cassileth BR, Cassileth PA, eds. *Clinical Care of the Terminal Cancer Patient.* Philadelphia, Pa: Lea & Febiger; 1982:15.

22. Bruera E, MacDonald N. Nutrition in cancer patients: an update and review of our experience. *J Pain Symptom Manage.* 1988;3:133-140.

23. Cancer. In: *Manual of Clinical Dietetics.* 6th ed. Chicago, Ill: American Dietetic Association; 2000:235-252.

24. DeWys WD, Kubota TT. Enteral and parenteral nutrition in the care of the cancer patient. *JAMA.* 1981;246:1725-1727.

25. Nixon DW, Lawson DH, Kutner M. Hyperalimentation of the cancer patient with protein-calorie undernutrition. *Cancer Res.* 1981;41:2038-2045.

26. Holden C. Anorexia in the terminally ill cancer patient: the emotional impact on the patient and the family. *Hospice J.* 1991;7:73-84.

27. Ganzini L, Goy ER, Miller LL, Harvath TA, Jackson A, Delorit MA. Nurses' experiences with hospice patients who refuse food and fluids to hasten death. *N Engl J Med.* 2003;349:359-365.

28. Jacobs S. Death by voluntary dehydration—what the caregivers say. *N Engl J Med.* 2003;349:325-326.

29. McCann RM, Hall WJ, Groth-Juncker A. Comfort care for terminally ill patients: the appropriate use of nutrition and hydration. *JAMA.* 1994;272:1263-1266.

30. Zerwekh JV. Do dying patients really need IV fluids? *Am J Nurs.* 1997;97:26-30.

31. White KS, Hall JC. Ethical dilemmas in artificial nutrition and hydration: decision-making. *Nurs Case Manage.* 1999;4:152-157.

32. Nutrition and hydration: assessment, evidence, and ethical issues. In: *Comprehensive Course in Medical Direction: Palliative Care Curriculum.* Columbia, Md: American Medical Directors Association; in press.

33. Bruera E, Franco JJ, Maltoni M, Watanabe S, Suarez-Almazor M. Changing pattern of agitated impaired mental status in patients with advanced cancer: association with cognitive monitoring, hydration, and opioid rotation. *J Pain Symptom Manage.* 1995;10:287-291.

34. Holden CM. Nutrition and hydration in the terminally ill cancer patient: the nurse's role in helping patients and families cope. In: Gallagher-Allred C, O'Rawe Amenta M, eds. *Nutrition and Hydration in Hospice Care: Needs, Strategies, Ethics.* Binghamton, NY: The Haworth Press, Inc; 1993:15-35.

35. Grauer PA. Appetite stimulants in terminal care: treatment of anorexia. In: Gallagher-Allred C, O'Rawe Amenta M, eds. *Nutrition and Hydration in Hospice Care: Needs, Strategies, Ethics.* Binghamton, NY: The Haworth Press, Inc; 1993:73-83.

36. Dorner B. Don't let pain management complicate nutritional care. *Nurs Homes Long Term Care Manage.* Sept 2002:46-51.

37. Hall JC. Choosing nutrition support: how and when to initiate. *Nurs Case Manage.* 1999;4:212-220.

38. Guenter P, Jones S, Roberts Sweed M, Ericson M. Delivery systems and administration of enteral nutrition. In: Rombeau JL, Rolandelli RH, eds. *Clinical Nutrition: Enteral and Tube Feeding.* 3rd ed. Philadelphia, Pa: WB Saunders Co; 1997:240-267.

39. McCamish MA, Crocker NJ. Enteral and parenteral nutrition support of terminally ill patients: practical and ethical perspectives. In: Gallagher-Allred C, O'Rawe Amenta M, eds. *Nutrition and Hydration in Hospice Care: Needs, Strategies, Ethics.* Binghamton, NY: The Haworth Press, Inc; 1993:107-129.

40. Hall JC. *Best Practice Guidelines for Tube Feeding: A Nurse's Pocket Manual.* Columbus, Ohio: Ross Products Division, Abbott Laboratories; 1997:8.

41. American Society for Parenteral and Enteral Nutrition Board of Directors and Task Force on Standards for Specialized Nutrition Support for Hospitalized Adult Patients. Standards for specialized nutrition support: adult hospitalized patients. *Nutr Clin Pract.* 2002;17:384-391.

42. Boisaubin EV. Legal decisions affecting the limitation of nutritional support. In: Gallagher-Allred C, O'Rawe Amenta M, eds. *Nutrition and Hydration in Hospice Care: Needs, Strategies, Ethics.* Binghamton, NY: The Haworth Press, Inc; 1993:131-147.

43. Drew Kidd K, Lane MP. Maximizing foodservice in an inpatient hospice setting. In: Gallagher-Allred C, O'Rawe Amenta M, eds. *Nutrition and Hydration in Hospice Care: Needs, Strategies, Ethics.* Binghamton, NY: The Haworth Press, Inc; 1993:85-106.

44. Finucane TE, Christmas C, Travis K. Tube feeding in patients with advanced dementia. *JAMA*. 1999;282:1365-1370.

45. Gillick MR. Rethinking the role of tube feeding in patients with advanced dementia. *N Engl J Med*. 2000;342:206-210.

46. Lewis L. Should patients with advanced dementia be tube fed? *Caring Ages*. 2001;2(7):17-18.

47. Michell SL, Kiely DK, Gillick MR. Nursing home characteristics associated with tube feeding in advanced cognitive impairment. *J Am Geriatr Soc*. 2003;51:75-79.

48. Mitchell SL. Financial incentives for placing feeding tubes in nursing home residents with advanced dementia. *J Am Geriatr Soc*. 2003;51:129-131.

49. Mitchell SL, Teno JM, Roy J, Kabumoto G, Mor V. Clinical and organizational factors associated with feeding tube use among nursing home residents with advanced cognitive impairment. *JAMA*. 2003;290:73-80.

50. Robinson BE. Tube feeding in patients with advanced dementia [letter]. *JAMA*. 2000;283:1563.

51. Keller HH, Gibbs AJ, Boudreau LD, Goy RE, Pattillo MS, Brown HM. Prevention of weight loss in dementia with comprehensive nutritional treatment. *J Am Geriatr Soc*. 2003;51:945-951.

52. Lynn J, Childress JF. Must patients always be given food and water? *Hastings Center Rep*. 1983;13(Oct):17-21.

53. Lo B, Jonsen AR. Ethical decisions in the care of the patient terminally ill with metastatic cancer. *Ann Intern Med*. 1980;92:107-111.

54. O'Sullivan Maillet J, Potter RL, Heller L. Position of the American Dietetic Association: ethical and legal issues in nutrition, hydration, and feeding. *J Am Diet Assoc*. 2002;102:716-726.

55. Aring DC. Intimations of mortality: an appreciation of death and dying. *Ann Intern Med*. 1968;69:137.

56. White KS, Hall JC. Ethical dilemmas in artificial nutrition and hydration: initiation vs withholding. *Nurs Case Manage*. 1999;4:85-89.

57. American Medical Directors Association. *Altered Nutritional Status Clinical Practice Guideline*. Columbia, Md: American Medical Directors Association; 2001.

58. President's Commission for the Study of Ethical Problems in Medicine and Biomedical and Behavioral Research. *Deciding to Forego Life-Sustaining Treatment*. No. 83-600503. Washington, DC: US Government Printing Office; 1983.

59. *Brophy v New England Sinai Hospital, Inc*, 497 NE 2d 626 (Mass 1986).

60. *Cruzan v Director, Missouri Department of Health*, 497 US 261 (1990).

61. Dunn H. *Hard Choices for Loving People*. 4th ed. Herndon, Va: A&A Publishers; 2001.

62. Council on Scientific Affairs and Council on Ethical and Judicial Affairs. Persistent vegetative state and the decision to withdraw or withhold life support. *JAMA*. 1990;263:426-430.

63. Smucker W. Palliative care in a nursing home: policies, procedures, and outcomes. Presented at the American Medical Directors Association 24th Annual Symposium, March 16, 2001, Atlanta Marriott Marquis Hotel, Atlanta, Ga.

64. Dorner B. When a resident won't eat. *Provider*. June 1997:61-64.

CHAPTER
26

Litigation and Liability Issues

Litigation is becoming a topic that all too often involves dietetics professionals. Health care professionals are no longer regarded with awe. Instead, when harm has allegedly occurred, a claimant's lawyer may join every party, including all health care providers, in an effort to increase the possibility of recovery. Jurors are then asked to consider the conduct of the health care providers, including dietetics professionals.

Current research documents that the incidence of nutrition litigation in the long-term-care industry has dramatically increased in recent years (1,2). Several law firms suggest that nutrition is a central issue in more than 50% of all litigation involving assisted-living and skilled nursing facilities (3). In today's legal arena, lawsuits involving weight loss, pressure ulcers, dehydration, and malnutrition are common. In an unpublished October 5, 1999, report for Ross Products Division, Abbott Laboratories, S. Sheridan, P. Hahn, and T. Malkoff indicate that the recovery for residents whose pressure ulcers were caused by poor nutrition alone was almost five times higher than the recovery for residents whose pressure ulcers were caused by poor pressure management alone.

The increase in nutrition-related recovery rates and litigation is a double-edged sword for individuals practicing medical nutrition therapy (MNT). Nutrition is receiving increased attention from the Centers for Medicare & Medicaid Services (CMS), attorneys, long-term-care corporations, legal nurse consultants, and clinical staff. On a positive note, the increased attention sets the stage for improvement and recognition of the role of dietetics professionals in improving quality of life and quality of care for the residents, thus reducing the overall risk of litigation to the facility. At the same time, however, the increased attention has also placed dietetics professionals at risk for professional and personal litigation, which increases stress and financial risks.

ELEMENTS FOR SUCCESSFUL LITIGATION

As a general matter, for litigation to be successful, several criteria must be met, including the following (4):

- Harm occurred to the resident (ie, negative outcome has occurred and this is reported in the clinical record documentation).
- Facility was responsible for poor care delivery.
- Harm was preventable.
- Facility knew or should have known that something bad could happen.
- There was a "duty" breach to the resident, in that something that should have been done was either poorly done or was not done at all.
- The conduct, whether by mistake or omission, caused or contributed to the harm. ("But for you, the resident would not have had a pressure ulcer, unintentional weight loss, dehydration, etc.")

Liability, insurance coverage laws, reduction in reimbursement rates, tort reform, and financial burdens reduce the amount of coverage that many long-term-care providers carry and/or can afford. If a facility has only a $250,000 policy, a plaintiff's attorney may look for other "deep pockets" that will return viable and substantial recovery rates. The dietetics professional may be seen as another "pocketbook" to contribute to the recovery that the plaintiff's counsel seeks.

OPTIMAL PROTECTION

Dietetics professionals should protect themselves in many ways for optimal safety, including aggressive financial planning and adequate malpractice insurance. Liability insurance helps to protect personal and professional assets. There are many companies that offer professional liability insurance on a national basis. It is important to obtain an insurance plan that meets the professional, financial, and personal needs of the person obtaining the insurance. Additionally, many institutions and corporations carry "umbrella policies" that may cover "all" employees, and it is important for dietetics professionals to know whether they are included in such coverage. Contractors, subcontractors, and independent consultants are at a greater risk for lawsuits than is an employee, who is usually insulated from risk by the employer. By joining the dietetics professional in litigation instituted against a facility, the facility may attempt to share its losses. In any event, a professional liability policy can provide needed protection, security, and peace of mind. Adequate protection is well worth what is usually a proportionately reasonable fee.

In circumstances in which one's net worth is substantial (eg, exceeding $1 million personally or jointly), professional liability, an umbrella policy, and legal financial planning are necessary. The personal and jointly held assets of the dietetics professional and his/her family can be at risk if the dietetics professional is sued individually. There are many ways to protect finances. For example, "tenants by entirety" may be a method to protect business, professional, personal, and joint assets. It is strongly recommended that, if at a high risk for litigation, dietetics professionals plan aggressively for both financial and liability concerns. Consultation with an attorney who practices in the area of financial or estate planning may be necessary in those cases in which there are significant assets and complicating factors (5).

STAYING CURRENT IN THE FIELD

Additionally, all dietetics professionals can reduce the risk of litigation by keeping abreast of regulatory and practice standards in their prospective fields. The dietetics professional who, for example, receives calls or referrals from the nursing facility staff but does not address or document a plan of care clearly and in a timely manner may be found to have deviated from the standards of care in the community. Such a deviation could attract the

attention of a jury and could be seen to have caused or contributed to the damages alleged (3). Documentation is a key to avoiding litigation. The medical records, Minimum Data Set (MDS), Resident Assessment Instrument (RAI) process, and care plan should be primary tools of clinical care and communication (6).

Dietetics professionals must also stay updated on nutritional concerns, such as enteral feedings, all types of wounds, nutrition treatments, hydration, and current MNT protocols for older adults. Generally, the "gold standard" of care in the skilled nursing environment is the Omnibus Budget Reconciliation Act of 1987 (OBRA '87, also referred to as Chapter 483 of the CFR 42) (7). The final regulation or the Interpretative Guidelines for surveyors published by the Health Care Financing Administration (HCFA; predecessor to CMS) provide structure and govern facilities participating in the Medicare and Medicaid programs (8). Current MNT protocols, federal and state regulations, practice acts, and the facility's organizational policies and procedures also are considered standards of care. In acute-care and hospital-affiliated skilled nursing facilities, Joint Commission on Accreditation for Healthcare Organizations (JCAHO) regulations may be regarded as another standard. Dietetics professionals are expected to implement appropriate standards of treatment, assessment, and monitoring systems, based on any such standards of care. Additionally, the contractual agreement may set the standard of care for a contracted employee or independent contractor.

For example, assume that the contract of a registered dietitian (RD) with "ABC" facility states that the consultant RD or licensed dietitian will evaluate all significant weight losses and dialysis residents monthly, and that a resident was hemodialized three times a week for an entire calendar year and lost 45 pounds during that period. Assume, as well, that there was no documentation from the RD. The clinical record in this instance confirms a deviation from the standard of care. If the dietetics professional's deviation from the standard of care can be linked as a causation factor for a negative outcome, then the dietetics professional is at risk for litigation, stress, professional and financial losses, and, in extreme cases, criminal allegations.

More than ever before, today's legal environment exposes dietetics professionals to the risk of litigation. Dietetics professionals need to embrace the opportunity for positive changes in roles, image, and financial status. Those practicing in long-term care must realize that they are the nutrition experts and thus take on related responsibilities. They must provide state-of-the-art advice, documentation, education, and consultation.

CURRENT INDUSTRY STANDARDS

The following are some current industry standards of care that may help to clarify the role of dietetics professionals in minimizing the risk of MNT litigation in the nutrition care and assessment of older adults:

1. Address visceral nutritional status (prealbumin, hemoglobin and hematocrit, albumin, total lymphocyte count) (9).

2. Address somatic nutritional status (physical attributes) (10).

3. Address hydration status (needs, input and output, laboratory test results, risks).

4. Make appropriate nutrition recommendations based on current MNT protocols, specifically related to weight loss, enteral feedings, pressure ulcers, and hydration.

5. Address nutrition needs of residents with pressure ulcers and other wounds.

6. Make recommendations that follow standards of practice.

7. Individualize recommendations for each resident.

8. Make clear, concise statements that identify whether or not the nutrition, energy, protein, vitamin, mineral, and fluid needs are being met.

9. Document issues in quality assurance (QA) monthly reports. (QA reports are often not discoverable; ie, cannot be subpoenaed for use.)

10. Chart weights in a nonaccusatory manner that does not implicate the facility in any wrong doing or negligence.

11. Address all care plans with nutritionally related information.

12. Make sure care plans match nutrition needs and status as reflected in the assessment and progress notes.

13. Include laboratory analyses (hemoglobin, hematocrit, prealbumin, albumin, BUN, etc).

14. Include the diagnosis with the diet order.

15. Ensure that the physician's orders for diet prescriptions match the dietetics professional's documentation.

16. Liberalize diets with physicians' consent; avoid restricted diets.

17. Make sure recommendations comply with state, JCAHO, federal regulations, and facility process procedures (ie, enteral feedings/dehydration, complete assessments).

18. Do not just sign off charts; one's license, finances, and reputation are at risk.

19. Document on all high-risk residents.

20. Keep a detailed list of residents documented on each visit.

21. Keep a facility tracking list of all high-risk residents and dates of documentation.

22. Include waivers or consider education sheets for noncompliant residents.

23. Tell the story in the chart.

24. Document resident refusal/noncompliance.

25. Document education of families and residents, as well as an explanation of risks/negative outcomes. Consider including time spent with the resident and/or family on controversial areas.

26. Document family/resident's refusal to follow recommendations.

27. Keep a resident referral list.

Adherence to all these standards will place the dietetics professional in a relatively strong position. Where one or more of the standards have not been followed, however, an argument can be made that the professional's care was negligent or that the failure to follow a particular standard contributed to harm to a patient.

Demonstrating that all these standards were followed, however, can be difficult 2 to 3 years after care was given, when the chart is cold. Documentation is therefore critical. This is especially true in the case of certain residents or families about whom the practitioner feels uncomfortable. The practitioner should get a sense of the resident and whether documentation needs to be a paragraph or a page. In those cases in which the practitioner is uncomfortable with a resident or family, it may help to develop a "trigger" that will bring back memories from the time in question.

Remember the following when treating residents' nutrition needs:

- Appropriate documentation is a key to avoiding litigation.

- If it is not documented, it was not done.

- Accuracy is a must.

- Use appropriate documentation techniques, terminology, and legible penmanship.

SUMMARY

Many lawsuits are avoidable. Be aware of all state and federal rules and regulations and of those residents who are at risk. Adherence to RD referral policies is a must, and immediate assessment on high-risk admissions must be made either in person, by fax, or by teleconference. Unhappy families are more likely to sue. Excellent food service, customer care, and communication with the family are premium "anti-lawsuit" techniques. Associating with facilities that have excellent survey records and positive customer/resident satisfaction rates minimizes the risk of nutritional litigation for dietetics professionals. Inadequate hours and coverage, poor survey records, and inadequate facility nutritional monitoring systems for weights, laboratory tests, hydration, and pressure ulcers increase the risk that the dietetics professional might be a potential codefendant.

Dietetics professionals must protect themselves. They should stay current on professional information, research, and other relevant matters; use and expand their available resources; and always work in well-respected facilities. Additionally, they should supervise actively and establish their own standards of practice. They should never tolerate illegal behaviors or acts. By understanding the dietetics professional's role in resident care, one can minimize the potential for legal action.

Note: It is not the intent of this chapter to provide legal advice but only to suggest some practical considerations for coping with and reducing the risks of litigation. For actual advice and guidance in the planning or litigation areas discussed above, the reader should seek professional consultation with a competent financial planner, insurance professional, or attorney.

REFERENCES

1. Hogstel MO, Cox LC, Walker C. Limiting litigation in long-term care. *Ann Long-Term Care.* 2003;11:27-32.
2. Bourdon TW, Dubin SC. Aon Risk Consultants, Inc. Long-term care general liability and professional liability actuarial analysis. February 28, 2002. Available at: http://www.ahca.org/brief/aon_ltcanalysis.pdf. Accessed March 3, 2003.
3. Krisztal R. *Nursing Home Negligence III: Asserting Claims and Defending Nursing Homes.* Eau Claire, Wisc: Professional Education Systems; 2001.
4. Keeton WP, Prosser WL. *Prosser and Keeton on the Law of Torts.* 5th ed. Eagen, Minn: West Group Publishing; 1984:30.
5. National Association of Financial and Estate Planners Web site. Available at: http://www.NAFEP.com/ Accessed March 24, 2004.
6. Centers for Medicare & Medicaid Services Web site. Available at: http://www.cms.hhs.gov. Accessed March 24, 2004.
7. Levine JM. The role of the expert in evaluating nursing home care. In: Krisztal R, Levine JM, eds. *Nursing Home Litigation: Pretrial Practice and Trials.* Tucson, Ariz: Lawyers and Judges Publishing Co; 2001:55-73.
8. Levine JM. Medical and legal aspects of physical and chemical restraints. *Am Jurisprudence Trials.* 2000;75:1-49.
9. Litchford M. Practical Applications in Laboratory Assessment of Nutritional Status. Greensboro, NC: Case Software; 2002.
10. Nutrition assessment of adults. In: *Manual of Clinical Dietetics.* 6th ed. Chicago, Ill: American Dietetic Association; 2000:3-38.

CHAPTER

27

Quality Management

A recent trend in health care has been to base care processes on evidence and research. Dietetics professionals have therefore been encouraged to seek data on outcomes to validate the nutrition care they provide, instead of relying on anecdotal information to guide their work. This chapter discusses information and tools that help dietetics professionals to become more accountable for the outcomes of the care they provide. It uses the example of a medical nutrition therapy (MNT) protocol to highlight aspects of the monitoring and evaluation step of the nutrition care process, and it provides understanding of the outcomes management system component of the Nutrition Care Process and Model as it pertains to the care of older adults (1) (see Figure 27.1).

Evidence-based practice is the conscientious, explicit, and judicious use of the current best evidence in making decisions about the care of individual patients (2). It requires knowledge of the scientific literature, clinical training, experience, and knowledge of the individual resident (see Box 27.1). When dietetics professionals recommend a liberalized diet as the nutrition intervention for a resident with type 2 diabetes, they are implementing evidence-based practice. This is because (1) they are considering the latest research, in which there is much evidence for liberalizing the diet of an individual in a residential setting; (2) they are acting on their clinical expertise and completing a nutrition assessment and nutrition diagnosis of this resident; and (3) they are considering the values of this resident, which is critically important in long-term care.

NUTRITION MONITORING AND EVALUATION

Nutrition monitoring and evaluation is the fourth step of the Nutrition Care Process and Model (see Figure 27.1). *Monitoring* specifically refers to the review and measurement of the resident's status at a scheduled (preplanned) follow-up point, with regard to nutrition diagnosis, intervention plans/goals, and outcomes. *Evaluation* is the systematic comparison of current findings with previous status, intervention goals, or a reference standard. Monitoring and evaluation use selected outcome indicators (markers) that are relevant to the resident's defined needs, nutrition diagnosis, nutrition goals, and disease state. Recommended times for follow-up, as well as relevant outcomes to be monitored, can be found in ADA's Evidence-Based Guides for Practice (3-6), MNT protocols, and other evidence-based sources.

The purpose of monitoring and evaluation is to determine the degree to which progress is being made and goals or desired outcomes of nutrition care are being met. It is more than just "watching" what is happening; it requires an active commitment to measuring and recording the appropriate outcome indicators (markers) relevant to the nutrition diagnosis and intervention strategies. Progress should be monitored, measured, and evaluated on a planned schedule until discharge. Data from this step are used to create an outcomes management system.

KEY CONCEPTS IN OUTCOMES MANAGEMENT SYSTEMS

Effectively and efficiently implementing the Nutrition Care Process and Model for older adults involves interfacing with other processes. For example, having

Figure 27.1

ADA Nutrition Care Process and Model. Shaded areas represent the Nutrition Care Process.

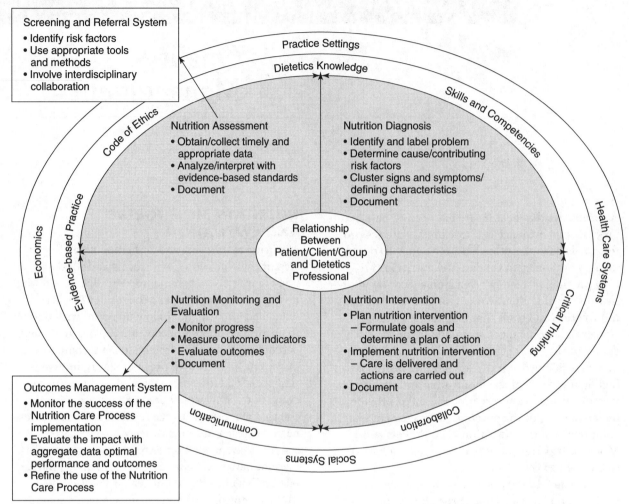

Box 27.1   American Dietetic Association Medical Nutrition Therapy
Evidence-Based Guides for Practice, Protocols, and Practice Guidelines

Although each client is unique, taking a standard approach to his/her condition can help provide optimal nutrition care, reduce legal risks, and lower health care costs. Medical nutrition therapy (MNT) protocols and practice guidelines (ie, American Dietetic Association MNT Evidence-Based Guides for Practice) are a great resource for providing a standardized nutrition care process of evidence-based nutrition care (3-6).

The American Dietetic Association MNT Evidence-Based Guides for Practice are supported by scientific evidence, not just tradition or intuition. This makes for better, more consistent patient care. This information allows clients to become informed consumers and helps them to participate more fully

in the decisions related to their care. It also encourages families to get involved with these decisions.

The dietetics professional's employer benefits because evidence-based MNT guides for practices can reduce costs in at least three ways:

1. By shortening lengths of stay through use of better-defined appropriate interventions.

2. By identifying the optimal assessment and treatment and avoiding the treatments of undocumented benefit.

3. By providing a consistent nutrition care process that supports meeting and exceeding regulatory and accreditation standards.

the appropriate height and weight to complete a nutrition assessment or reassessment involves a good process in a facility for obtaining accurate weights. When we link the process for obtaining accurate weights to the nutrition care process, we are describing a *system,* a series of linked processes designed to produce a given outcome. Data are collected on individual residents to provide information about that particular resident, so that the best care can be provided to that resident. Data are also collected across groups of residents with similar characteristics, so that the best care is consistently provided systematically and so that needs can be identified to improve the care. Systems thinking is not easy. It is an unnatural act. It is more common for individuals to see the parts, not the whole; the trees, not the forest. Yet, mastering the art of improvement requires a deep and fundamental understanding that parts are connected in a system.

An individual "trying harder" within a current system may achieve some short-term improvement; however, that change does not represent a new level of capability. For example, a dietetics professional may believe that clients at high risk for unintended weight loss should be provided with an in-depth nutrition assessment, but this belief alone will not guarantee that the assessment will occur. Instead, a system must be designed to ensure that the desired clinical care is a routine part of every client encounter. Appropriate systems are the only way to ensure that the right thing happens at the right time to the right patient each and every time.

Unintentional variation is defined as unplanned variation in the process of care that can lead to a suboptimal outcome. Such variation is present in all systems and is caused by inadequate processes within a system. Because most variation within a system is unplanned, it goes unidentified unless it is measured. Data should be monitored and evaluated, to help design and implement consistently standardized processes and systems for quality care that prevent avoidable negative outcomes. Sometimes good outcomes are not possible for certain individuals. A negative outcome does not necessarily mean that there was poor quality of care provided. The key is to demonstrate that quality care was provided, because process and systems are in place to ensure that the right thing happens at the right time to the right patient each and every time; and if the outcome was negative, it was unavoidable. (Box 27.2 contains more on this important distinction between avoidable and unavoidable negative outcomes).

Outcomes management links care processes and resource use with outcomes. It is a systems approach that requires an infrastructure in which outcomes for the population served are routinely assessed, summarized, and reported. Outcomes management aims to collect, organize, and evaluate data in a timely manner, so that performance can be adjusted and quality of care improved. Quality necessarily involves both processes and outcomes. Measuring the relationship between the process and the outcome is essential for quality improvement, and the success of quality improvement initiatives will be reflected in measurable improvements in outcomes (7).

OUTCOMES MANAGEMENT IN ACTION

As previously described, when evaluating outcomes, one must also evaluate the process of care by which the outcome is measured. The following is an example of how this happens in practice.

First, a way to evaluate the effectiveness of the process of care provided is chosen. This can be done by collecting data on the client's adherence to MNT. The progress note of the MNT protocol (Figure 27.2) and the section recording adherence to MNT should be examined (8). By aggregating the data across a group of client's scores in this area, data will be available on the process of care. The process indicator is the total number of individuals who score "good" or "excellent" divided by the total number of individuals receiving MNT for unintended weight loss. This is a process measure of the effectiveness of the MNT protocol, one way to tell whether the protocol as implemented by the dietetics professional does what it is designed to do.

In Facility A, of 10 clients provided with MNT, eight (80%) had adherence scores of good to excellent. To complete the analysis of the effectiveness of the protocol, this process indicator must be compared with outcomes indicators. To show a positive picture of protocol effectiveness, there must be a positive correlation of the process indicator with the outcome indicators.

Outcomes data on unintended weight loss should be collected from the same individuals from whom data on adherence to MNT were collected. For an unintended weight-loss MNT protocol, maintaining or increasing weight is the expected positive outcome indicator of effectiveness. The outcome indicator is defined as the total number of individuals whose weight is maintained or increased divided by the total number of individuals receiving

Box 27.2 Avoidable and Unavoidable Negative Outcomes

When a resident's health declines or does not improve as one might expect it to, gather detailed information to determine whether this outcome was avoidable or unavoidable. To collect data, conduct multiple observations; engage in ongoing dialogue with the direct care-giving staff, the resident, and his or her family; and review records targeted to clarify and validate information. The goal of this investigation is to determine the following:

- Does the facility have a continuous ongoing process for consistently providing individualized care and services for the resident? (Obtain this information through ongoing observations and dialogue with residents, their families, and staff.)

- Has the facility completed a comprehensive, appropriate, and adequate assessment of the resident that identifies the resident's baseline status and potential for improvement?

- Has the facility identified and assessed risk factors that may have contributed to the resident's decline or failure to improve? (Such factors include the natural progression of the resident's medical conditions.)

- Does the facility develop appropriate care plans and consistently implement interventions identified in those plans to forestall disease progression and address risks, needs, and strengths of the resident?

- Does the facility conduct ongoing evaluation of the outcomes of care, determining whether the resident reached his/her goals, declined, or improved? If the resident's health declines or shows no improvement, are alternate care and service interventions tried and adapted as needed for the resident?

Assessment, interventions, the resident's individual baseline functional status, and the natural history of the disease states should all be considered when evaluating whether decline or failure to improve are avoidable. Surveyors and providers should not assume that factors such as age or chronic disease inevitably result in a resident's decline or failure to maintain the level of functioning. Instead, they should always look for the possibility and opportunity for positive responses to appropriate interventions.

If any of the following are found, then the decline was likely *avoidable:*

- Assessments are incomplete or inaccurate, or are not conducted in an ongoing, individualized, comprehensive manner.

- Interventions are not ongoing, are incompletely implemented, or do not adhere to accepted standards of practice.

- The facility lacks an ongoing process for evaluating the resident's response and outcomes to the care and services being provided.

- Reassessment and revision of interventions are not tied to the resident's response and outcomes (unless all reasonable options have been aggressively attempted and exhausted).

Decline is likely *unavoidable* when all probable contributors to potential decline (such as the underlying disease and other medical conditions, aging, psychosocial factors, activity level, medications, and treatments) have been identified, comprehensively assessed, and addressed through care-planning, continuous implementation of interventions, and evaluation of responses to all attempted interventions; and/or when there is a steadfast refusal of care despite ongoing efforts to counsel the resident and offer alternative treatments.

MNT for unintended weight loss. In Facility A, 10 clients were provided with MNT; nine (90%) maintained or gained weight.

The analysis of this situation shows a positive trend in the process indicator correlated with a positive trend in the outcome indicator, which means that the protocol is effective. It is important to capture all the cues/strategies that make the protocol effective. Examples of cues/strategies are as follows:

(*a*) assessments are completed in a timely manner, (*b*) referrals are communicated to the dietetics professional, and (*c*) eating assistance is provided consistently when indicated. The dietetics professional should note these cues/strategies; if reinforced, they will happen consistently. They are part of the system of interlinking processes that support the positive outcomes. What if there were a situation in Facility B in which the process does what it is

Figure 27.2

Nutrition progress notes form for prevention of unintentional weight loss MNT protocol. Adapted from Medical nutrition therapy protocols. In: American Dietetic Association. *Medical Nutrition Therapy Across the Continuum of Care: Supplement 1.* Chicago, Ill: American Dietetic Association; 1997:10, with permission from American Dietetic Association.

NUTRITION PROGRESS NOTES
Prevention of Unintentional Weight Loss

Other Diagnosis: _____

Client's Name: _____
Phone Number: _____
Medical Record #: _____
DOB:_____ Gender: M/F
Ethnic Background (optional): _____
Referring Physician: _____

Outcomes of Medical Nutrition Therapy (MNT)

Expected outcome	Intervention provided to meet goal (Intervention = self-management training plus client verbalizes/ demonstrates)			Goal reached (Check indicates goal reached)		
Session	1 (60 min)	2 (30 min)	3 (30 min)	Date:_____ 1	Date:_____ 2	Date:_____ 3
Clinical Outcomes				Value	Value	Value
Albumin (g/dL)				_____	_____	_____
Hgb (g/dL)				_____	_____	_____
Hct (vol %)				_____	_____	_____
BUN (mg/dL)				_____	_____	_____
Creatinine (mg/dL)				_____	_____	_____
Blood pressure (mm Hg)				___/___	___/___	___/___
Height _____Weight_____				_____lb	_____lb	_____lb
BMI (kg/m^2)				_____	_____	_____
Functional Outcomes						
• Verbalizes improved tolerance to activities						
• Increases activity level (ADLs)						
• Maximizes food intake through cueing, self-help devices, or feeding assistance						
MNT Goal						
kcal _____ Protein _____g				_____kcal	_____kcal	_____kcal
Fluid _____mL				_____g pro	_____g pro	_____g pro
				_____mL	_____mL	_____mL
Vitamins/minerals to meet RDA				_____	_____	_____
QOL score						
Behavioral Outcomes						
• Consumes nutrient-dense foods and snacks/supplements						
• Consumes > 30-35 kcal/kg				_____kcal/kg	_____kcal/kg	_____kcal/kg
• If necessary, alternative nutrition support provided to prevent further weight loss and reduce complication						
• Free from signs/symptoms of vitamin/mineral deficiencies						
• Consumes 90%-100% of meals, snacks, and supplements without distress				_____%	_____%	_____%
• Consumes foods and drugs at appropriate time				_____ dose	_____ dose	_____ dose
• Verbalizes food/drug interaction Drugs _____				_____ dose	_____ dose	_____ dose
Overall Compliance Potential				E G P*	E G P*	E G P*
• Comprehension				E G P*	E G P*	E G P*
• Receptiveness				E G P*	E G P*	E G P*
• Adherence						

Intervention: D-Discussed, R-Reinforced,/Reviewed, ≠ - Not reviewed, ✓- Outcome achieved *, N/A- Not applicable. Key for Compliance Potential: E=excellent, G=Good, P=Poor

designed to do, as indicated by the process indicator of adherence with the protocol, but when it is correlated with the outcome indicator of unintended weight loss, it is found that weight was not maintained or did not increase consistently?

In Facility B, of 10 clients provided MNT, eight (80%) had adherence scores of good to excellent (process indicator of 80%), but only 5 (50%) maintained or gained weight (outcome indicator).

If this were to occur, having data on both process of care and outcomes will point the dietetics professional in the right direction to initiate an improvement. It gives the dietetics professional information that a change is needed in the process of care. Dietetics professionals should not mistakenly try to defend what they were doing, just because the process indicators had positive results. If the overall outcomes are not being met, then these processes are not effective in achieving the positive outcomes. Pairing process indicators with outcomes indicators gives the complete picture of the effectiveness of the MNT/nutrition care process. This example is about weight loss, but the same concepts could be applied to other nutrition care services.

INITIATING AN IMPROVEMENT PROJECT

Quality assurance (QA) has been around for decades. The QA approach does not look at the whole process of care provided; rather, it focuses on only those outcomes that are unacceptable. This does not improve quality, because it does not correlate process with outcome. Quality improvement recognizes that the entire output of the process provides a basis for action. Quality improvement is about improving the process of care, so that more of the outcomes are on target (9).

Continuing with the above example, with dietetics professionals at Facility B using an MNT protocol as the way of providing the nutrition care process for preventing weight loss, data for a quarter show the following trend:

- Month 1: 10 clients were provided MNT, eight (80%) of whom had adherence scores of good to excellent (process indicator), but only five (50%) of whom maintained or gained weight (outcome indicator).

- Month 2: 20 clients were provided MNT, 18 (80%) of whom had adherence scores of good to excellent (process indicator), but only 10 (50%) of whom maintained or gained weight (outcome indicator).

- Month 3: 15 clients were provided MNT, 14 (93.3%) of whom had adherence scores of good to excellent (process indicator), but only six (40%) of whom maintained or gained weight (outcome indicator).

Dietetics professionals bring data for a quarter trended over time and information to the quality assessment and assurance (QA&A) committee for support of a quality improvement approach to weight-loss prevention. A quality improvement team is initiated. The quality improvement team will use a quality improvement problem-solving model, called Plan-Do-Study-Act (PDSA). The following are some highlights of the PDSA cycle and quality improvement tools used by this team. The PDSA cycle helps teams move from hunches and theories to knowledge and action. It is doubly effective not only because it speeds the design, testing, and implementation of individual changes that lead to improvement but also because it creates knowledge, which can be used to develop new ideas for change (see Figure 27.3).

THE PLAN-DO-STUDY-ACT

Plan

A team can be chartered (Box 27.3) to develop a "weight wellness" component to the current unintended weight loss MNT protocol. A charter serves as a clear communication tool and link with the QA&A committee, providing a focus for the improvement team, which is clearly defined and finite in scope. During the "planning" phase, possible problems that might prevent achieving the goal and potential solutions to the problems are identified. To produce lasting improvement, potential solutions need to produce systems changes. Three tools useful in the planning phase include brainstorming, the Affinity Diagram, and the Cause and Effect Diagram.

Do

The "do" phase is focused on implementing process improvement. These modifications should be implemented once the baseline data are collected, the process steps for improvement are identified, and planned process step modifications have been determined. Initially, the new actions are implemented for a short period of time on a small scale or trial basis.

Facility B chooses two process improvement actions to implement. The first process improvement action implemented is weekly transdisciplinary rounds, involving the review of the clinical links of the MDS-based nutrition/eating quality

Figure 27.3

The improvement model: PDSA cycle (the continual improvement or Shewhart Cycle).

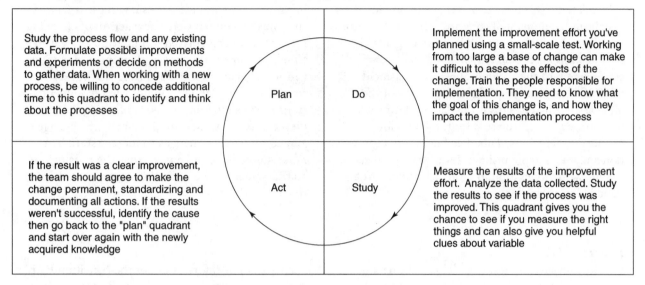

Study the process flow and any existing data. Formulate possible improvements and experiments or decide on methods to gather data. When working with a new process, be willing to concede additional time to this quadrant to identify and think about the processes

Implement the improvement effort you've planned using a small-scale test. Working from too large a base of change can make it difficult to assess the effects of the change. Train the people responsible for implementation. They need to know what the goal of this change is, and how they impact the implementation process

If the result was a clear improvement, the team should agree to make the change permanent, standardizing and documenting all actions. If the results weren't successful, identify the cause then go back to the "plan" quadrant and start over again with the newly acquired knowledge

Measure the results of the improvement effort. Analyze the data collected. Study the results to see if the process was improved. This quadrant gives you the chance to see if you measure the right things and can also give you helpful clues about variable

Plan   Do   Act   Study

Box 27.3   Team Charter Example

Team Title: Weight Wellness

Purpose of the Team
- To identify, develop, and implement weight wellness strategies for the MNT protocol.
- To implement actions that positively affect the Quality Measure—unintended avoidable weight loss.

Background Information
- Significant avoidable unintended weight loss in long-term care has negative consequences. When significant avoidable unintended weight loss is high, the impact will be noted in residents' quality of life and in the quality of service provided.
- The facility has identified prevention of significant avoidable unintended weight loss as a high-priority issue.
- The facility has implemented actions to address the problem. Actions have not resulted in a process for significant weight-loss prevention that is consistently below the facility benchmark of 4%.
- The current weight-loss prevention MNT protocol emphasizes that the weight variance committee will follow the resident after the weight loss has been identified as significant. This is a quality-assurance approach focusing on the outlier. A

quality-improvement approach looks to reduce the variation.

Expected Outcomes
- A process that will decrease the incidence of significant avoidable unintended weight loss
- Clear priority set of new options/strategies identified
- Communication/education plan implemented to promote strategies

Expected Completion: December 2005

Resources
- Team meetings and conference calls
- E-mail for written communication
- Work hours for affected staff for training to implement changes

Constraints
- Federal and state regulations, accreditation standards
- Facility budgets

Sponsor: Facility QA&A Committees

Team Members: Dietetic technicians registered, registered dietitian, director of nursing services, staff nurse, nursing assistant

indicator domain for each resident. Clinical links are a mapping of quality indicators that are clinically related to each other and that can provide insight into a domain of care (10). The residents to investigate should be chosen by reviewing a facility's *Resident Level Quality Indicator Report,* which states which of these clinical links each resident triggers. Residents may trigger only some of the clinical links listed. This is the data tool for the team to gather information for the Nutrition/ Eating (Weight Loss, Tube Feeding, Dehydration) domain. (See sample resident-level quality indicator report, with circles around residents who might be included in a sample.)

Figure 27.4 shows the documentation tool that the facility team uses during the rounds (10). The improvement team identifies key success factors that must accompany this new action of checking for care problems related to nutrition and eating: timely documentation, care planning of any intervention changes identified during the weekly rounds, and implementation of the recommendations that result from the above findings. The dietetics professional will document the change and communicate changes to dietary staff. The nurse supervisors will ensure that the nursing staff assigned to the individual is aware of the recommendations.

Figure 27.4

Quality indicator clinical links. This is the data tool for the team gathering information for the Nutrition/Eating (Weight Loss, Tube Feeding, Dehydration) Domain. Clinical links are a mapping of quality indicators that are clinically related to each other that can provide insight into a domain of care. To find the residents to investigate, review the facility's *Resident Level Quality Indicator Report,* which identifies the clinical links a resident triggers. A resident may only trigger some of the clinical links listed. Data are from reference 10 (p 23).

Resident Name:_____   Date:_____

NUTRITION/EATING Clinical Links

Symptoms of Depression	Use of 9+ Medications	Incidence of Cognitive Impairment	Fecal Impaction	Bedfast Residents	Decline in Late Loss ADLs	Psychotropic Drug Use	Daily Physical Restraints	Pressure Sores

Key success factors for the results of the investigation and actions below are timely documentation, care planning of intervention changes, and implementation of recommendations that result from above findings.

Investigation:
Example: Resident AB has been receiving nine or more medications for over a year but depression is new this last quarter. The psychologist is currently monitoring, and in the last week the resident's primary Certified Nursing Assistant has described the resident's reluctance to feed herself.

Actions:
Example: AB's current weights indicate no weight loss, but due to the changes in these clinical links the interdisciplinary team will monitor weight weekly for the next month.

The second process improvement action implemented is meal rounds for all residents, which focuses on environmental and food considerations. The meal rounds would be done a minimum of 5 days a week, including at least 1 weekend day (three lunch meals, two dinner meals). The meal rounds would include dietary staff trained in completing meal rounds. This provides the dietary staff an opportunity to see the whole picture, not just from the perspective of preparing meals. The form the facility used for the meal rounds can be found in Figure 27.5. The dietetics professional would be responsible for documenting in the resident's chart.

Figure 27.5
Weight wellness form.

Meal rounds for all residents should focus on environmental and food considerations 5 days per week (3 lunch meals, 2 dinner meals).

The environmental and food considerations for meal rounds to observe include (but should not be limited to)

1. Offering of alternatives to residents who are not eating
2. Encouraging consumption of liquids and tracking their consumption
3. Eating assistance
4. Positioning
5. Resident's tolerance of food consistency
6. Resident provided supplements at mealtime (and is not consuming meal)
7. Distractions at mealtime
8. Resident is not satisfied with meals
9. Updating of resident's preferences on tray card
10. Adaptive equipment
11. Resident eats less than 75%
12. Use of dentures and glasses as indicated

Date: _____

Resident name: _____

Concern observed: _____

Action:

Forward to RD/DTR
- -
Date: *10-22-03*

Resident name: *AB*

Concern observed: *Food preferences not accurate on tray card, resident does not eat fish and was served fish.*

Action:
Food preferences updated on computer and in care plan.

Forward to RD/DTR

As with the transdisciplinary rounds, the key success factors for meal rounds are timely documentation, care planning of intervention changes, and implementation of recommendations that result. These strategies are supplements to the individualized Nutrition Care Process, which is delineated by the MNT protocol. They are meant to enhance the effectiveness of the protocols (act as cues), not replace the in-depth assessment; to personalize interventions that the dietetics professional will continually monitor; and to provide further evaluation as appropriate for each resident.

Study

An important tool in the study phase is the run chart.

A run chart is a simple graphic representation that displays data in the order in which they occur and shows a characteristic of a process over time. It is often known as a line chart or a line graph outside the quality management field. To create a run chart, a commercial spreadsheet software program, such as Microsoft Excel, can be used. Run charts are used to understand the trends and shifts in a process or variation over time or to identify decline or improvement in a process over time. In a run chart, events, shown on the y axis, are graphed against a time period on the x axis. The following are steps for constructing a run chart.

1. Deciding what to measure: What needs to be measured and in what unit? Measurements must be taken over a period of time.

2. Gathering data: The data must be collected in a chronological or sequential order. The collection of data may start at any point and end at any point. Ideally, there should be a minimum of 15 data points, but as a general rule, the more points, the better.

3. Organizing data: Once the data are in place, they can be divided into two sets of values x and y. The values for x represent time, and the values for y represent the items to be measured.

4. Creating the graph: The appropriate scale should be used to make the points on the x and y axes. This can be done by hand or by computer. Then the data points are plotted on the chart (the x values vs the y values) in the order in which they became available, and the points are connected with lines between them. The average line can be drawn to evaluate the movement of the data points relative to the average.

5. Interpreting data: After the horizontal and vertical lines are drawn to segment data, the data are interpreted and conclusions as to what action to take are drawn. Some possible outcomes are trends in the chart or cyclical patterns in the data. The key is to look for trends and not to focus on individual plot points. A trend is when six consecutive jumps in the same direction indicate that something was introduced into the process to cause a fundamental improvement (11).

The run chart in Figure 27.6 is an example for the outcome indicator: the number of residents with avoidable unintended weight loss for Facility B where before the improvement project, weight was not maintained or did not increase consistently. To have a complete picture of the data regarding Facility B changes related to the transdisciplinary rounds and meal rounds, a run chart should also be constructed for the process indicators, including the number of transdisciplinary rounds per month occurring as scheduled and the number of meal rounds occurring per month as scheduled.

Act

The PDSA cycle is repeated several times until the interventions achieve the desired goals (Figure 27.7, multiple cycles). The use of several small cycles of PDSA implemented in a rapid fashion is known as rapid-cycle improvement. After a change is made, data are collected on a small sample to see if the change worked. The change is then adapted, abandoned, or adopted, and then another is tested. Multiple small changes are often more effective than trying to make a major improvement with a single change. It allows the group to try things quickly, to see what works, and to change what does not work. It also provides for "early wins," which motivate the group to continue the process until goals are eventually achieved (12).

The next steps are to monitor and provide positive reinforcement of the improvement strategies (cues). This requires observing the process in action. Steps to take include the following:

- Clarify policy and procedure.
- Educate staff.
- Add strategies as a consistent part of MNT protocol.

Figure 27.6

Significant weight-loss run chart trend at a facility. Data plotted over time on a run chart is a way to depict fundamental improvement. Seven or more data points below the mean indicate that new strategies are a true improvement. This chart shows a trend of eight data points below the mean after new strategies of preventing significant weight loss were put in place.

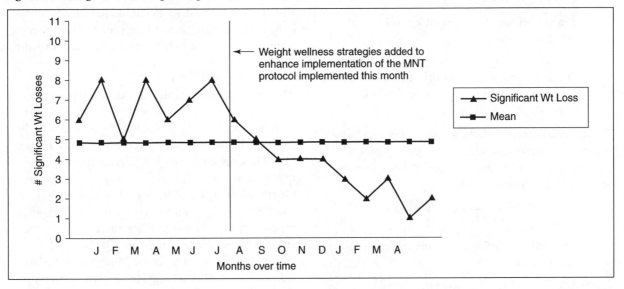

Figure 27.7

The improvement model: testing changes with repeated use of PDSA cycle.

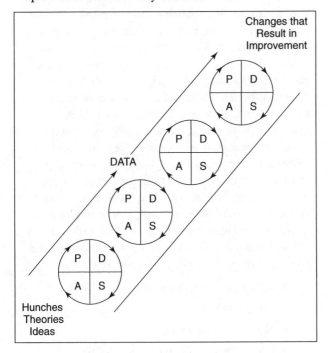

- Include strategies in orientation of new employees.
- Review individual residents during grand rounds.
- Implement care plan interventions.

Combining standardization of the process and flexibility is critical to having a successful CQI system. Standardization is necessary to meaningfully compare clinical outcomes. Flexibility is necessary to accommodate the uniqueness of individual residents.

PITFALLS TO AVOID WHEN EMBARKING ON A QUALITY IMPROVEMENT PROJECT

The dietetics professional should become familiar with the pitfalls that can occur at each step of the PDSA cycle *before* starting a CQI project.

Plan

Failure to document the actual process is an important pitfall that should be avoided. The failure to reflect reality may result from a variety of causes, such as the following:

- The process is described as an "ideal" process and not as it actually happens.

- Team members are reluctant to describe parts of the process that might expose weaknesses in their areas.

- Rework loops are seen as small and unimportant and are overlooked.

- Team members truly do not know how the process operates.

- Team members fail to evaluate the information gathered and to identify cause(s) of the problem, which may not be the root cause(s).

To avoid this pitfall, the strategy of asking "why" five or more times can be applied, which should uncover links in a causal chain until the "root cause" of the problem is uncovered.

- First ask, "Why"—what caused this problem?

- Then ask, "Why" again to uncover the cause of the cause.

- Ask "Why" until the actionable level is reached.

Root cause should not be taken to mean the last link in the causal chain. It should refer to the network of factors (below the surface), which, taken together, produced the problem (on the surface).

Do

Mistakes that can compromise the "Do" step include the following:

- A failure to document unexpected observations

- A failure to communicate with everyone what the change involves

- Trying to tackle everything at once

Study

In "Study" step, caution should be taken to avoid the following pitfalls:

- Leaving data unanalyzed. Collecting data is only the beginning. Analyzing the data collected over time, to draw conclusions about the performance of a process or the nature of an outcome, is what is important.

- Failing to ensure that everyone collecting data is using the same definitions about the indicator. The definitions must be consistent, so that data are valid.

Act

It is important to follow through with the "Act" step. One should not redo the Plan and Do steps before gathering data again to evaluate the effectiveness of the solution. This would be doing Plan-Do/Plan-Do activity. Changes should not be added before data are gathered to support further changes or before concluding that something does not work.

IMPROVEMENT TOOLS

The above example highlighted some improvement tools used for quality improvement. Additional information about these tools and how to use them can be found in the resources listed at the end of this chapter.

A key resource that can provide training for quality improvement is the Quality Improvement Organization (QIO). QIOs work within each state and US territory to ensure the quality, effectiveness, efficiency, and economy of health care services provided to Medicare beneficiaries. QIOs have been contracted by the Centers for Medicare and Medicaid Services (CMS), to provide support to nursing facilities. The QIOs use innovative strategies to lead nursing facilities toward an "ideal" quality improvement culture, through training and education that speak to a primary motivation of nursing facilities today: the desire to improve clinical and organizational systems. QIOs offer materials and technical support to nursing facilities, including current clinical information and ideas to achieve the progressive organizational structure that will support the implementation of sustainable quality improvement models. The QIOs partner with state Survey and Certification Agencies (SSCAs), fiscal intermediaries and carriers, trade associations, other professional groups, state agencies, patient advocacy organizations, and academic faculty to achieve acceptance and credibility with nursing facilities, as well as to minimize duplicative quality improvement efforts. These partnerships also aid the QIOs in dissemination of material and assist the QIOs in implementing quality improvement models. QIO and partners sponsor statewide or regional workshops, collaboratives, and train-the-trainer sessions on the following:

- Public reporting QIs

- Using MDS QIs

- Quality improvement

- Clinical topics related to MDS QIs

Dietetics professionals should discuss QIOs with facility administrators and use local QIOs as a resource for improvement projects.

TABLE 27.1. Quality Improvement vs Scientific Outcome Research

	Quality Improvement	Scientific Outcomes Research
Purpose	• To monitor the quality of care delivered • To increase the probability of achieving desired outcome	• To determine whether the intervention results in the expected positive outcomes with minimal negative effects
Sample	• Single-facility sites • Single group	• Multiple sites • Comparison groups
Generalizability	• Results apply only to the specific agency involved in the project; they may not be generalizable to other facilities without further research	• The generalizability of the results depends on the strength of the research design and is often more broadly generalizable

OUTCOMES RESEARCH

CQI projects can be extended to outcomes research projects (13) (see Table 27.1). Outcomes research involves methodologically sound collection and analysis of health-related data on the application and results of therapeutic intervention in a specific population. Patient-centered outcomes are important, as are clinical outcomes. Most outcomes research still focuses on mortality and morbidity rates (Do test-group patients live longer? Do they show significant improvements in physiologic measures of health status? Are there untoward side effects or complications?). Relatively few research studies have assessed outcomes in terms of health-related quality of life (HQOL), disability, or patient satisfaction. Patient-centered measurement, such as HQOL, can change treatment practices by identifying relatively neglected areas of major concern to patients. These measures can develop better services from the patient's perspective. Illness-specific measures of HQOL (based on self-report) can be systematically decomposed to reveal the areas of key importance to patients, which typically differ from those of doctors. Thus, HQOL measures can play a diagnostic as well as an outcome-measurement role.

THE FUTURE

Clinical measures, cost efficiency, HQOL, and client satisfaction measures will approach equal status (14). HQOL and other psychometric tests will play a major diagnostic role, to identify issues and areas most important to the patient and to target services/treatments to them.

ADA is currently finalizing a Nutrition Care Quality of Life tool, which will be available in the near future. A research article reporting the initial steps in the development of the Nutrition Quality of Life tool can be found in the July 2003 *Journal of the American Dietetic Association.* (14). The draft version is also available (15).

POSITIONING NUTRITION SERVICES IN TODAY'S HEALTH CARE ENVIRONMENT

An aggregate data analysis involves the experiences of multiple patients. Examination of these data offers insights into practice patterns. Aggregate data analysis permits benchmarking against competitors, national standards, and other institutions, as well as development of quality enhancement initiatives.

Key elements to remember for using data to improve processes and outcomes of care are as follows:

- Keep measurement simple: think big and start small.

- More data are not necessarily better data: seek usefulness, not perfection, in measures.

- Write down the operational definition of measures.

- Use a balanced set of process and outcome measures.

- Build measurement into daily work and job descriptions.

- If possible, use available data.

To understand sources of resistance to change, dietetics professionals should consider the following:

- People always do what makes sense to them, in their context, at the time.

- Every system is perfectly designed to get what it actually gets.

- If different results are desired, different processes must be used to create them.

- The ultimate judges of the quality of one's work are the individuals who are served (16).

SUMMARY

Organizations will soon begin to truly compete over the quality of services they provide and the achievement of client outcomes, not unlike the way many organizations currently compete over the price of their services. In such an environment, organizations and health care professionals who raise their level of quality will be rewarded, whereas those who do not will face a less certain future or may even be forced out of business. Adding to growing market pressures, the Centers for Medicare and Medicaid Services (CMS), the Joint Commission on Accreditation of Healthcare Organizations (JCAHO), the National Council for Quality Assurance (NCQA), and other regulatory bodies are intensifying their focus on quality improvement. Taken together, these pressures suggest that, in the future, the clinical and economic interests of dietetics professionals will depend heavily on their ability to improve quality. Thus, to advance as a profession in the years ahead, dietetics professionals will need good data on measures of quality that are linked to the nutrition care process, and they will need to know how to use these data to continuously improve the quality of the nutrition care process and outcomes (17).

Dietetics professionals must develop skills in quality improvement and not depend on health care organizations alone to provide all the necessary experiences to develop these skills. The ADA Code of Ethics, the Standards of Professional Practice, and the Professional Development Portfolio are tools to assist dietetics professionals to assess their competence in quality improvement. Dietetics professionals can use these tools to evaluate and develop an education plan on the application of quality improvement methods. Dietetics professionals must keep pace with, if not lead, efforts to improve quality.

In daily practice, the dietetics professional can show evidence of success and value by consistently using the Nutrition Care Process and Model. The methods and tools presented in this chapter will aid in modeling a systematic, evidence-based quality improvement approach to quality care.

REFERENCES

1. Lacey K, Pritchett E. Nutrition care process and model: ADA adopts a road map to quality care and outcomes management. *J Am Diet Assoc.* 2003;103:1061-1072.

2. Sackett DL, Rosenberg WMC, Gray J, Haynes RB, Richardson WS. Evidence-based medicine: what it is and what it isn't. *Br Med J.* 1996;312:71-72.

3. American Dietetic Association. *Medical Nutrition Therapy Evidence-Based Guides for Practice: Hyperlipidemia Medical Nutrition Therapy Protocol* [CD-ROM]. Chicago, Ill: American Dietetic Association; 2001.

4. American Dietetic Association. *Medical Nutrition Therapy Evidence-Based Guides for Practice: Nutrition Practice Guidelines for Type 1 and 2 Diabetes Mellitus* [CD-ROM]. Chicago, Ill: American Dietetic Association; 2001.

5. American Dietetic Association. *Medical Nutrition Therapy Evidence-Based Guides for Practice: Nutrition Practice Guidelines for Gestational Diabetes Mellitus* [CD-ROM]. Chicago, Ill: American Dietetic Association; 2001.

6. American Dietetic Association. *Medical Nutrition Therapy Evidence-Based Guides for Practice: Chronic Kidney Disease (Non-dialysis) Medical Nutrition Therapy Protocol* [CD-ROM]. Chicago, Ill: American Dietetic Association; 2002.

7. Splett P. *Developing and Validating Evidence-Based Guides for Practice: A Tool Kit for Dietetics Professionals.* Chicago, Ill: American Dietetic Association; 2000.

8. American Dietetic Association. Medical nutrition therapy protocols. In: *Medical Nutrition Therapy Across the Continuum of Care: Supplement 1.* Chicago, Ill: American Dietetic Association; 1997.

9. Nelson EC, Splaine ME, Godfrey MM, Kahn V, Hess A, Batalden P, Plume SK. Using data to improve medical practice by measuring processes and outcomes of care. *Jt Comm J Qual Improv.* 2000;26:667-685.

10. *The Facility Guide for the Nursing Home Quality Indicators.* Madison, Wisc: Nursing Home Quality Indicators Development Group, Center for Health Systems Research and Analysis; 1999.

11. Carey RG, Lloyd RC. *Measuring Quality Improvement in Healthcare: A Guide to Statistical Process Control Applications.* Milwaukee, Wisc: ASQ Quality Press; 2001.

12. Berwick DM. Developing and testing changes in delivery of care. *Ann Intern Med.* 1998;128:651-656.

13. Eck LH, Slawson DL, Williams R, Smith K, Harmon-Clayton K, Oliver D. A model for making outcomes research standard practice in clinical dietetics. *J Am Diet Assoc.* 1998;98:451-457.

14. Barr JT, Schumacher GE. The need for a nutrition-related quality-of-life measure. *J Am Diet Assoc.* 2003;103:177-180.

15. American Dietetic Association Foundation and National Education and Research Center for Outcomes Assessment in Healthcare. Nutrition Quality of Life (draft). Available at: http://www.bouve.neu.edu/index_publications.html. Accessed March 3, 2004.

16. Nelson EC, Batalden PB, Mohr JJ, Plume SK. Building a quality future. *Front Health Serv Manage.* 1998;15:3-32.

17. Joint Commission on Accreditation of Healthcare Organizations. *Comprehensive Accreditation Manual for Long-term Care.* Oakbrook Terrace, Ill: Joint Commission on Accreditation of Healthcare Organizations; 2002.

ADDITIONAL RESOURCES

Agency for Healthcare Research and Quality
http://www.ahrq.gov

AHRQ is one of 11 agencies governed by the Department of Health and Human Services. It is a lead agency charged with supporting research designed to improve the quality of health care, reduce its cost, improve patient safety, decrease medical errors, and broaden access to essential services. AHRQ sponsors and conducts research that provides evidence-based information on health care outcomes, quality, cost, use, and access. The information on this Web site helps health care decision makers—patients and clinicians, health system leaders, and policy makers—make more informed decisions and improve the quality of health care services.

American Dietetic Association Quality, Outcomes and Coverage Team
http://www.eatright.org/Public/Government Affairs/98_7996.cfm

American Health Quality Association
http://www.ahqa.org

The AHQA works collaboratively with health care practitioners, health plans, and hospitals to analyze health care patterns, identify opportunities for improvement, and interpret and share information about current science and best practices with physicians, hospitals, and health plans.

Institute for Healthcare Improvement
http://www.ihi.org

IHI offers resources and services to help health care organizations make dramatic and long-lasting improvements that enhance clinical outcomes and reduce costs. Specific goals that IHI works toward include improved health status, better clinical outcomes, reduced costs that do not compromise quality, greater access to care, an easier-to-use health care system, and improved satisfaction for patients and communities.

Institute of Medicine
http://www.iom.edu/iom/iomhome.nsf?OpenDatabase

IOM's mission is to advance and disseminate scientific knowledge to improve human health. The Institute provides objective, timely, authoritative information and advice concerning health and science policy to government, the corporate sector, the professions, and the public. IOM's Board on Health Care Services focuses on issues of health care organization, financing, effectiveness, workforce, and delivery, with special emphasis on quality, costs, and accessibility of care.

Joint Commission on Accreditation of Healthcare Organizations
http://www.jcaho.org

JCAHO evaluates the quality and safety of care for nearly 17,000 health care organizations. To maintain and earn accreditation, organizations must have an extensive on-site review by a team of JCAHO health care professionals, at least once every 3 years. The purpose of the review is to evaluate the organization's performance in areas that affect care. Accreditation may then be awarded based on how well the organizations meet JCAHO standards.

National Association for Healthcare Quality
http://www.nahq.org

The NAHQ is dedicated to improving the quality of health care and to supporting the development of professionals in health care quality. Use of the site requires membership.

National Council of Quality Assurance
http://www.ncqa.org

NCQA is best known for its work in assessing and reporting on the quality of US managed care plans, through accreditation and performance measurement programs.

National Guideline Clearinghouse
http://www.guideline.gov

NGC is a comprehensive database of evidence-based clinical practice guidelines and related documents, produced by the Agency for Healthcare Research and Quality (AHRQ) in partnership with the American Medical Association (AMA) and the American Association of Health Plans (AAHP).

The Quality Tools Cookbook
http://www.sytsma.com/tqmtools/tqmtoolmenu.html

A step-by-step guide to using quality improvement tools, examples.

Scott and White Memorial Hospital
http://www.sw.org/sw/portal/_pagr/107/_pa.107/116?previewURL=iwcontent/public/quality/en_us/html/quality_tools.jsp

Search "quality improvement" for quality improvement tools, examples.

CHAPTER 28

Federal Regulations

With the passage of the Omnibus Budget Reconciliation Act (OBRA) of 1987, Congress changed the total assessment and process for all facilities certified to participate in the Medicare or Medicaid programs. Specifically, OBRA 1987 and the federal regulations created new standards, one of which was the Resident Assessment Instrument (RAI), including the Minimum Data Set (MDS). Effective understanding of regulations, resident assessment, comprehensive care planning, and clinical documentation provides the foundation for expert professional practice, quality resident care, and regulatory compliance in nursing facilities.

RESIDENT ASSESSMENT INSTRUMENT

The RAI helps the nursing facility staff to gather specific, detailed information on a resident's strengths and needs that must be addressed in the individualized care plan. Interdisciplinary use of the RAI promotes the identification of these strengths and needs. The RAI uses clinical, competent observations, skills, and expertise from the interdisciplinary team to develop the individualized care plan (1,2). The care plan assists staff members to evaluate goal achievement and to revise these individual care plans accordingly, by enabling the facility to track changes in the resident's status. As the process of problem identification is integrated with sound clinical interventions, the care plan becomes each resident's unique path toward achieving or maintaining his or her highest practicable level of well-being.

The RAI Process

The RAI is a problem-identification model that includes steps similar to other models of these types. It contains three basic components: (*a*) the MDS; (*b*) resident assessment protocols (RAPs) (composed of triggers, trigger legends, RAPs analysis, and RAPs summary sheet); and (*c*) utilization guidelines. Clinicians in the health care arena are educated on the problem identification process as a part of the curriculum. The RAI easily fits into this model, providing structure and standardized approaches for problem identification. The steps generally include the following:

1. Assessment (MDS/other)
2. Decision making (RAPs/other)
3. Care plan development
4. Implementation of the care plan
5. Evaluation (care plan, approaches, overall status of resident)

Minimum Data Set

The MDS (2,3) is a core set of clinical and functional status elements, including common definitions and coding categories. This forms the foundation of the comprehensive assessment for all residents of long-term-care facilities certified to participate in Medicare or Medicaid.

The MDS is an assessment tool but does not provide a comprehensive assessment. It does not include detailed descriptions of all factors necessary for care planning and evaluation. The MDS is used for preliminary screening, to identify potential resident problems, strengths, and/or preferences. When completing the MDS, the assessor indicates whether or not a factor is present after obtaining the information from the resident's record, the resident, direct care staff, licensed professionals, the physician, and the resident's family.

The information contained in the MDS is the basis for Quality Indicator (QI) reports. For certain clinical situations, if the MDS indicates the presence of a potential resident problem, need, or strength, the assessor may need to investigate and document the resident's condition in more detail using RAPs.

The dietetics professional completing any section of the MDS must sign, date, and indicate the sections of assessment completed. It is the facility's responsibility to ensure that all participants in the assessment have the requisite knowledge to complete an accurate comprehensive assessment. The RN coordinator is required to sign, to certify that the MDS is complete.

Data collected from MDS assessments are also used for the Medicare reimbursement system as well as for many state Medicaid reimbursement systems. These data reflect the acuity level of the resident, including diagnosis, treatments, and an evaluation of the resident's functional status.

Section K: Oral/Nutritional Status is specific to nutrition services. However, there is information throughout the MDS that may be relevant for the dietetics professional to aid in further analyzing the resident's condition. Table 28.1 is the item-by-item MDS guide for dietetics professionals (4). Table 28.2 summarizes the different types of assessments that are federally mandated (5). Table 28.3 is a summary of RAI assessment schedules (5).

Beginning in 1998, Medicare reimbursement under the Prospective Payment System (PPS) for extended care facilities moved from a reimbursement system, based on self-reported costs, to one that imposes fixed rates of reimbursement on the facility. Rates are set based on Centers for Medicare & Medicaid Services (CMS) Resource Utilization Groups (RUGs). This requires that the dietetics professional stay informed about the most effective reimbursement for the resident (3,6). The Medicare PPS for skilled nursing facilities' schedules are presented in Tables 28.4 and 28.5.

A federal requirement, codified at 42 CFR §483.20(b)(1), stipulates that facilities use an RAI that has been specified by the state. This requirement also mandates that facilities encode and electronically transmit the MDS data from the facility to the state MDS database. The specific requirement for transmission is §483.20(f). (Resident assessment is covered in §483.20.)

Triggers

Triggers are resident-specific responses for a single element or a combination of MDS elements. The triggers identify the residents who have developed or are at risk for developing a specific problem that requires further evaluation using the RAPs (1).

Trigger Legend

The trigger legend is a worksheet summary of all of the triggers for the 18 RAPs. It is not a required form but aids the interdisciplinary team in identifying those RAPs triggered in the MDS process.

RAPs Analysis

RAPs are structured, problem-oriented frameworks for organizing MDS information and for examining additional clinically relevant information about an individual. The RAPs help to identify social, medical, and psychological problems and form the basis for individualized care planning.

RAP Summary Sheet

The RAP Summary Sheet documents which RAPs have been triggered, the specific location of information where the RAP decision making can be found (eg, registered dietitian [RD] nutrition progress note dated 9/12/03), and whether or not to proceed in care planning for that area.

Utilization Guidelines

Utilization guidelines provide information on when and how to use the RAI. These guidelines aid the assessor in evaluating the problem and in determining whether or not to continue to care plan the item triggered. The following examples illustrate when the team may not proceed to care planning from a triggered RAP:

1. *Dehydration:* Resident does not consume all fluids provided. The dietetics professional calculates fluid requirements and can justify that the resident does not need to consume all fluids provided. Resident calculated needs are 1,200 mL or 30 mL/kg; resident received 1,800 mL daily. Resident shows no signs or symptoms of dehydration.

2. *Nutrition:* Resident leaves more than 25% of food uneaten. The dietetics professional documents that this 100-lb, 90-year-old woman consumes only 50% of most meals. The dietetics professional calculates an average of 1,800 to 2,000 kcal in the regular diet. If the resident's basal energy expenditure and total daily

TABLE 28.1 Item-by-Item Minimum Data Set (MDS) Guide for the Dietetics Professional

MDS Section	Issues Dietetics Professionals Should Keep in Mind
Section AC. Customary Routine	Options included in "Eating Patterns" section: • Distinct food preferences • Eats between meals all or most days • Use of alcoholic beverage(s) at least weekly • None of the above
Section A. Identification and Background	Advanced directives: feeding restriction option
Section B. Cognitive Patterns	• Does the resident have difficulty in making decisions about food? • Is the resident forgetful about mealtimes? • Does the resident have altered thought processes affecting the ability to feed himself?
Section C. Communication/ Hearing	• When you are speaking to the resident, does he or she have hearing aids in? • Do you need to communicate with the family for information? • Does the resident understand others? • Do you need to use written communication?
Section D. Vision Pattern	• Is resident able to see tray? • Does the resident have tunnel vision, impaired peripheral vision, or vision limited on one side?
Section E. Mood and Behavior Patterns	• Does the resident fear that food is poisoned? • Does the resident have a fear of swallowing? • Does the resident resist assistance? • Is the resident depressed, anxious, sad, or apathetic? • Does the resident refuse to eat? • Is resident's behavior disruptive? • Does the resident pace or wander? • Has the resident withdrawn from activities?
Section F. Psychosocial Well-being	• Does the resident easily interact with others? • Does the resident eat in rehab dining area? • Does the resident refuse to eat in dining room? • Does the resident eat out occasionally? • Does the resident request meals in room? • Is the resident able to choose table mates?
Section G. Physical Functioning Abilities **NOTE:** If the dietetics professional does not complete item G(h), he or she must make sure it is accurate.	• What is the resident's self-feeding ability? • Does the resident need self-help devices? • Dining locations • Examine body control problems—contractures, range of motion, lack of dexterity, partial or total loss of ability to position self, locomotion/ambulation
Section H. Continence	• Does the resident have frequent urinary tract infections? • Does the resident have frequent fecal impactions? • Does the resident have frequent diarrhea? • Does the resident have a catheter or ostomy?

continued

Section I. Disease Diagnoses	• Diabetes • Cardiac disease: congestive heart failure, hypertension, peripheral vascular disease • Musculoskeletal conditions: arthritis, fractures, osteoporosis • Neurological disease: cerebral palsy, cerebrovascular accident, dementia, Parkinson's disease • Depression • Chronic obstructive pulmonary disease • Macular degeneration • Infections
Section J. Health Conditions	• Weight changes • Dehydration—intake is less than recommended; resident has clinical signs of dehydration • Insufficient fluid in last 3 days • Edema, fever, internal bleeding, shortness of breath, vomiting • Pain • End-stage disease
Section K. Oral/ Nutritional Status	• What are chewing/swallowing problems related to? • What is mouth pain related to? • What caused weight/height changes? • What are the resident's calculated nutrition needs vs intake? • Are the approaches appropriate? • What is the rationale for the diet order, portion size?
Section L. Oral/ Dental Status	• Condition of teeth, fit of dentures/partials • Can the resident suck through a straw? • Can the resident swallow when asked? • Is there a difference in ability to swallow thin/thick liquid?
Section M. Skin Condition	• Does the resident have a stasis or pressure ulcer? • Is there a resolved/closed pressure ulcer? • Are there other skin problems/lesions? • Does the resident's nutritional status/intake increase the risk for impaired skin? • What are the nutritional interventions for wound care?
Section N. Activity Pursuit Patterns	• Does the resident actively participate in the Dining Committee?
Section O. Medications	• Does the resident take medications that may contribute to nutritional conditions (antacids, antibiotics, antihypertensives, anticonvulsants, anti-ulcer drugs, cardiac glycosides, diuretics, insulin, oral diabetic medications, laxatives, psychotropics, vitamins/minerals) • Possible food/drug interactions of routine medications • Changes in medications and/or doses in last 90 days
Section P. Special Treatments/Procedures	• Recent hospitalizations • Special treatments—chemotherapy, dialysis, ventilators, intravenous therapy, fluid restriction/forced fluids, special dementia unit, radiation, transfusion, ostomy • Abnormal laboratory test results—glucose, electrolytes, protein stores, iron stores, lipids, blood urea nitrogen/creatinine
Section Q. Discharge Potential	• Is resident capable of providing own meals (procuring, preparation, etc)? • Is diet instruction needed? (Should be completed with competency demonstrated.)

Source: Data are from reference 4 (pp 29-36).

TABLE 28.2 Federally Mandated Assessments

Type of Assessment	Timing of Assessment	Regulatory Requirement CMS "F" Tag
Admission (Initial) Assessment (Comprehensive)	Must be completed (VB2) by the 14th day of the resident's stay.	42 CFr 483.20(b)(4)(i)/F 273
Annual Reassessment (Comprehensive)	Must be completed (VB2) within 366 days of the most recent comprehensive assessment.	42 CFr 483.20(b)(4)(v)/F 275
Significant Change in Status Reassessment (Comprehensive)	Must be completed (VB2) by the end of the 14th calendar day following determination that a significant change has occurred.	42 CFr 483.20(b)(4)(iv)/F 274
Quarterly Assessment (State-mandated subset or MPAF)	Set of MDS items, mandated by State (contains at least CMS established subset of MDS items). Must be completed every 92 days.	42 CFr 483.20(b)(5)/F 276
Significant Correction of a Prior Full Assessment	Completed (VB2) no later than 14 days following determination that a significant error in a prior full assessment has occurred.	42 CFr 483.20/F 287
Significant Correction of a Prior Quarterly Assessment	Completed (R2b) no later than 14 days following determination that a significant error in a prior Quarterly assessment has occurred.	42 CFr 483.20/F 287

Source: Reprinted from Centers for Medicare & Medicaid Services. Revised Long Term Care Resident Assessment Instrument User's Manual Version 2.0. December 2002. Chapter 2: The Assessment Schedule for the RAI (p 3). Available at: http://www.cms.hhs.gov/medicaid/mds20/rai1202ch2.pdf. Accessed March 11, 2004.

expenditure have been calculated, the justification can note that this resident does not need the energy provided in the regular diet if no weight loss is occurring. Small portions may be recommended. However, even if this is not addressed on the overall plan of care, it must still be addressed in the nutrition progress notes, so that all members of the team are aware of the decreased overall intake.

3. *Nutrition mechanically altered diet:* The dietetics professional documents that a resident requires ground meat, because the resident refuses to wear dentures after having them realigned and readjusted. The resident continues to request ground meat, consumes 75% of this food group, and shows no weight loss or signs of nutrition problems related to texture modification. Again, this would be covered in the progress notes, but progression to the care plan is not necessary.

During this phase of the process, the team begins to develop the overall plan of care. Comprehensive care plans must be developed and reviewed within 7 days of completion of the RAI. The care plan must address the medical, nursing, and psychosocial needs identified in the assessment.

TABLE 28.3 RAI Assessment Schedule Summary

Record Type	Completion	Care Plan Completion (VB4)	Submit to State by No Later Than:
Admission	By VB2, no later than day 14.	VB2 + 7 days	VB4 + 31 days
Annual Assessment	Completed within 366 days of most recent comprehensive assessment (VB2 to VB2)	VB2 + 7 days	VB4 + 31 days
Significant Change in Status	Must be completed by the end of the 14th calendar day following determination that a significant change has occurred.	VB2 + 7 days	VB4 + 31 days
Significant Correction of Prior Full Assessment	Must be completed within 14 days of identification of a major, uncorrected error in a prior comprehensive assessment.	VB2 + 7 days	VB4 + 31 days
Quarterly	R2b, no later than 14 days after the ARD, 92 days from R2b to R2b.	N/A	R2b + 31 days
Significant Correction of Prior Quarterly Assessment	Must be completed within 14 days of the identification of a major uncorrected error in a prior quarterly assessment.	N/A	R2b + 31 days
Discharge Tracking Form	Date of event at R4 + 7 days.	N/A	R4 + 31 days
Reentry Tracking Form	Date of event at A4a + 7 days.	N/A	A4a + 31 days
Correction Request Form	Date at AT6, no later than 14 days after detecting an inaccuracy in an MDS record that has been accepted in state MDS database.	N/A	AT6 + 31 days

Source: Reprinted from Centers for Medicare & Medicaid Services. Revised Long Term Care Resident Assessment Instrument User's Manual Version 2.0. December 2002. Chapter 2: The Assessment Schedule for the RAI (p 22). Available at: http://www.cms.hhs.gov/medicaid/mds20/rai1202ch2.pdf. Accessed March 11, 2004.

TABLE 28.4 SNF Medicare Prospective Payment System Assessment Schedule

Medicare MDS Assessment Type	Reason for Assessment (AA8b Code)	Assessment Reference Date*	Assessment Reference Date Grace Days†	Number of Days Authorized for Coverage and Payment	Applicable Medicare Payment Days
5-day	1	Days 1-5*	6-8	14	1 through 14
14-day	7	Days 11-14	15-19	16	15 through 30
30-day	2	Days 21-29	30-34	30	31 through 60
60-day	3	Days 50-59	60-64	30	61 through 90
90-day	4	Days 80-89	90-94	10	91 through 100

*If a resident expires or transfers to another facility before the 5-day assessment has been completed, the facility will still need to prepare an MDS as completely as possible for the RUG-III Classification and Medicare payment purposes. Otherwise, the days will be paid at the default rate. The Assessment Reference Date must also be adjusted to no later than the date of discharge.

†Grace Days: A specific number of grace days (ie, days that can be added to the Medicare assessment schedule without penalty) are allowed for setting the Assessment Reference Date (ARD) for each scheduled Medicare assessment.

Source: Reprinted from Centers for Medicare & Medicaid Services. Revised Long Term Care Resident Assessment Instrument User's Manual Version 2.0. December 2002. Chapter 2: The Assessment Schedule for the RAI (p 27). Available at: http://www.cms.hhs.gov/medicaid/mds20/rai1202ch2.pdf. Accessed March 11, 2004.

TABLE 28.5 Medicare MDS Assessment Schedule for SNFs

Codes for Assessments Required for Medicare	Assessment Reference Date (ARD) Can be set on any of the following days	Grace Period Days ARD can also be set on these days	Billing Cycle Used by the business office	Special Comment
5 day AA8b = 1 AND Readmission/ Return AA8b = 5	Days 1-5	6-8	Set payment rate for days 1-14	• If a resident transfers or expires before the Medicare 5-day assessment is finished, prepare an MDS as completely as possible for the RUG Classification and proper Medicare payment, or bill at the default rate. • RAPS must be completed only if the Medicare 5-day assessment is dually coded as an Admission assessment or SCSA.

continued

14 Day AA8b = 7	Days 11-14	15-19	Set payment rate for days 15-30	• RAPS must be completed only if the 14-day assessment was dually coded as an Admission or Significant Change in Status Assessment • Grace period days do not apply when RAPS are required on a dually coded assessment, eg, Admission assessment.
30 Day AA8b = 2	Days 21-29	30-34	Set payment rate for days 31-60	
60 Day AA8b = 3	Days 50-59	60-64	Set payment rate for days 61-90	
90 Day AA8b = 4	Days 80-89	90-94	Set payment rate for days 91-100	• Be careful when using grace days for a Medicare 90-day assessment. The completion of the Quarterly (R2b) must be no more than 92 days after the R2b of the prior OBRA assessment.
Other Medicare Required Assessment (OMRA)	• 8-10 days after all therapy (PT, OT, ST) services are discontinued and resident continues to require skilled care. • The first non-therapy day counts as day 1.	N/A	Set payment rate effective with the ARD	• Not required if the resident has been determined to no longer meet Medicare skilled level of care. • Establishes a new nontherapy RUG Classification. • Not required if not previously in a RUG-III Rehabilitation group.
Significant Change in Status Assessment (SCSA)	Completed by the end of the 14th calendar day following determination that a significant change has occurred.	N/A	Set payment rate effective with the ARD	• Could establish a new RUG Classification and remains effective until the next assessment is completed.

NOTE: Significant correction assessments are not required for Medicare assessments that have not been combined with an OBRA assessment.

Source: Reprinted from Centers for Medicare & Medicaid Services. Revised Long Term Care Resident Assessment Instrument User's Manual Version 2.0. December 2002. Chapter 2: The Assessment Schedule for the RAI (p 29). Available at: http://www.cms.hhs.gov/medicaid/mds20/rai1202ch2.pdf. Accessed March 11, 2004.

INTERDISCIPLINARY CARE PLAN

Developing an effective nutrition plan of care for a resident requires the dietetics professional to be cognizant of all aspects of the resident's physiological, psychological, and sociological status. Use of the MDS and the RAPs culminates in designing a care plan that is individualized for each resident.

In the integrated health care network (ie, acute, subacute, extended care, and home care), there are some organizational differences, but the basics of care planning remain the same—to enhance the resident's outcome and quality of life. As an integral member of the interdisciplinary health care team, the dietetics professional needs to share information from one setting to another, to assist in the integration of the best nutrition services for the resident who moves across the continuum of care. The service must provide recognized nutrition care protocols that are cost effective.

A plan of care for the resident begins on the first day of admission to the facility. Facilities use an "interim care plan" until a comprehensive care plan has been developed. The facility has up to 14 days to complete the MDS and an additional 7 days to complete the comprehensive care plan.

Care plans are implemented in all areas of the health care continuum and allow an integrated approach involving the resident, facility staff, the resident's family or guardian, and the physician. The care planning process involves four steps (1,2).

1. Assessment: identifying the resident's strengths and weaknesses
2. Planning
   - Formulating problem/needs statements
   - Developing measurable goals
   - Planning intervention/approaches
3. Implementation
4. Evaluation and reassessment

The goal of care planning is to develop a course of action designed to maintain or return the resident to the best possible state of health. The dietetics professional develops the nutrition component using the interdisciplinary format in the facility. In general, each resident's care plan should include the following (7,8):

- Problems or needs that must be addressed, to attain and maintain the resident at the highest practicable physical, mental, and psychosocial well-being.

- Realistic goals, in terms of resident understanding, if possible. Goals must be realistic and measurable, must be stated in terms of expected behaviors, must be changed as the resident's condition changes, must have an anticipated date of completion or attainment, and must designate responsibility.

- Interventions/approaches to solve problems and satisfy needs. These must state what is to be done and by whom for each specified problem. In describing an intervention, words such as "encourage, understand, or reassure" should be avoided. Each statement should start with a verb such as "provide" (eg, "Provide a cup with a large handle and teach resident how to use it to reach the goal of self-feeding and drinking.").

- Implementation is carried out as stated on the care plan. It is essential that the timing, repetitions, and sequencing be followed precisely by the designated persons, to ensure consistency of implementation.

- An evaluation/reassessment of the resident is an essential part of the care plan.

- A discharge plan developed in accordance with facility protocol.

The care plan is a part of each resident's medical record. It must be accessible to all who are involved in the care of the resident, including the resident and the resident's family or guardian. It is reviewed regularly, to ensure that the approaches to improve or maintain the resident's state of health are effective. In care planning, the simplest terminology possible should be used in writing the care plan, to ensure that all members of the team understand the plan.

IMPLEMENTING THE CARE PLAN

One of the most effective methods for planning resident care is the interdisciplinary team conference. The interdisciplinary team conference offers an excellent opportunity for developing a coordinated plan for each resident. It allows each discipline to share assessments and to gain a greater understanding of the total needs of the resident. Much can be learned by carefully listening to and questioning other team members. Team cooperation is particularly important, because implementing the goals often involves more than one discipline. For example, when one of the goals is weight loss, the RD develops a personalized diet plan and counsels the resident; the dietetic technician or dietary manager makes sure that the food is served correctly and offers support; the activities director plans activities to increase the resident's energy expenditure, to include an exercise program commensurate with the resident's physical health; and the nursing staff provides support and reinforcement to the resident.

Nursing often is the appropriate discipline to chair the interdisciplinary team conference, because of frequent contact with the other disciplines. It is advisable that all the disciplines meet as a team at regularly scheduled intervals. The physician has ultimate responsibility for the health care of the resident and may be invited to the conference but generally is not asked to chair the team (7,8).

Each discipline should come to the conference prepared to share assessment data. Since the conference is usually prescheduled, the dietetics professional can prepare by collecting and updating the nutrition assessment data and developing tentative plans for dealing with the problem(s) identified.

After the interdisciplinary team conference, the chair of the team follows with written information. Many of these items will be suggestions and recommendations made by the disciplines, including the dietetics professional, at the conference. The nutrition care recommendations most often will be found in the progress summary of the assessment and will have been discussed during the team conference. If the RD is unable to attend the care conference, the recommendations should be disseminated at the interdisciplinary team conference by the dietetics designee, such as the dietetic technician or the dietary manager who signs the plan.

The facility is ultimately responsible for the overall care of its residents, including their nutrition care. The role of the dietetics professional is to identify problems and concerns. These procedures ensure that recommendations made by the dietetics professional are included in the care plan if the RD cannot attend the conference.

The goal of the care plan is to develop a course of action designed to attain or maintain the resident's highest practicable physical, mental, and psychosocial well-being. The resident's care plan should include the following items:

- Problems and needs
- Realistic goals
- Interventions and approaches
- Implementation
- Evaluation/reassessment
- Discharge plans

Because the care planning process is interdisciplinary, problems may be individually addressed or combined with others (eg, pressure ulcers and nutrition). The goals should be resident oriented, realistic, and measurable. Interventions or approaches state what will be done to attain the goal, when it will be done, and who is responsible for seeing that it is done. The approaches should be individualized, practical, and understandable.

The care-planning process should be oriented to preventing avoidable decline, should manage risk factors, and should build on the resident's strengths. Care plans are evaluated/reassessed at least every 90 days. If the goal is not met, changes to the care plan should be revised, to be more realistic and achievable. If the problem has been resolved, this should also be reflected in the care plan, along with the date of resolution. The care plan should be reflective of the resident's status or condition at the present time.

Although the facility staff develops the care plan, the resident and/or their responsible party (eg, family, guardian) are also part of this process. Care plan meetings are held on a quarterly basis, and the resident or responsible party should be invited to attend this meeting.

DISCHARGE PLANNING

Nursing homes do admit residents for short-term rehabilitation. These residents, and sometimes residents with longer stays, return to home or former residences, or are transferred to another nursing facility. Education from the various disciplines and services from outside agencies (eg, home health agencies, home-delivered meals) may need to be put in place before discharge. Although nursing and social services coordinate the move, the dietetics professional is an integral part of the discharge process. Once the resident has been discharged, the social worker is responsible for a follow-up call, to see how the former resident is doing in the new setting.

Discharge planning is an important activity in any health care setting. The discharge potential needs to focus on what happens to the resident before that resident can be safely discharged. This discharge potential should appear in the plan of care. Reasons for discharge planning include the following:

- Need to design written diet instructions that are required for reference and reinforcement.

- Need to contact nutrition support programs in advance and make arrangements for home-delivered meals.

- Need to provide a source of dietary information on nutritional status, explaining the degree of, and the resident's response to, nutrition intervention to other health care facilities where the patient is to be discharged. This information can save the admitting facility time and prevent it from trying approaches that were previously unsuccessful. The nutrition discharge summary also can highlight a problem, such as weight loss, that might not be readily apparent to the admitting facility.

- Need to provide opportunity to reinforce the principles of nutrition learned while the resident was in the facility. Residents returning to the home setting have a written reminder of the nutrition services offered by the facility.

A summary of the resident's nutritional status and problems while in one facility is valuable information for the facility that receives the resident and helps the dietetics professional to develop an effective nutrition care plan sooner than would otherwise be possible (8). It also provides continuity of care and may, therefore, enhance the resident's quality of life.

SURVEY PROCESS

Long-term care facilities volunteer to participate in the federally funded Medicare and/or Medicaid programs. Skilled nursing facilities (SNFs) and nursing facilities (NFs) must be in compliance with the requirements codified in 42 CFR Part 483, Subpart B, to receive payment under the Medicare and/or Medicaid programs. To certify an SNF or NF, an initial health survey must be completed, along with a Life Safety Code Survey. The facility is then reviewed periodically, in a recertification survey. These are unannounced surveys conducted by the state survey agency, which is contracted by the federal government to do the surveys, and may occur on any day or at any time during the 24-hour period.

The health or standard survey (recertification survey) is a periodic, resident-centered inspection that gathers information about the quality of services furnished in a facility. Survey frequency requires that each SNF or NF be subjected to a standard survey no later than 15 months after the last day of the previous standard survey and that the statewide average interval between standard surveys not exceed 12 months. A complaint survey, or an abbreviated standard survey, focuses on a specific issue that has been identified by the survey agency. These surveys gather information primarily through resident-centered techniques focused on facility compliance with the requirements for participation. They are the result of complaints received by the state agency. The complaint survey concentrates on a particular area of concern. However, the survey team can expand an abbreviated or complaint survey to a standard survey if they find evidence that warrants a more extensive review.

In addition to the initial, recertification, or complaint surveys that the state agency conducts within the specified time, CMS must also conduct Federal Monitoring Surveys (FMS), to review the state agency performance (ie, 5% of total facilities per state with a minimum of 5 surveys). There are two types of FMS: (1) the Federal Oversight Support Survey (FOSS), which is conducted at the same time as the state agency survey; and (2) the Comparative Survey (look-behind survey), which is conducted by the CMS Region Office (RO) or designated contractors under the authority of CMS-Central Office or the RO, within 2 months of the state agency exit.

The survey procedures can be found in Appendix P of the State Operations Manual (SOM) (9) and consists of the following tasks:

- Task 1: Off-site Survey Preparation
- Task 2: Entrance Conference/On-site Preparatory Activities
- Task 3: Initial Tour
- Task 4: Sample Selection
- Task 5: Information Gathering
  - 5A: General Observations of the Facility
  - 5B: Kitchen/Food Service Observation
  - 5C: Resident Review
  - 5D: Quality of Life Assessment
  - 5E: Medication Pass
  - 5F: Quality Assessment and Assurance Review
  - 5G: Abuse Prohibition Review

- Task 6: Information Analysis for Deficiency Determination
- Task 7: Exit Conference

The objectives of the Off-site Survey Preparation are to analyze various sources of information available about the facility, to identify concerns and potential residents for review in Phase 1 of the survey. The sources of information used include the following:

- Quality Indicator (QI) Reports (further discussion follows)
- OSCAR Report 3—History Facility Profile for the past four standard surveys
- OSCAR Report 4—Full Facility Profile, based on the first day of the last standard survey
- Results of Complaint Investigations
- Information from the State Ombudsman Office
- Preadmission Screening and Resident Review Reports (PASRR)
- Other information

QI Reports, from the Standard Analytic Reporting System of the CMS National Resident Assessment Data Base, are reports generated from MDS data that are available to each individual facility as well as to state and federal survey agencies. The QIs are to be used as indicators of potential problems or concerns that warrant further investigation. They are not determinations of facility compliance with the long-term-care requirements. These reports include the following items:

- Facility Characteristics: demographic information about the resident population.
- Quality Indicator Profile: facility status for each of the MDS-based QIs, as compared to a peer group of facilities in the state. The higher the percentile rank, the greater potential there is for a care concern in the facility. A QI is flagged if it is at or above the 90th percentile or is one of the three sentinel events—dehydration, fecal impaction, or low-risk pressure ulcers. It excludes residents who have only an initial MDS record in the system.
- Resident Level Summary: resident-specific QI information for all residents in the system (initial, annual, significant change or quarterly MDS).

Any QI that is a sentinel event, is flagged at the 90th percentile or above, or is at the 75th percentile or above is selected as a concern. Other information from the sources listed above may also be added to the concerns. Residents with these concerns will be preselected from the Resident Level Summary Report, for possible resident reviews during Phase 1.

On entering the facility, the team coordinator introduces the team and conducts an Entrance Conference. The purpose of this conference is to review the survey process and facility-specific reports (OSCAR Reports and QIs), and to hand out forms to be completed with specific time frames before the end of the survey.

While the Entrance Conference is being conducted, the rest of the survey team begins the Initial Tour. This provides the team with an initial review of the facility, residents, and staff. The team will try to meet as many residents as possible. They will obtain an initial evaluation of the total environment, including the kitchen. The team will confirm or invalidate preselected concerns and/or add concerns observed on-site.

The team will then meet to review their observations, select areas of concern, and finally choose Phase 1 residents for comprehensive and focused reviews. Phase 2 sample selection is based on concerns found during Phase 1. Closed records are also included in the Phase 2 sample.

Resident reviews include review of the medical record (eg, the physician order, discipline-specific notes, MDSs, care plans) and interviews with residents, family/guardians, and staff about the care and services that the resident had received and/or is receiving. There is also a group interview with cognitively aware residents, giving them the opportunity to voice their opinions and concerns about the quality of care and the quality of life in their present residence.

Observations of the residents and staff are made throughout the survey. These areas include resident rooms, dining rooms, activities, common living area, laundry, housekeeping, and maintenance areas. Treatments may be observed if applicable. The medication pass is also observed during the survey. Abuse Prohibition and the Quality Assessment/Assurance reviews are completed in Phase 2.

There is a more extensive tour of the kitchen during the survey, in which storage, food preparation, tray delivery, and the dishroom sanitation are examined. This is when the Kitchen/Food Service Observation Form is completed. (See Figure 28.1 [10].)

Figure 28.1

Kitchen/Foodservice Observation Form. Reprinted from Department of Health and Human Services, Centers for Medicare and Medicaid Services. Form CMS-804 (7-95). Available at: http://www.cms.hhs.gov/forms/cms804.pdf. Accessed March 9, 2004.

KITCHEN/FOOD SERVICE OBSERVATION

Facility Name: _____   Surveyor Name: _____

Provider Number: _____   Surveyor Number: _____   Discipline: _____

Observation Dates/Times: _____

Instructions:

Use the questions below to focus your observations of the kitchen and the facility's storage, preparation, distribution and service of food to residents. Initial that there are no identifiable concerns or note concerns and follow-up in the space provided. All questions relate to the requirement to prevent the contamination of food and the spread of food-born illness. (F371 This tag is not all inclusive.)

LIST ANY POTENTIAL CONCERNS FROM OFFSITE SURVEY PREPARATION: _____

_____

FOOD STORAGE

1. Are the refrigerator and freezer shelves and floors clean and free of spillage, and foods free of slime and mold?

2. Is the freezer temperature 0 degrees F or below and refrigerator 41 degrees F or below (allow 2-3 degrees variance)? Do not check during meal preparation.

3. Are refrigerated foods covered, dated, labeled, and shelved to allow air circulation?

4. Are foods stored correctly (e.g., cooked foods over raw meat in refrigerator, egg and egg rich foods refrigerated)?

5. Is dry storage maintained in a manner to prevent rodent/pest infestation?

FOOD PREPARATION

6. Are cracked eggs being used only in foods that are thoroughly cooked, such as baked goods or casseroles?

7. Are frozen raw meats and poultry thawed in the refrigerator or in cold, running water? Are cooked foods cooled down safely?

8. Are food contact surfaces and utensils cleaned to prevent cross-contamination and food-borne illness?

FOOD SERVICE/SANITATION

9. Are hot foods maintained at 140 degrees F or above and cold foods maintained at 41 degrees F or below when served from tray line?

10. Are food trays, dinnerware, and utensils clean and in good condition?

11. Are the foods covered until served? Is food protected from contamination during transportation and distribution?

12. Are employees washing hands before and after handling food, using clean utensils when necessary and following infection control practices?

13. Are food preparation equipment, dishes and utensils effectively sanitized to destroy potential food borne illness? Is dishwasher's hot water wash 140 degrees F and rinse cycle 180 degrees F or chemical sanitation per manufacturer's instructions followed?

14. Is facility following correct manual dishwashing procedures (i.e., 3 compartment sink, correct water temperature, chemical concentration, and immersion time)?

NOTE: If any nutritional concerns have been identified (such as weight loss) by observation, interviews or record review, check portion sizes and how that type of food is prepared (see guidelines at 483.35). If any concerns are identified regarding meals that are not consistent in quality see guidance at Task 5B and at 483.35.

LADLES: $\frac{1}{4}$ C = 2 oz., $\frac{1}{2}$ C = 4 oz., $\frac{3}{4}$ C = 6 oz., 1 C = 8 oz.

SCOOPS: #6 = $\frac{2}{3}$ C., #8 = $\frac{1}{2}$ C., #10 = $\frac{2}{5}$ C., #12 = $\frac{1}{3}$ C., #16 = $\frac{1}{4}$ C.

THERE ARE NO IDENTIFIED CONCERNS FOR THESE REQUIREMENTS: (Init.) ____

Document concerns and follow-up on back of page.

Form CMS-804 (7-95)

continued

KITCHEN/FOOD SERVICE OBSERVATION

Tag/Concerns	Source*	Surveyor Notes (including date/time)

*Source: O = Observation, RR = Record Review, I = Interview

Throughout the survey, team members exchange information to determine compliance with the regulations. All facility staff, including members of the dietary department, may be asked questions concerning resident care, abuse, and disaster protocols.

During Task 6, the survey team privately discusses their findings and systematically reviews the regulations found in Appendix PP of the SOM, to determine whether a deficiency exists. The team should have gathered all information and confirmed with interviews if there was a deficient practice. For example, according to the care plan, weights were to be taken weekly. However, there is no evidence that weights were taken. The survey team verified by asking the staff how often weights were to be taken and recorded. Staff identified the procedure as being based on monthly weights, not weekly weights.

The team coordinator conducts an exit conference with facility staff and residents, reviewing team findings and areas of concern but not giving specific deficiency tags. Final determination of deficiencies with scope and severity are decided at the state agency.

If a facility is issued a Statement of Deficiency or CMS-2567, the facility must submit a Plan of Correction (PoC), which must contain the following:

- How the facility is going to fix the problem for the residents cited in the CMS-2567.

- How the facility is going to fix the problem for those residents presently in the facility that have the same problem or are at risk for developing the problem.

- How the facility is going to ensure that the problem does not happen for new residents or for those residents that presently do not have the problem. Generally this is done with a staff in-service.

- Who is responsible for monitoring that it doesn't happen again.

- How the corrective action(s) will be monitored to ensure that the deficient practice will not recur (ie, what quality assurance program will be put in place).

EXAMPLE

Residents 1, 2, and 3 were not given assistive devices to help them in eating their meals in accordance with their plan of care.

Plan of Correction

The facility needs to determine where the problem is by asking the following questions:

- Is nursing not notifying dietary about the adaptive equipment?

- Is occupational therapy (OT) not notifying nursing/dietary?

- Is dietary being notified but not marking the cards?

- Is the dietary aide able to read the cards?

Part 1: For Specific Residents

Resident #1 refuses to use the spoon with the built-handle. The care plan has been revised to reflect the resident's wishes.

Resident #2's diet card now indicates that this resident needs a special cup for all liquids.

Resident #3 has been discharged from the facility.

Part 2: For All Residents That Use Adaptive Equipment

All residents who use adaptive equipment for feeding have been assessed for their use or acceptance. The specific adapted equipment needed for eating/feeding has been written on the resident's tray card.

Part 3: How Not to Recur

OT/Nursing will be given inservice training on the proper procedure for ordering or notifying the dietary department about residents needing adaptive equipment.

Part 4: Monitoring

The foodservice manager will be responsible for the card notations and for ensuring that a system is in place for keeping track of adaptive equipment. The dietetics professional will monitor, or the staff development nurse will do weekly care plan/implementation audits. (This all depends on where the problem is.)

The facility is also offered one opportunity to question cited deficiencies through an Informal Dispute Resolution (IDR). If the facility disagrees with the results of the IDR, they may request a hearing before an administrative law judge of the Department of Health and Human Services, Departmental Appeal Board.

SUMMARY

There are many tasks included in the survey protocols, from evaluating the physical plant to resident interviews, chart reviews, and care plan evaluations. The regulations and the accompanying guidance to surveyors stress the importance of accurate, timely assessments as the basis of care planning. The dietetics professional must pay close attention to the resident assessment regulations, to ensure quality resident care as well as positive survey results.

REFERENCES

1. *MDS 2.0 RAI User's Manual.* Marblehead, Mass: HCPro; 2003.

2. State Operations Manual. Centers for Medicare & Medicaid Services, Department of Health and Human Services. Available at: http://www.cms.hhs.gov/manuals/pub07pdf/pub07pdf.asp. Accessed June 20, 2003.

3. Peck L. Adapting to PPS: the business realities, an interview with Malcolm H. Morrison. *Nursing Homes.* 1998;47(4):13-17.

4. Centers for Medicare & Medicaid Services. Revised Long Term Care Resident Assessment Instrument User's Manual Version 2.0. December 2002. Chapter 1: Resident Assessment Instrument. Available at: http://www.cms.hhs.gov/medicaid/mds20/rai1202ch1.pdf. Accessed March 11, 2004.

5. Centers for Medicare & Medicaid Services. Revised Long Term Care Resident Assessment Instrument User's Manual Version 2.0. December 2002. Chapter 2: The Assessment Schedule for the RAI. Available at: http://www.cms.hhs.gov/medicaid/mds20/rai1202ch2.pdf. Accessed March 11, 2004.

6. Fisher C. Crossing over to PPS: providers seek opportunities under new payment system. *Provider.* 1998;24:28-30, 33-34.

7. March CS. *The Complete Care Plan Manual for Long-Term Care.* Revised ed. Chicago, Ill: American Hospital Association; 1997.

8. Carson CH, Gerwick CL. *Guidelines for Nutrition Care.* Overland Park, Kan: Nutrition Education Center; 2002.

9. Appendix P. State Operations Manual. Centers for Medicare & Medicaid Services, Department of Health and Human Services. Available at: http://www.cms.hhs.gov/manuals/pub07pdf/AP-P-PP.pdf. Accessed March 9, 2004.

10. Department of Health and Human Services, Centers for Medicare & Medicaid Services. Kitchen/food service observation form. Form CMS-804 (7-95). Available at: http://www.cms.hhs.gov/forms/cms804.pdf. Accessed March 9, 2004.

ADDITIONAL RESOURCES

MDS 2.0 Manuals and Forms
http://cms.hhs.gov/medicaid/mds20/man-form.asp

State Operations Manual and other CMS manuals
Centers for Medicare & Medicaid Services
http://www.cms.hhs.gov

To find State Operations Manual, click on Manuals; click on Paper-Based Manuals; click on Pub 7.

APPENDIX

A

Subjective Global Assessment Summary

History

1. Weight change

   Overall loss in the past 6 months: amount = _____ kg _____ %

   Change in the past 2 weeks: _____ increase

                                  _____ no change

                                  _____ decrease

2. Dietary intake change (relative to normal)

   _____ no change

   _____ change

   duration: _____ weeks

   type: _____ suboptimal solid diet   _____ full liquid diet

            _____ hypocaloric liquids   _____ starvation

3. Gastrointestinal symptoms (persisting for > 2 weeks)

   _____ none   _____ nausea   _____ vomiting

   _____ diarrhea   _____ anorexia

4. Functional capacity

   _____ no dysfunction (eg, full capacity)

   _____ dysfunction

   duration: _____ weeks

   type: _____ working suboptimally

            _____ ambulatory

            _____ bedridden

Physical Examination

For each trait, specify a rating as follows: 0 = normal, 1+ = mild, 2+ = moderate, 3+ = severe.

   _____ loss of subcutaneous fat (triceps, chest)

   _____ muscle wasting (quadriceps, deltoids)

   _____ ankle edema

   _____ sacral edema

   _____ ascites

Subjective Global Assessment Rating (Select one):

   _____ A = well nourished

   _____ B = moderately (for suspected of being) malnourished

   _____ C = severely malnourished

Source: Reprinted with permission from Detsky AS, McLaughlin JR, Baker JP, Johnston N, Whittaker S, Mendelson RA, Jeejeebhoy KN. What is subjective global assessment of nutritional status? *JPEN J Parenter Enter Nutr.* 1987;11:8-13.

APPENDIX

B   Mini Nutritional Assessment

NESTLÉ NUTRITION SERVICES

Nestlé

Mini Nutritional Assessment
MNA®

Last name: First name: Sex: Date:

Age: Weight, kg: Height, cm: I.D. Number:

Complete the screen by filling in the boxes with the appropriate numbers.
Add the numbers for the screen. If score is 11 or less, continue with the assessment to gain a Malnutrition Indicator Score.

Screening

A Has food intake declined over the past 3 months due to loss of appetite,
digestive problems, chewing or swallowing difficulties?
0 = severe loss of appetite
1 = moderate loss of appetite
2 = no loss of appetite   ☐

B Weight loss during the last 3 months
0 = weight loss greater than 3 kg (6.6 lbs)
1 = does not know
2 = weight loss between 1 and 3 kg (2.2 and 6.6 lbs)
3 = no weight loss   ☐

C Mobility
0 = bed or chair bound
1 = able to get out of bed/chair but does not go out
2 = goes out   ☐

D Has suffered psychological stress or acute disease
in the past 3 months
0 = yes   2 = no   ☐

E Neuropsychological problems
0 = severe dementia or depression
1 = mild dementia
2 = no psychological problems   ☐

F Body Mass Index (BMI) (weight in kg) / (height in m)^2
0 = BMI less than 19
1 = BMI 19 to less than 21
2 = BMI 21 to less than 23
3 = BMI 23 or greater   ☐

Screening score (subtotal max. 14 points)   ☐☐
12 points or greater   Normal – not at risk – no need to complete assessment
11 points or below   Possible malnutrition – continue assessment

Assessment

G Lives independently (not in a nursing home or hospital)
0 = no   1 = yes   ☐

H Takes more than 3 prescription drugs per day
0 = yes   1 = no   ☐

I Pressure sores or skin ulcers
0 = yes   1 = no   ☐

Ref.   Guigoz Y, Vellas B and Garry P.J. 1994. Mini Nutritional Assessment: A practical assessment tool for
grading the nutritional state of elderly patients. *Facts and Research in Gerontology*. Supplement
#2:15-59.
Rubenstein LZ, Harker J, Guigoz Y and Vellas B. Comprehensive Geriatric Assessment (CGA) and the
MNA: An Overview of CGA, Nutritional Assessment, and Development of a Shortened Version of the
MNA. In: "Mini Nutritional Assessment (MNA): Research and Practice in the Elderly". Vellas B, Garry
P.J and Guigoz Y, editors. Nestlé Nutrition Workshop Series. Clinical & Performance Programme, vol.
1. Karger, Bâle, in press.

J How many full meals does the patient eat daily?
0 = 1 meal
1 = 2 meals
2 = 3 meals   ☐

K Selected consumption markers for protein intake
• At least one serving of dairy products
(milk, cheese, yogurt) per day?   yes ☐ no ☐
• Two or more servings of legumes
or eggs per week?   yes ☐ no ☐
• Meat, fish or poultry every day   yes ☐ no ☐
0.0 = if 0 or 1 yes
0.5 = if 2 yes
1.0 = if 3 yes   ☐ . ☐

L Consumes two or more servings
of fruits or vegetables per day?
0 = no   1 = yes   ☐

M How much fluid (water, juice, coffee, tea, milk…) is consumed per day?
0.0 = less than 3 cups
0.5 = 3 to 5 cups
1.0 = more than 5 cups   ☐ . ☐

N Mode of feeding
0 = unable to eat without assistance
1 = self-fed with some difficulty
2 = self-fed without any problem   ☐

O Self view of nutritional status
0 = views self as being malnourished
1 = is uncertain of nutritional state
2 = views self as having no nutritional problem   ☐

P In comparison with other people of the same age,
how does the patient consider his/her health status?
0.0 = not as good
0.5 = does not know
1.0 = as good
2.0 = better   ☐ . ☐

Q Mid-arm circumference (MAC) in cm
0.0 = MAC less than 21
0.5 = MAC 21 to 22
1.0 = MAC 22 or greater   ☐ . ☐

R Calf circumference (CC) in cm
0 = CC less than 31   1 = CC 31 or greater   ☐

Assessment (max. 16 points)   ☐ ☐ . ☐

Screening score   ☐ ☐

Total Assessment (max. 30 points)   ☐ ☐ . ☐

Malnutrition Indicator Score

17 to 23.5 points   at risk of malnutrition   ☐

Less than 17 points   malnourished   ☐

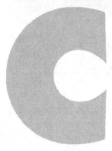

APPENDIX

Nutrition Risk Assessment

Instructional Guide for
Nutrition Risk Assessment

Nutrition risk is determined by the presence of characteristics that are associated with an increased likelihood of poor nutritional status. This includes various non-acute or chronic diseases and conditions, unintended weight change, inadequate or inappropriate food/fluid intake, dependency, disability, chronic medication use, and abnormal lab values. The Nutrition Risk Assessment form is designed for use in nursing facilities and can be used as the assessment form.

Frequency: The Nutrition Risk Assessment form should be completed on the same cycle as the Minimum Data Set (MDS) as follows:

(I)   Initial, upon admission as part of nutrition assessment

(Q)   Quarterly, with each care plan review if nutrition changes are identified in the MDS

(SC) With each significant change in condition, if nutrition-related

(R)   Readmission

(A)   Annual review

Data collection: The Nutrition Risk Assessment data will be collected by a registered dietitian (RD); dietetic technician, registered (DTR); or as appropriate, the certified dietary manager (CDM).

Form completion: The Nutrition Risk Assessment form will be completed, signed, and dated by a qualified dietetic professional (ie, RD, DTR).

Procedures

1. Complete the top of the form as indicated. The "assessment type" is determined by the frequency (see Frequency above).

2. After reviewing the resident's medical record, interviewing the resident and/or family, monitoring the resident's actual dining performance (eg, intake, positioning), and discussing with pertinent staff members, evaluate each resident for individual risk factors. Circle the description/terms that apply to the resident. Use the comment column to specify details of the assessment.

3. Record the appropriate number in the point column for each risk factor. The total for each risk factor cannot exceed three points.

4. If the resident falls into more than one category within a risk factor, assign the points for the most severe level. For example, if DM is controlled, but the resident receives dialysis, assign 3 points.

5. Total the number of points, determine the resident's Overall Risk Category, and record on the bottom of the form.

    0-2 points = No/Low Risk
    3-7 points = Moderate Risk
    ≥ 8 points = High Risk

6. If the resident is identified to be at MODERATE or HIGH RISK for ANY risk factor, follow the appropriate Strategies/Interventions that follow and document in nutrition progress notes and care plan. Strategies/Interventions are guides to consider using in view of residents' identified needs.

7. The nutrition professional must communicate with the interdisciplinary team to coordinate care for residents at risk.

8. File the Nutrition Risk Assessment form in the Nutrition Section of the clinical record or in the appropriate section identified by the facility and communicate recommendations to appropriate team members.

9. Do not count vitamin and mineral supplements as medications. Use progress notes to document needs.

10. Document lab values obtained within the past quarter.

Nutrition Risk Assessment Strategies/Interventions
Weight Status

Rationale: Unintended weight changes are prevalent among extended care residents and may lead to negative health outcomes. Along with evaluating the resident's accurate annual height and routine weight, the RD should review the medical record, interview the resident and/or the resident's family, and monitor the resident's dining performance. (MDS references J, K, E)

Strategies	Interventions To Consider
1. Communicate with nursing concerning residents with change in weight status.	1. Reweighing resident to verify weight change. 2. Consulting with nursing to identify possible causes.
2. Develop facility-wide weight policy.	1. Weighing on admission. 2. Weighing weekly for first month after admission. 3. Weighing residents with significant weight changes weekly for 4 weeks. 4. Instructing STNAs on how to accurately weigh residents. 5. Using consistent protocol when weighing. 6. Calibrating scales monthly.
3. Track weight trends.	1. Assisting in developing weight-tracking form. 2. Reviewing weights and communicating weight changes with nursing. 3. Alerting physician to unintended weight changes. 4. Identifying eating habits, food preferences, and consumption.
4. Determine possible causes of weight change. • Review for clinical signs, symptoms, and causes of malnutrition. • Review for increased nutrient needs. • Review lab tests indicating undernutrition. • Review clinical conditions that may cause unintended weight loss. • Review medications that cause anorexia, altered taste, and psychosocial needs.	1. Ordering high-calorie diet. 2. Determining a need for increased protein and calorie diet. 3. Offering nutrient-dense foods. 4. Observing for needed assistance in dining room. 5. Evaluating need for adaptive devices. 6. Encouraging exercise to increase appetite. 7. Offering appropriate substitutions at mealtimes.
5. Review multidisciplinary assessment.	1. Reviewing diet order to see if change in food consistency, liberalization, or fluid status might be warranted. 2. Assessing calorie and fluid needs. 3. Evaluating need for speech therapy screening. 4. Discussing advance directives with interdisciplinary team. 5. Communicating with STNAs assisting resident.
6. Review advance directives. Verify wishes and decision regarding placement of tube feeding with resident/family.	1. If advance directives indicate comfort care only, RD may consider implementing aggressive comfort care measures to maximize quality of life. 2. If advance directives agree to placement of feeding tube, RD completes nutrition assessment and discusses recommendations with nursing who follows-up with MD.
7. Review and complete RAI.	1. Completing/reviewing MDS. 2. Completing RAPs. 3. Developing overall plan of care in cooperation with interdisciplinary team. 4. Determining if care plans are developed to provide consistent intervention by appropriate staff. 5. Determining if care plan has been implemented in accordance with professional standards of practice and changes. 6. Monitoring, reassessing, documenting, and modifying care plan. 7. Charting progress and changes as needed.

Nutrition Risk Assessment Strategies/Interventions
Oral/Nutrition Intake — Food

Rationale: If food intake is inadequate, unplanned weight loss can occur. Monitoring food intake is essential, and poor intake requires in depth assessment, monitoring, and intervention. (MDS references AC, K)

Strategies	Interventions To Consider
1. Communicate with nursing concerning changes in food intake.	1. Reviewing meal intake records. 2. Reviewing changes in resident's food intake with staff.
2. Develop a procedure on meal intake.	1. Estimating caloric requirements of resident based on individual needs. 2. Interviewing resident/family to obtain diet history, food allergies/intolerances, food preferences, cultural concerns. 3. Observing intake during meals.
3. Review risk factors for decreased intake based on the MDS.	1. Completing nutritional sections of MDS. 2. Weighing resident on admission/significant change, and as needed for monitoring. 3. Reviewing weight and relationship to UBW. 4. Using consistent weighing protocols. 5. Evaluating diet order for appropriateness. 6. Evaluating present intake based on individual needs. 7. Reviewing medical record for losses of nutrients. 8. Monitoring mental status. 9. Identifying residents who need assistance in preparing (opening cartons, cutting) and consuming foods. 10. Reviewing lab tests, if available. 11. Reviewing possible impact of medication on intake.
4. Determine possible causes of poor food intake, identify appropriate interventions, and monitor status of interventions.	1. Considering consistency modifications. 2. Exploring resident's cultural attitude toward food, identifying preferences, and providing favorite/comfort foods. 3. Scheduling routine snacks 3x/day or administer at least 6 small feedings if agreeable with resident. 4. Individualizing meal plan according to resident's wishes to encourage compliance. 5. Instructing STNA and family on importance of adequate nutrition intake. 6. Involving resident/caregiver/family in establishing intake goals. 7. Evaluating if resident/family may be restricting or exceeding calorie needs. 8. Arranging for foods to be provided at activities and in social setting. 9. Encouraging exercise to stimulate appetite and maintain muscle mass. 10. Discouraging medication passes in dining room during meal service. 11. Establishing mealtime routine in positive dining experience.
5. Review Advance Directives.	1. Verifying with resident/family wishes and placement for tube feeding. (Refer to Nutrition Therapy for Palliative Care if tube feeding not desired.)
6. Review and complete RAI.	1. Completing/reviewing MDS. 2. Completing RAPs. 3. Developing overall plan of care in cooperation with interdisciplinary team. 4. Determining if care plan interventions are developed to provide consistent intervention by appropriate staff. 5. Determining if the care plan has been implemented in accordance with professional standards of practice. 6. Monitoring, reassessing, documenting and modifying care plan. 7. Charting progress and changes as needed.

Nutrition Risk Assessment Strategies/Interventions
Oral/Nutrition Intake — Fluid

Rationale: Water accounts for 50%-60% of total body weight. Humans can survive only a few days without water. Water regulates body temperature and is a medium for transport of nutrients and metabolic waste. Maintenance of fluid balance is essential to basic health and recovery from illness. (MDS references AC, J, K)

Strategies	Interventions To Consider
1. Communicate with nursing and physician changes in hydration status.	1. Suggesting I/O when fluid or electrolyte imbalance occurs. 2. Consulting with nursing or physician to identify possible causes.
2. Develop a policy for hydration and fluid that addresses potential causes of dehydration.	1. Estimating fluid requirements per kg of body weight adjusted for clinical condition. 2. Monitoring weight of residents on diuretics. 3. Identifying and monitoring high-risk patients. 4. Identifying interdisciplinary team responsibilities; monitoring and documenting care.
3. Review risk factors for dehydration based on the MDS.	1. Completing areas of MDS that relate to hydration. 2. Monitoring status of rehydration therapy. 3. Weighing resident as clinical condition requires. (See Weight Status Strategies/Interventions.) 4. Observing clinical health and physical signs of hydration status. 5. Monitoring I/O if applicable. 6. Reviewing lab test if available to confirm hydration status.
4. Determine possible causes of dehydration and identify appropriate interventions: • Review other potential risk factors for dehydration. • Review for volume deficit. • Review for volume excess.	1. Individualizing hydration plan according to resident's wishes to encourage compliance. 2. Instructing STNA/family on importance of adequate hydration and interventions to meet fluid requirements. 3. Arranging for fluids to be provided at activities and in a social setting. 4. Observing resident in dining environment. 5. Exploring cultural attitude toward fluids. 6. Reviewing resident's medications to assess possible impact on fluid electrolyte balance.
5. Review advance directives.	1. Verifying with resident/family wishes and placement for tube feeding. (Refer to Nutrition Therapy for Palliative Care if tube feeding not desired.)
6. Review and complete RAI.	1. Completing/reviewing MDS. 2. Completing RAPs. 3. Developing overall plan of care in cooperation with interdisciplinary team. 4. Determining if care plans are developed to provide consistent intervention by appropriate staff. 5. Determining if care plan has been implemented in accordance with professional standards of practice and changes. 6. Monitoring, reassessing, documenting, and modifying care plan. 7. Charting progress and changes as needed.

Nutrition Risk Assessment Strategies/Interventions
Medications—Nutrition-Related

Rationale: Interactions between drugs and nutrients may alter drug or nutrient disposition, action, or toxicity. Drugs taken by older adults for disease and/or symptom management may impose a particularly high risk of causing drug and nutrient interactions. Since residents often take several medications and because other factors affect an individual's response to medications, nutrient and drug interactions need to be addressed by the interdisciplinary team. (MDS reference O)

Strategies	Interventions To Consider
1. Communicate with nursing and appropriate staff concerning medication regimen.	1. Reviewing medical record for routine drug use. 2. Interviewing resident and family. 3. Discouraging medication passes in dining room during meal service.
2. Evaluate nutrition implications of current medications and effect aging has on drugs prescribed. • Loss of appetite • Taste/smell dysfunction • Dry or sore mouth • Appetite stimulation or weight gain • Epigastric distress • Nausea • Diarrhea • Gastrointestinal gas • Constipation • Fluid loss • Mental status change	1. Identifying and documenting drugs that may impair senses or cause diuresis, anorexia, catabolism, nausea, vomiting, dry mouth, constipation, diarrhea, dysphagia, dypsia. 2. Identifying and documenting drugs that may stimulate appetite or cause edema or weight gain. 3. Identifying and documenting drugs that may have drug-nutrient interactions (DNIs) when compounded by alcohol use or pose significant risk when taken with alcohol. 4. Identifying and documenting potential DNIs caused by diet changes. 5. Identify and document drugs that may alter functional, cognitive, or emotional status. 6. Identifying and documenting side effects of drugs that may be reduced by altering timing and/or content of meals and snacks. 7. Reviewing possible side effects with interdisciplinary team and discussing recommendations with physician.
3. Review and complete RAI.	1. Completing/reviewing MDS. 2. Completing RAPs. 3. Developing overall plan of care in cooperation with interdisciplinary team. 4. Determining if care plan interventions (alternative fluid schedules, fluid options, etc) are developed to provide consistent intervention by appropriate staff. 5. Determining if care plan has been implemented in accordance with professional standards of practice. 6. Monitoring, reassessing, documenting, and modifying care plan. 7. Charting progress and changes as needed.

Nutrition Risk Assessment Strategies/Interventions
Relevant Conditions and Diagnoses

Rationale: Nutrition plays a role in many of the leading causes of death in the US, including illnesses common in residents, such as heart disease, cancer, stroke, hypertension, and diabetes mellitus. Nutrition risk assessment is the first step in developing and providing disease-specific nutrition care options that are customized to meet the needs of the residents served. (MDS references E, H, I, J, M, P)

Strategies	Interventions To Consider
1. Communicate with nursing concerning changes in relevant conditions and diagnosis, causes of changes, and overall evaluation of the resident's condition	1. Reviewing medical record. 2. Interviewing resident/family, investigating status prior to admission. 3. Reviewing with interdisciplinary team any significant change at moderate risk. (See Nutrition Risk Assessment form.) 4. Review with interdisciplinary team any significant change of condition/diagnosis placing resident at high risk. (See Nutrition Risk Assessment form.)
2. Evaluate nutrition implications for current relevant conditions and diagnoses	1. Determining history of weight changes. 2. Determining previous treatment modalities. 3. Reviewing labs in light of diagnosis/condition. 4. Reviewing diet order, consistency, and overall intake including changes in fluid status. 5. Reviewing medications and potential drug-nutrient interactions. 6. Observing resident in current care setting. 7. Assessing edema, skin turgor, pressure ulcer/sore and making appropriate nutrition interventions. 8. Recommending nutrition intervention as appropriate, eg, liberalized diet based on resident's needs, alterations for food intolerances, enteral support, vitamin/mineral supplement.
3. Review and complete RAI.	1. Completing/reviewing MDS. 2. Completing RAPs. 3. Developing overall plan of care in cooperation with interdisciplinary team. 4. Determining if care plan is developed to provide consistent intervention by appropriate staff. 5. Determining if care plan has been implemented in accordance with professional standards of practice. 6. Monitoring, reassessing, documenting, and modifying care plan. 7. Charting progress and changes as needed.

Nutrition Risk Assessment Strategies/Interventions
Physical and Mental Functioning

Rationale: Physical and mental functioning play a significant role in the motivation and capacity of older persons to achieve and maintain nutritional health. Although numerous approaches, including feeding assistance and dietary supplementation, may be effective, proper assessment and intervention must be the first step to effective care. Assessment with appropriate intervention is key for identifying physical and mental conditions that may affect physical and emotional well-being and functional effectiveness. The involvement of the health care team is critical to improved nutritional health. (MDS references A, B, E, G, L, P)

Strategies	Interventions To Consider
1. Communicate with nursing and all other disciplines involved in changes related to physical and mental functioning.	1. Reviewing medical record. 2. Interviewing resident and family. 3. Investigating status in previous living environment.
2. Develop restorative dining program.	1. Assessing resident's ability to eat independently. 2. Evaluating dining environment. 3. Using a team approach to determine restorative potential.
3. Evaluate for physical functioning abilities using the restorative dining program.	1. Observing resident in appropriate care setting. 2. Observing for depression, anxiety, sadness. 3. Identifying resident's general orientation: time, place, person. 4. Identifying what kind of assistance resident needs and why. 5. Identifying percentage of meal resident is eating without assistance. 6. Identifying total percentage of meal eaten. 7. Identifying need for use of adaptive devices. 8. Identifying time required for resident to finish meal. 9. Identifying need for special positioning devices. 10. Identifying physical and/or verbal cues resident needs to initiate and continue with meal. 11. Monitoring resident's response to program.
4. Evaluate oral status.	1. Reviewing guidelines for assessing oral cavity. 2. Completing oral cavity assessment. 3. Reviewing need for mechanically altered diet. 4. Reviewing multidisciplinary assessment.
5. Evaluate for signs and symptoms of dysphagia.	1. Educating caregivers on warning signs of dysphagia. 2. Consulting with speech language pathologist. 3. Altering food/fluid consistencies as appropriate.
6. Evaluate conditions and therapies associated with compromised nutrition and oral status.	1. Reviewing for polypharmacy, major surgery, poor dentition, cranial/facial abnormalities, disorder of taste/smell, salivary dysfunction, immunocompromising conditions.
7. Evaluate communicative barriers (vision, speech, hearing, cognitive status).	1. Educating staff on limitations of resident (plate placement, use of communication board, side of hearing deficit, etc). 2. Providing appropriate cues as needed. 3. Developing standardized tray setup. 4. Consulting with appropriate rehabilitation therapist.
8. Review and complete RAI.	1. Completing/reviewing MDS. 2. Completing RAPs. 3. Developing overall plan of care in cooperation with interdisciplinary team. 4. Determining if care plan is developed to provide consistent intervention by appropriate staff. 5. Determining if care plan has been implemented in accordance with professional standards of practice. 6. Monitoring, reassessing, documenting, and modifying care plan. 7. Charting progress and changes as needed.

Nutrition Risk Assessment Strategies/Interventions
Lab Values

Rationale: Laboratory assessment can be prudently used to confirm suspected nutrition-related problems identified by clinical diagnosis, observation, history, and physical examination. Laboratory tests are recommended when plan of care warrants. (MDS reference P)

Strategies	Interventions To Consider
1. Communicate with nursing and appropriate staff concerning laboratory results.	1. Reviewing clinical diagnosis, history, and physical. 2. Determining whether requesting labs would affect outcome.
2. Evaluate nutrition implication of current lab results and effects of aging process.	1. Reviewing nutrition indications of lab data. 2. Identifying and documenting medications that could cause abnormal lab results. 3. Recommending and documenting changes in diet that could improve lab values. 4. Reviewing lab data with multidisciplinary team and recommending lab draws as appropriate. Before requesting labs, consider the following: 5. Will the outcome actually change the nutrition care plan? 6. Is the test cost-effective? 7. Is the nutrition goal for the resident consistent with treatment and advance directives?
3. Review and complete RAI.	1. Completing/reviewing MDS. 2. Completing RAPs. 3. Developing overall plan of care in cooperation with interdisciplinary team. 4. Determining if care plan (alternative fluid schedules, fluid options, etc) is developed to provide consistent intervention by appropriate staff. 5. Determining if care plan has been implemented in accordance with professional standards of practice. 6. Monitoring, reassessing, documenting, and modifying care plan. 7. Charting progress and changes as needed.

Nutrition Risk Assessment Strategies/Interventions
Risk Factor: Skin Conditions

Rationale: Pressure ulcers and other wounds are among the most challenging problems faced by caregivers in nursing facilities because of the frequency of occurrence and the cost to the resident and the facility physically, emotionally, and financially. Poor nutritional status is a risk factor for development of pressure ulcers; healing can be augmented with aggressive nutritional support. The cause of pressure ulcers is multifactorial and intervention is best accomplished through an interdisciplinary team. (MDS reference M)

Strategies	Interventions To Consider
1. Communicate with nursing concerning all residents with skin impairments.	1. Reviewing skin assessment. 2. Reviewing medical record frequently for healing of pressure ulcers.
2. Review risk factors for pressure ulcers.	1. Completing and/or updating skin risk assessment with nursing. 2. Documenting factors that place resident at risk for impaired skin. 3. Reviewing medical treatments, laboratory values, and medications that may contribute to risk for pressure ulcers. 4. Reviewing lab values placing resident at possible risk for pressure ulcer development and poor healing.
3. Develop a skin care team.	1. Developing and implementing interdisciplinary pressure sore/ulcer protocol that includes: 2. Nursing measures such as skin checks, turning/positioning, applying barrier cream, offering fluids, and ordering specialty mattress. 3. Nutrition measures such as determination of calories, protein, fluid, vitamin and mineral needs. 4. Medical measures such as debridement, surgery, if medically appropriate. 5. Referring to AHCPR Guidelines for suggestions on nutrition assessment and intervention. 6. Assisting skin care team in staff education related to pressure ulcer etiology, risk prevention, and treatment. 7. Setting up restorative dining program. 8. Providing family/resident education and counseling. 9. Involving therapists as needed.
4. Observe resident in dining environment.	1. Completing eating/dining performance evaluation. 2. Placing interventions into care plan. 3. Moving to appropriate dining environment. 4. Providing adequate devices as needed.
5. Review advance directives.	1. Verifying with family wishes for continued care and treatment. 2. If advance directives indicate comfort care only, skin and/or interdisciplinary team may consider implementing comfort care measures to maximize quality of life; follow-up with MD.
6. Review and complete RAI.	1. Completing/reviewing MDS. 2. Completing RAPs. 3. Developing overall plan in cooperation with interdisciplinary team. 4. Determining if care plans are developed to provide consistent intervention by appropriate staff. 5. Determining if care plan has been implemented in accordance with professional standards of practice and changes. 6. Monitoring, assessing, documenting, and modifying care plan. 7. Charting progress and changes as needed.

Nutrition Risk Assessment

Name _____ Adm date _____ Rm _____ Assess type _____

DOB _____ Age _____ Sex: M F Advance directive _____ Physician _____

Diagnosis _____

Ht (in) _____ Wt (lb) _____ Wt (kg) _____ Usual body wt range _____ BMI _____

BEE _____ Activity factor _____ Injury factor _____ Total cal _____ Total protein _____ g (_____ g/kg)

Total fluids _____ mL (_____ mL/kg) Fluid restriction _____

Diet order _____ Food allergies/sensitivities _____

Supplement/snacks _____ Cultural/religious preferences _____

Risk Factor	No/Low Risk (0 pts)	Moderate Risk (1 pt)	High Risk (3 pts)	MDS Ref	Pts	Comments
Weight status; loss or gain	BMI 19-27 No weight change	<5% wt change in 30 days; <7.5% within 90 days; or <10% within 6 mo	BMI <19 or >27 ≥5% wt change in 30 days; ≥7.5% in 90 days; or ≥10% within 6 mo	J, K, E		
Oral/nutrition intake; food	Intake meets 76%-100% of estimated needs	Intake meets 26%-75% of estimated needs	Intake meets ≤25% of estimated needs	AC, J, K		
Oral/nutrition intake; fluids	Consumes 1,500-2,000 mL/day	Consumes 1,000-1,499 mL/day	Consumes <1,000 mL/day	AC, J, K		
Medications; nutrition-related	0-1 drugs/day	2-4 drugs/day	5 or more drugs/day	O		
Relevant conditions and diagnoses	HTN, DM, heart disease, or other controlled diseases/ conditions	Anemia, infection, CVA (recent), fracture, UTI, alcohol abuse, drug abuse, COPD, edema, surgery (recent), osteoporosis, hx of GI bleed, food intolerances and allergies, poor circulation, constipation, diarrhea, GERD, anorexia, Parkinson's	Cancer (advanced), septicemia, liver failure, dialysis, ESRD, Alzheimer's, dementia, depression, dehydration, dysphagia, radiation/chemo, active GI bleed, chronic nausea, vomiting, ostomy, gastrectomy, fecal impaction, uncontrolled diseases or conditions	E, H, I, J, M, P		
Physical and mental functioning	Ambulatory, alert, able to feed self, no chewing or swallowing problems	Out of bed w/assistance, motor agitation (tremors, wandering), limited feeding assistance, supervision while eating, chewing or swallowing problems, teeth in poor repair, ill-fitting dentures or refusal to wear dentures, edentulous, taste and sensory changes, unable to communicate needs	Bedridden, inactive, total dependence, extensive or total assistance or dependence while eating, aspirates, tube feeding, TPN, mouth pain	A, B, E, G, L, P		
Lab values	Albumin and other nutrition-related lab values WNL	Albumin 3.0-3.4 g/dL, 1-2 other nutrition-related labs abnormal	Albumin less than 3.0 g/dL, 3-5 other nutrition-related labs abnormal	P		
Skin conditions	Skin intact	Stage I/II pressure ulcers or skin tears not healing, hx of pressure ulcers, stasis ulcer, fecal incontinence	Stage III/IV pressure ulcers or multiple impaired areas	M		

Overall Risk Category: 0-2 points: NO/LOW RISK   3-7 points: MODERATE RISK   ≥8 points: HIGH RISK

Total Points: _____   Overall Risk Category: _____

Signature: _____   Date: _____

INDEX

absorption, nutrient, 6, 54, 75, 125, 159, 221
    food-drug interactions, 154–155
accessory apartments, 23
acetate, 231
acetylcysteine, 38
acid-inhibiting agents, 6
activities of daily living (ADL), 12, 22, 23, 24
acute disease, 12–13
ADA. *See* American Dietetic Association (ADA)
adaptive eating disorders, 80
adaptive equipment, 215, 294
adjusted weight, 113
ADL. *See* activities of daily living (ADL)
Administration on Aging, 8, 26
adult day care, 30
Adult Treatment Panel III (ATP III) guidelines, 34–35
African Americans, 1, 28, 110
African immigrants, 110
Agency for Health Care Policy and Research, 13, 185
Agency for Healthcare Research and Quality, 279
age-related macular degeneration, 3
ageusia, 89
AIDS, 76, 245
    weight loss, 206
alanine aminotransferase (ALT), 136, 138
albumin, serum, 9, 147–148, 220
albuterol, 38
alcohol, 46
    abuse, 13–14
    drug interactions, 159–160
alcoholic liver disease, 52
alcoholism, GI symptoms and, 66
alfalfa, 168
Alliance for Aging Research, 8
allopurinol, 76, 78
aloe, 168
alpha glucosidase inhibitors, 48

alpha-linolenic acid, 5
alpha-sympathomimetics, 6
alpha-tocopherol, 36
ALS. *See* amyotrophic lateral sclerosis (ALS)
ALT. *See* alanine aminotransferase (ALT)
alternative medicine. *See* complementary and
    alternative medicine (CAM)
Alzheimer's disease, 3, 8, 16, 85, 86, 91, 255
American Academy of Family Physicians, 220
American Cancer Society, 100
American Dietetic Association (ADA), 220, 257
    Evidence-Based Guides, 265
    *Medical Nutrition Therapy Across the Continuum
    of Care,* 269
    Quality Outcomes and Coverage Team, 279
American Health Quality Association, 279
American Heart Association, 34–35
American Medical Directors Association, 13, 199
American Psychiatric Association, 15
American Society on Aging, 15
amino acids. *See* protein
amlodipine, 3
amoxicillin, 75
amoxicillin potassium, 75
amputation, 113, 115
amyotrophic lateral sclerosis (ALS), 80, 246
anabolic agents, 208
anemia, 13, 74–79
    in chronic kidney disease, 60–61
    classifications, 74–77
    definitions, 74
    implications for practice, 77–78
    lab tests, 74, 75, 76, 77, 137
    medications, 75
anemia of chronic disease, 76, 136
    lab tests, 76, 137
angelica, 169

ano-rectum, 2
anorexia, 1, 202, 253. *See also* weight loss
  drugs associated with, 206
  medications, 3
anthropometrics, 53, 107, 108–117
antibiotics, 6
antibiotic therapy, 32
anticholinergic effects. *See* medications, side
  effects
anticoagulation therapy, 158
antiepileptic agents, 6
antioxidants, 3
appetite, 1–2, 9, 64, 66
  medications and, 2, 6
  stimulants, 205–206, 207–208
apraxia, 215
ARD. *See* Assessment Reference Date (ARD)
arginine, 190
aromatherapy, 166
arterial insufficiency, 190
ascites, 52–53
ascorbic acid, 231
  drug interactions, 156
aspartame, 82
aspartate aminotransferase, 136, 138–139
aspiration, 211, 227
aspirin, 75, 76
Assessment Reference Date (ARD), 286
assisted living, 23–24
asthma, 38
atherosclerosis, 34
ATP III guidelines. *See* Adult Treatment Panel III
  (ATP III) guidelines
Axid, 3
ayurveda, 166
azotemia, 229, 237

Balanced Budget Act of 1997, 31
barbiturates, 6
Barrett's esophagus, 67
basal energy expenditure, 118–120
bed-bound client, 216–217
belching, 251
beta carotene deficiency, 4
beta-sympathomimetics, 6
biguanide, 47
bilberry, 169
biotin, 5, 231
black cohosh, 169
blood loss anemia, 74
blood sugar, appetite stimulants and, 207.
  See also glucose

blood urea nitrogen (BUN), 61, 138, 139–140, 199
BMI. *See* body mass index (BMI)
board and care homes, 24
body composition, 3–4, 115, 155, 219
body mass index (BMI), 3–4, 8, 112–113
  amputees, 113
body weight, 106, 112, 114, 115–116, 117. *See also*
  weight loss
  amputation, 113, 115
Braden Scale, 185, 186–187
bromide, 38
bronchodilators, 161
built-up flatware, 215
bumetanide, 75
BUN. *See* blood urea nitrogen (BUN)

cachexia, 100
caffeine, 17, 160–161, 162
CAGE questions, 13, 14
calcium, 5, 59, 159, 231
  drug interactions, 156
cancer, 100–103
  enteral feeding, 102
  metabolic components of, 100
  nutrition requirements, 101–103
  oral feedings, 102
  parenteral feeding, 102
  symptoms, 102
  treatment modalities, 101
capsicum, 170
carbidopa, 82
carbohydrates, 5, 45, 221
cardiomyopathy, 36
cardiovascular disease, 34–41, 91
cardiovascular system, 4
care plans, 248, 288–290. *See also* nutrition care
case studies, 151–152
catabolic state, 203, 208
catecholamines, 203
cat's claw, 170
ceftriaxone, 75
Center for Mind/Body Studies, 184
Center for Science in the Public Interest, 17
Centers for Disease Control and Prevention, 26
Centers for Medicare & Medicaid Services (CMS),
  196, 202, 261, 276, 290
central nervous system (CNS), 90
cerebral vascular accident (CVA), 34, 36
chamomile, 170
chasteberry, 171
chemosensory loss. *See* olfactory perception;
  taste perception

chemotherapy, 101
chewing, 122
Child and Adult Care Food Program (CACFP), 28, 30
Chinese Americans, 110–111
chiropractic, 166
chloride, 231
choking, 211. *See also* dysphagia
cholecystokinin, 1, 64
cholesterol, 34, 35, 42
    lab tests, 138, 149–151
cholestyramine, 6
choline, 5
chromium, 5, 231
chronic disease, 12–13, 138. *See also specific diseases*
chronic heart failure (CHF), 36
chronic hepatitis virus, 52
chronic kidney disease (CKD), 57–62, 66
    anemia, 60–62
    nutrition recommendations, 59
    renal failure, 13
    stages of, 58
chronic obstructive pulmonary disease (COPD), 37
cimetidine, 78
Cipro, 3
ciprofloxacin, 3
circulating hormones, 100
cirrhosis, 52
claudication, 34
clonidine, 75
clostridium difficile bacteria, 125
CMS. *See* Centers for Medicare & Medicaid Services (CMS)
CMS National Resident Assessment Data Base, 291
Cockcroft-Gault formula, 57
cognitive impairment, 85, 125, 217, 282
colchicine, 6, 76
collagen, 125
College of Maharishi Ayurveda Health Spa, 184
colon, 2
combination drugs (type 2 diabetes), 48
Commodity Credit Corporation (CCC), 28
Commodity Supplemental Food Program (CSFP), 29
community-based nutrition services, 26–33
    adult day care, 30
    Child and Adult Care Food Program (CACFP), 28
    congregate nutrition services, 27
    Eldercare Locator, 27
    Emergency Food Assistance Program (TEFAP), 29
    Food and Nutrition Service (FNS), 28
    Food Stamp Program, 28–29
    home-delivered meals, 27
    homemaker services, 30
    older Americans nutrition program, 26–27
    Seniors Farmers' Market Nutrition Program (SFMNP), 28
complementary and alternative medicine (CAM), 162, 165–184
    nutrition and, 167
    resources, 184
    therapy categories, 165–166
concentrated-energy diet, 249
congregate nutrition services, 27, 30
conjugated estrogen, 3
constipation, 14–15, 71, 80, 124, 251
contaminated food detection, 91
continence, 14, 282
continuing care retirement community (CCRC), 23
Cooperative Extension System (CES), 29
COPD. *See* chronic obstructive pulmonary disease (COPD)
copper, 4, 5, 190, 231
    drug interactions, 157
coronary artery bypass grafts (CABG), 34, 86
coronary artery disease (CAD), 12, 34
coronary heart disease (CHD), 12, 34, 36
correctional facilities, 30–31
cortisol, 203
Coumadin, 3
Council for Responsible Nutrition, 17
cranial nerves, 96, 97
creatinine, 138, 140
creatinine clearance (CrCl), 57
Crohn's disease, 76
cutout cup, 215
CVA. *See* cerebral vascular accident (CVA)
cyprohedtadine, 206
cytokine activity, 100

DASH. *See* Dietary Approaches to Stop Hypertension (DASH)
data collection, 13, 202, 262, 267
deficient erythropoiesis anemia, 75
dehydration, 196–197, 200, 221, 229, 237, 253. *See also* hydration status
dementia, 85–88, 125, 212
dental problems. *See* dentition
dental professionals, 97
dentition, 1, 9, 94–99, 122, 124, 127
dentures, 94, 98
depression, 15–16, 85, 125
DETERMINE, 30, 104, 105
DHEA, 171

diabetes, 2, 42–51
 aging and, 42–43
 appetite stimulants and, 207
 complications, 43
 diabetic wounds, 194
 diagnosis, 43
 drug therapy, 47–49
 gastrointestinal symptoms and, 66
 interventions, 43–44
 nutrition therapy, 43–47
Diagnostic and Statistical Manual of Mental Disorders, 13
diarrhea, 68, 124, 125, 158, 251
Dietary Approaches to Stop Hypertension (DASH), 12–13, 36
dietary reference intake (DRI), 80, 220
Dietary Supplement Health and Education Act (DSHEA), 167
dietary supplements, 17. *See also* minerals; vitamins
dietitians/dietetics professionals, 219
 alternative medicine and, 167
 home care and, 31
 industry standards, 263
 insurance for, 262
 oral health and, 94–95
 referrals to, 247
 role of, 246, 258
 staying current in the field, 262–263
diflunisal, 75
digoxin, 3
Dilantin, 3
discharge planning, 289–290
diuretics, 6
diverticular disease, 71–72
documentation, 258, 263–264
 federal regulations, 282–287
dong quai, 171
D-penicillamine, 6
DRI. *See* dietary reference intake (DRI)
dronabinal, 206
drug-nutrient interactions, 6–7, 38, 121–122, 154–164, 205. *See also* medications
drug receptors, age-related changes, 155
drug therapy, 47–49. *See also* medications
 "inherited therapy," 155
dry mouth. *See* xerostomia
Duragesic, 3
dycem/nonslip materials, 215
dying process, 245, 248
dysgeusia, 89
dyspepsia, 1
dysphagia, 1, 9, 66, 80, 211–212, 246, 255
 screening, 96, 97

eating-disabled clients. *See* rehabilitation of eating-disabled clients
eating habits, 106
 positioning, 215–217
 wheelchair-bound clients, 215
eating independence, 215
echinacea, 172
ECHOs. *See* elder cottages housing opportunities (ECHOs)
edema, 52–53
edentulism, 1–2, 95, 98
EER. *See* estimated energy requirement (EER)
EFAD. *See* essential fatty acid deficiency (EFAD)
Eldercare Locator, 27
elder cottages housing opportunities (ECHOs), 23
eldertonic, 206, 207
electrolyte balance, 196, 198, 229
electromagnetic field (EMFs), 166
electronic benefits transfer (EBT), 28–29
emboli, 86
Emergency Food Assistance Program (TEFAP), 29
enalapril maleate, 3
endocrine system, 4
endogenous opioids, 1
end-stage renal disease (ESRD), 60
energy, 59, 189, 220
 needs, 101, 117–120
 therapies, 166
enteral feeding, 102, 221–229, 262
 access issues, 222–224
 contraindications for, 222
 drug-nutrient interactions, 155–159
 formula selection, 224–225
 indications for, 222
 intolerance, 158
 medications, 159
 pharmaceutical incompatibilities, 157–158
 pharmacokinetic incompatibilities, 158
 pharmacologic incompatibilities, 158
 physical incompatibilities, 155, 157
 physiologic incompatibilities, 158
ephedra, 172
ERPs. *See* event-related brain potentials (ERPs)
esophageal reflux, GI symptoms and, 66
esophagus, 2
 motility, 64
essential fatty acid deficiency (EFAD), 241
estimated energy requirement (EER), 5
ethical issues
 nutrition support, 221
 palliative care clients, 255–257
 weight loss, 208

ethnic diets, 110–111
evening primrose oil (EPO), 173
event-related brain potentials (ERPs), 90
excessive hemolysis anemia, 75
eyes, 127

face, 128
facial nerves, 96
famotidine, 3
fasting plasma glucose (FPG), 43, 47
fat, 45, 221
    recommended dietary allowance, 5
fecal impaction, 14. *See also* constipation
Federal Monitoring Surveys (FMS), 290
Federal Oversight Support and Survey (FOSS), 290
Federal Poverty Income Guidelines, 29
federal regulations, 280–295
Federal Trade Commission (FTC), 17
feeding limitations, 124
feeding model, 223
feeding tubes, 122, 208, 222, 224, 226, 246, 255.
        See also enteral feeding
    complications, 226–229
    monitoring, 226, 228
felodipine, 161, 162
fennel, 173
fentanyl transdermal, 3
ferritin, 74, 75
fiber, 5, 14–15, 45
finger food diet, 213–214
flavonoids, 161
flavor enhancement, 91–92
flaxseed, 174
fluid balance, 196, 198, 221
fluid intake, 9–10, 52–53, 59, 189, 197, 221
    parenteral feeding, 231
    requirements, 120, 121, 122, 200
fluid overload, 237
fluoride, 5
folacin, 156
folate, 5, 8, 74, 140–141
folate antagonists, 76
folic acid, 4, 6, 36, 54, 231
Food and Drug Administration, 17, 184
Food and Nutrition Board, 27
Food and Nutrition Service, 28, 29
food-drug interactions. *See* drug-nutrient
        interactions; medications
food intake, 1–2, 9–10, 204–205. *See also* oral
        nutrition intake
    food insufficiency, 26, 39
    pattern, 187

record, 123
    restricted, 1
food poisoning, 91
food preferences, 109
food service, 254
    monitoring, 294
    observation form, 292–293
    plan of correction, 294
Food Stamp Program, 28–29
formulas
    administration techniques, 226, 232–233
    enteral feeding, 224–226
    parenteral, 232
foster care, 24
FPG. *See* fasting plasma glucose (FPG)
functional status, 11–12, 106
furosemide, 3

GALT. *See* gut-associated lymphoid tissue (GALT)
garlic, 36, 174
gastric motility, 64
gastroesophageal reflux disease (GERD), 67–68
gastrointestinal problems, 13, 63–73, 128, 228–229
    gastrointestinal fluid loss, 196
    gastrointestinal obstruction, 252
    symptoms, 63
gastrointestinal tract, 1–2, 221
    aging and, 63–64
    complications, 228–229
    physiology, 2
gastroparesis, 13
genetic makeup, 8
GERD. *See* gastroesophageal reflux
        disease (GERD)
geriatrics, 155
GFR. *See* glomerular filtration rate (GFR)
ginger, 175
gingko biloba, 175
ginseng, 176
glomerular filtration rate (GFR), 57, 61
glossopharyngeal nerves, 96
glucosamine chondroitin, 176
glucose, 138, 141–142
glucose intolerance, 55
glutamine, 190
glycosylated hemoglobin (A_{1c}), 142–143
government regulations. *See* federal regulations
grapefruit juice, 161–162
green tea, 177
Guillain-Barré syndrome, 81
gums, 127
gut-associated lymphoid tissue (GALT), 64

hair, 127
Hamwi formula, 115
hand feeding, 255
hand-over-hand cueing, 217
Hard Choices for Loving People, 257
hawthorn, 177
HDL-C. *See* high-density lipoprotein
    cholesterol (HDL-C)
head, 4
Healthcare Financing Administration (HCFA),
    196, 202, 262
Health Professional's Guide to Popular Dietary
    Supplements, 184
hearing impairment, 16, 282
height, 117. *See also* stature
Helicobacter pylori bacteria, 125
hematocrit, 74, 143
hemodialysis, 61
hemoglobin, 74, 143–144
hepatic disease. *See* liver disease
hepatic encephalopathy. *See* portal systemic
    encephalopathy (PSE)
hepatitis B, 52
hepatitis C, 52
herbal therapies, 162, 168–183
Herb Research Foundation, 184
HHS. *See* hyperosmolar hyperglycemic state (HHS)
hiatal hernia, 67
high-density lipoprotein cholesterol (HDL-C), 34,
    35, 42, 138, 149–151
Hispanic Americans, 28, 110
Home and Hospice Care Survey (1998), 31
home care, 31
home-delivered meals, 27
home infusion services, 31–32
homemaker services, 30
home modification, 22
home nutrition support, 221. *See also* nutrition
    support
homeopathic medicine, 166
home therapy, 31–32
homocysteine levels, 8, 74, 77
hospice care, 24
housing, 22–33. *See also* nursing facilities
    options for independent older adults, 22–23
    options for older adults needing assistance, 23–24
H_2-receptor antagonists, 6
human immunodeficiency virus (HIV), 203
Huntington's disease, 85
hydralazine, 6
hydration status, 135, 196–201, 221, 256
hydrocortisone, 76

hypercalcemia, 239, 251
hypercapnia, 236
hyperglycemia, 42, 43, 55, 159, 236
hyperinsulinemia, 55
hyperkalemia, 159, 238
hypermagnesemia, 159, 240
hypernatremia, 159, 238
hyperosmolar hyperglycemic state (HHS), 43
hyperphosphatemia, 159, 241
hypertension, 12, 36
    chronic kidney disease and, 58
hypertriglyceridemia, 159, 237
hypoalbuminemia, 220
hypocalcemia, 239
hypochlorhydria
hypogeusia, 89
hypoglossal nerves, 96
hypoglycemia, 43, 159, 236
hypokalemia, 159, 238
hypomagnesemia, 159, 240
hyponatremia, 36, 53, 159, 238
hypophosphatemia, 159, 240
hyposmia, 90, 91–92
hypotonic dehydration, 197

IBD. *See* inflammatory bowel disease (IBD)
IBS. *See* irritable bowel syndrome (IBS)
ideal body weight (IBW), 115, 116
IgA. *See* immunoglobulin A (IgA)
immune system, 100
immunoglobulin A (IgA), 64
incontinence, 14, 282
infections, 227–228
inflammation, 3
inflammatory bowel disease (IBD), 65–66, 70–71
Informal Dispute Resolution, 294
information and referral services, 27
"inherited therapy," 155
inner lip plate, 215
Institute for Healthcare Improvement, 279
Institute of Medicine, 279
Institute of Noetic Sciences, 184
instrumental activities of daily living, 12
insulin, 46, 48
insurance, 261–262
interdisciplinary assessment clinics, 32
Interfaith Health Program, 184
International Association of Yoga Therapists/Yoga
    Research and Education Center, 184
involuntary weight loss (IWL), 202–209. *See also*
    anorexia; weight loss
iodine, 4, 5

ipratropium, 38
iron, 4, 5, 54, 159
    anemias and, 74–79, 137
    drug interactions, 157
    lab tests, 74, 144–145
    studies, 60
irritable bowel syndrome (IBS), 14, 65, 68–70
isoniazid, 6
isotonic dehydration, 196
Italian Americans, 111
IWL. *See* involuntary weight loss

Japanese Americans, 111
Joint Commission on the Accreditation of Healthcare
    Organizations (JCAHO), 163, 262, 279
Joint National Committee on Prevention,
    Detection, Evaluation and Treatment of High
    Blood Pressure (JNC7), 36
Journal of the American Medical Association, 96

kaempferol, 161
kava, 178
K-Dur, 3
kidney disease. *See* chronic kidney disease (CKD);
    renal disease
kidneys, age-related changes, 155
kidney transplant, 62
Korsakoff's psychosis, 91

laboratory assessment, 134–153
    alanine aminotransferase (ALT), 136, 138
    albumin, 107, 147–148
    anemia, 74, 75, 76, 77
    aspartate aminotransferase, 138–139
    blood urea nitrogen (BUN), 139–140
    case studies, 151–152
    cholesterol, 107, 149–151
    cost effectiveness, 136
    creatinine, 140
    equipment, 135
    ferritin, 74
    folate, 74, 140–141
    glucose, 141–142
    glycosylated hemoglobin (A$_{1c}$), 142–143
    hematocrit, 74, 143
    hemoglobin, 74, 143–144
    homocysteine levels, 74
    iron, 74, 144–145
    mean corpuscular volume (MCV), 74, 148
    methylmalonic acid, 74
    ordering tests, 134–136
    osmolality, serum, 145

potassium, 145–146
    prealbumin, 146–147
    protein, 137, 146–148
    sodium, 148–149
    total iron-binding capacity, 74
    triglyceride, 151
    vitamin B-12, 74, 148
LADA. *See* latent autoimmune diabetes in
    adults (LADA)
Lanoxin, 3
Lasix, 3
latent autoimmune diabetes in adults
    (LADA), 43
laxatives, 14, 66
LDL-C. *See* low-density lipoprotein
    cholesterol (LDL-C)
lean body mass, 101, 203, 219, 220
leptin, 64
levodopa, 75, 82
levothyroxine sodium, 3
Lewy bodies, 86
liability issues, 261–264
licorice root, 178
life expectancy, 8, 85, 89
Life Safety Code Survey, 290
linoleic acid, 5
lipids, 34, 35–36, 81, 91, 159. *See also* cholesterol
lips, 127
litigation, 261–264
liver, 2
    age-related changes, 155
    nutrition assessment, 52, 53
liver disease, 52–56
liver transplantation, 55
longevity, 1, 8
Lorcept, 3
low-density lipoprotein cholesterol (LDL-C),
    34, 149–151

macronutrients, 5, 230–231
magnesium, 5, 54, 159, 231
    drug interactions, 157
ma huang, 172
malnutrition, 91, 100, 104, 220
    gastrointestinal symptoms and, 66
    protein-energy malnutrition, 37, 57–58, 202, 203
    signs of, 127–129
malpractice insurance, 262
managed care organizations (MCOs), 125
manganese, 5, 231
manipulative and body-based alternative medicine,
    165–166

marinol, 207
massage, 166
MCV. *See* mean corpuscular volume (MCV)
MDRD. *See* Modification of Diet in Renal
    Disease (MDRD)
MDS. *See* Minimum Data Set (MDS)
meals on wheels, 27
mean corpuscular volume (MCV), 74, 76, 148
Medicaid, 29, 290. *See also* Centers for Medicare
    & Medicaid Services (CMS)
    waiver programs, 29–30
medical nutrition therapy (MNT), 31, 34, 44, 95, 134,
    261, 265, 266
    liver disease, 52
    oral health and, 94
    outcomes management, 267, 269
    renal disease, 57
Medicare, 29, 286, 290. *See also* Centers for Medicare
    & Medicaid Services (CMS)
medications
    administration, 227
    anorexia, 3
    appetite and, 2, 6
    B-12 levels and, 78
    crushing, 157–158
    folate antagonists, 76
    gastrointestinal symptoms and, 66
    hydration and, 198–199
    "inherited therapy," 155
    iron loss, 75
    nutrient requirements and, 6, 121–122
    parenteral feedings, 232
    polypharmacy pattern, 155
    side effects, 6–7, 38, 154–164, 205
    slow-release, 157–158
    sublingual, 158
    taste loss, 90
    xerostomia and, 94
Med Watch, 184
megace, 206, 207
megaloblastic anemia, 76–77, 137
megastrol acetate, 206
megavitamins, 162
meglitinides, 47
melatonin, 179
mental disorders, 251. *See also specific conditions*
menu development, 254
MEP Healthcare Dietary Services, 109
metabolic acidosis, 239
metabolic alkalosis, 239
metabolic syndrome, 34–35

metabolism, 86
    cancer and, 100
metaproterenol, 38
methotrexate, 6
methylmalonic acid, 74
micronutrients, 45, 190
    parenteral feeding, 230–232
mild cognitive impairment (MCI), 85. *See also*
    cognitive impairment
milk thistle, 179
mind-body interventions, 165
minerals, 5, 59, 221
    drug interactions, 156
    liver disease, 54
    supplements, 205
Minimum Data Set (MDS), 13, 202, 262, 280–287
Mini Nutritional Assessment (MNA), 9, 298–299
mixed dementia, 86
MNA. *See* Mini Nutritional Assessment (MNA)
MNT. *See* medical nutrition therapy (MNT)
Modification of Diet in Renal Disease
    (MDRD), 61
molybdenum, 5
monoamine oxidase inhibitors (MAOI), 160, 161
monoamines. *See* pressor amines
motor control, 212, 215
mouth, 127, 252
mucolytic, 38
multi-infarct dementia, 86
multiple sclerosis, 80–81, 85, 91
muscle wasting, 52
musculoskeletal system, 4, 128

nails, 128
naproxen, 75
narcotic analgesic, 3
naringenin, 161
National Academy of Sciences (NAS), 17, 27
National Association for Healthcare Quality, 279
National Association for Holistic Aromatherapy, 184
National Center for Complementary and Alternative
    Medicine, 165, 184
National Center for Health Statistics, 26
National Certification Commission for Acupuncture
    and Oriental Medicine, 184
National Cholesterol Education Program, 34–35
National Council of Quality Assurance, 279
National Council of the Aging, 220
National Dysphagia Diet, 211
National Guideline Clearinghouse, 279
National Heart, Lung, and Blood Institute, 13

National Institutes of Health (NIH), 17, 165
National Kidney Foundation Kidney Disease
    Outcomes Quality Initiative (NKF-K/DOQI), 57
National Research Council, 27
Native Americans, 111
naturopathic therapy, 166
nausea, 252
neck, 4, 128, 216
neomycin, 6
nerves/nervous system, 4, 96, 128
nettle, 180
neurological disease, 66, 80–84, 85
new admission nutrition questionnaire, 131
NHANES III survey, 26
niacin, 5, 231
nifedipine, 3, 75
NIH. *See* National Institutes of Health (NIH)
nitrofurantoin, 75
nitrogen balance, 208
nizatidine, 3
NKF-K/DOQI, 57
normoglycemia, 43
Norvasc, 3
nosey cup, 215
NSI. *See* Nutrition Screening Initiative (NSI)
nurse, role of, 246
Nurse Healers—Professional Associates
    International, 184
Nurses' Health Study, 81
nursing facilities, 24, 280–295
    chronic disease patients in, 12
    meal planning, 46 (*See also* food service)
nursing nutritional checklist, 130
nutrient absorption. *See* absorption, nutrient
nutrition. *See also specific diseases*
    absorption, 6, 54, 75, 125, 159, 221
    artificial, 256
    chemosensory loss and, 91
    interventions, 10, 203
    meaning of, 245–246
    with medications, 6–7
    monitoring, 265
    protocols, 203–204
    requirements, 4–6, 203, 220–221
    risk factors, 8–21, 104, 300–310
nutritional anemias, 75–77. *See also* anemia
nutrition assessment, 104–133, 219–220, 246–247, 265,
    266–267. *See also* nutrition risk
    food preferences, 109–111
    new admission nutrition questionnaire, 131
    nursing nutritional checklist, 130

nutritional status, 134
    quality management, 265–279
    screening, 39, 104, 106, 107, 220
nutrition care
    evaluation, 265
    goals, 246, 249, 258
    within health care, 277
    palliative care clients, 245–260
    plans, 288–290
    quality management, 265–279
    unintentional variation, 267
Nutrition Care Process and Model, 265, 266
nutrition counseling, 249
nutrition risk, 60, 122–129, 124
    assessment, 108, 122–129, 300–310
    cultural factors, 108
    DETERMINE, 104, 105
    oral factors, 95, 96
    psychological and social factors, 108, 124
Nutrition Screening Initiative (NSI), 12, 95, 104,
    106, 220
nutrition support, 219–244. *See also* enteral feeding;
    parenteral feeding

obesity, 117
    liver disease and, 54
OBRA. *See* Omnibus Budget Reconciliation
    Act (OBRA)
occlusion, 95–96
OGTT. *See* oral glucose tolerance test (OGTT)
older adults. *See also specific diseases; specific issues*
    common diseases of, 12
    demographics, 89
    housing options, 22–33
Older Americans Act, 8, 26, 27
Older Americans Nutrition Program, 26–27
olfactory perception, 3, 16, 89–93, 125, 126
omeprazole, 3
Omnibus Budget Reconciliation Act (OBRA),
    262, 280
oral cancer, 2, 16
oral cavity, 94
oral glucose tolerance test (OGTT), 43, 141
oral health problems, 16, 94–99, 252. *See also* dentition
Oral Health Risk Factor Checklist, 95
"oral invalids," 94
oral nutrition intake, 120–121, 250. *See also* fluid intake;
    food intake
oral nutrition risk factors, 95, 96
organ function, 3, 4
oropharyngeal dysphagia, 66–67

oropharynx, 2, 64
osmolality, serum, 145
osteoarthritis, 12, 219
osteopathic therapy, 166
osteopenia, 54
osteoporosis, 12, 219
outcomes management systems, 265–269
    in action, 267–270
    definition, 267
    negative outcomes, 268
    research, 277
outpatient clinics, 32
over-the-counter drugs, 17, 161
oxandrolone, 208
oxidase inhibitors, 160
oxidative stress, 8, 91
oxidized lipids, 91

PAB. *See* prealbumin (PAB)
PAL. *See* physical activity levels (PAL)
palliative care clients, 245–260
    clinical issues, 247
    ethical and legal issues, 255–257
    physiological intake issues, 247
    psychological issues, 247
    social issues, 247
pancreas, 2
pantothenic acid, 5, 231
paraplegics, 115
parathyroid hormone (PTH), 58
parenteral feeding, 102, 204, 221, 229–242, 254, 255
    complications, 235–242
    components of, 230–232
    formula selection, 232
    indications for, 229
    intravenous access, 229–230
    monitoring, 234, 235
    nutrition cycling rates, 235
    prescription, 233–234
Parkinson's disease, 3, 81–82, 85, 91
parosmia, 90
paroxetine, 3
Paxil, 3
PEG. *See* percutaneous endoscopic gastrostomy (PEG)
PEJ. *See* percutaneous endoscopic jejunostomy (PEJ)
PEM. *See* protein-energy malnutrition (PEM)
Pepcid, 3
percutaneous endoscopic gastrostomy (PEG), 224, 246
percutaneous endoscopic jejunostomy (PEJ), 224
periactin, 206, 207
periodontal disease, 1, 66
peripheral neuropathy, 190

peripheral parenteral nutrition (PPN), 32, 229
peripheral vascular disease, 34
peritoneal dialysis, 61
pernicious anemia, 76, 77, 137
personal service, 30
phantosmia, 90
pharmaceutical interventions, 205
pharmacokinetics, 154–155
phenobarbital, 76, 78
phenytoin, 3, 6, 76, 78, 158, 199
phosphorus, 5, 54, 59, 159, 231
    drug interactions, 157
physical activity, 47
    inactivity, 11–12
    skin condition and, 186
physical activity levels (PAL), 6
physical functioning, 124–125
physical therapy, 31–32
phytochemicals, 8
pioglitazone, 48
pirbuterol, 38
piroxicam, 75
Plan-Do-Study-Act (PDSA), 270–276
Plan of Correction, 294
plate guard, 215
Plendil, 161
pneumonia, 38, 40
polypharmacy pattern, 155, 198
polyunsaturated fatty acids (PUFA), 81
portal systemic encephalopathy (PSE), 53–54
positioning, eating, 215–217
potassium, 59, 138, 145–146, 159, 231
    drug interactions, 157
potassium chloride, 3
poverty, 1, 10–11, 28
PPN. *See* peripheral parenteral nutrition (PPN)
prealbumin (PAB), 146–147
predialysis patients, 61
prednisone, 35, 38
Premarin, 3
pressor amines, 160, 161
pressure ulcers, 185–194, 261
    guidelines for care, 188–194
    lab tests, 189
    nutrient needs and, 190
Pressure Ulcer Scale for Healing (PUSH), 189, 192–194
Pressure Ulcers in Adults: Prediction and Prevention, 185
Prilosec, 3
primidone, 6, 78
procainamide, 75
Procardia XL, 3
propylthiouracil, 75

prosthodontics, 95
protein, 45, 59, 101, 220
    catabolism, 208
    drug interactions, 157
    laboratory screening, 137, 146–148
    requirements, 5, 120, 121, 189
protein-energy malnutrition (PEM), 37, 57–58, 202, 203
proton pump inhibitors, 6
PSE. *See* portal systemic encephalopathy (PSE)
psychotropic drugs, 15
psyllium seed, 180
PTH. *See* parathyroid hormone (PTH)
PUFA. *See* polyunsaturated fatty acids (PUFA)
pulmonary system, 4
PUSH. *See* Pressure Ulcer Scale for Healing (PUSH)
pyridoxine, 4, 82
    drug interactions, 156

Qigong, 166
quadriplegics, 115
quality assessment and assurance, 270
quality assurance, 270
Quality Improvement Organization, 276
quality indicators, 196, 291
quality management, 265–279
    improvement tools, 276
    outcomes research, 276
    pitfalls, 275–276
    resources, 279
Quality Tools Cookbook, 279
quercetin, 161

radiation, 101
RAI. *See* Resident Assessment Instrument (RAI)
ranitidine HCl, 3
RDAs. *See* recommended dietary allowances (RDAs)
RDIs. *See* reference daily intakes (RDIs)
recommended dietary allowances (RDAs), 4–6, 5, 220
red blood cells, 74, 77
red clover, 181
refeeding syndrome, 229, 241
reference daily intakes (RDIs), 27
regulations. *See* federal regulations
rehabilitation of eating-disabled clients, 210–218
    adaptations, 215–217
    dining environment, 210–211
    personal needs, 211
    physical plant and equipment, 211
reiki, 166
remeron, 207
renal disease. *See* chronic kidney disease (CKD)
renal failure, 13

renal osteodystrophy, 58
renal replacement therapy, 57, 61
renal system, 4
Resident Assessment Instrument (RAI), 262, 280–285
resident assessment protocols (RAPs), 280–281
Resident Level Quality Indicator Report, 272
respite care, 24
retinoids, 3
retinol-binding protein, 9
retirement communities, 23
riboflavin, 4, 5, 231
Rilutek, 80
riluzole, 80
risk. *See also* nutrition risk
    dehydration, 198, 199
    pressure sores, 186–187, 188
    wound healing, 189
Risperdal, 3
risperidone, 3

saw palmetto, 181
SCALE instrument, 9
scoop dish, 215
Scott and White Memorial Hospital, 279
security issues, 22
selenium, 4, 5, 231
senile osteoporosis, 219
Seniors Farmers' Market Nutrition Program, 28
sensory impairment, 16, 125
sertraline HCl, 3
SGA. *See* Subjective Global Assessment (SGA)
side effects. *See* medications
sitting balance, 216
skeletal system, 128
skilled nursing facilities. *See* nursing facilities
skin, 3, 4, 125, 128
    conditions, 185–195
    friction and shear, 187
    moisture, 186
    pressure ulcers, 185–194, 261
    sensory perception, 186
small intestine, 2
smelling. *See* olfactory perception
social isolation, 11, 27
sodium, 36, 59, 231
    serum, 148–149, 159
SOM. *See* State Operations Manual (SOM)
soy, 36, 182
speech pathologists, 87
spoiled food detection, 91
St. John's wort, 182

stanol esters, 6
State Operations Manual (SOM), 290
stature, 108, 112
sterol esters, 6
stomach, 2
straws, 215
stress, 134, 203
subcutaneous fat, 125
Subjective Global Assessment (SGA), 11, 220,
    296–297
  liver disease, 52
sulfamethoxazole, 75, 76
sulfasalazine, 75, 76
sulfonylureas, 47
surgery, 101
Survey and Certification Agencies (SSCAs), 276
swallowing, 87, 122, 211–212
Synthroid, 3
systems thinking, 267

taste perception, 3, 16, 89–93, 125, 126, 127
  losses, 89–90
  nutrition and, 91–92
teeth. See dentition
TEFAP. See Emergency Food Assistance
    Program (TEFAP)
"tenants by entirety," 262
terbutaline, 38
terminal illness, 245–246
testosterone, 208
theophylline, 38
therapeutic diets, 124
therapeutic lifestyle changes (TLC), 34, 35
therapeutic touch, 166
thiamin, 5, 231
  deficiency, 4, 159
  drug interactions, 156
  side effects, 6
thiazide diuretics, 6
Third National Health and Nutrition
    Examination, 101
thirst perception, 198
TIBC. See total iron-binding capacity (TIBC)
TIPS. See transjugular intrahepatic portosystemic
    shunt (TIPS)
TLC. See therapeutic lifestyle changes (TLC)
TONE. See Trial of Nonpharmacologic
    Interventions in the Elderly (TONE)
tongue, 127
total iron-binding capacity (TIBC), 74, 75, 76
total parenteral nutrition (TPN), 32, 230, 254. See also
    parenteral feeding

trans fatty acids, 34
transjugular intrahepatic portosystemic shunt
    (TIPS), 54
transthyretin, 9
Treatment of Pressure Ulcers in Adults, 185
Trial of Nonpharmacologic Interventions in the
    Elderly (TONE), 36
triamterene, 76
trigeminal nerve, 96
triglyceride, 35, 151
trimethoprim, 75, 76
tryptophan, 157
tube feeding. See feeding tubes
tumor, 100
tyramine, 160, 161

unintentional variation, 267
universal cuffs, 215
urinary tract infections, 80
US Department of Agriculture (USDA), 28–29
US Department of Health and Human Services,
    17, 26
US Healthy Eating Index (HEI), 1
usual body weight, 115

vagus nerves, 96
valerian root, 183
vascular dysfunction, 3, 86
vasoactive amines, 160, 161
Vasotec, 3
venous insufficiency, 190
Vietnamese Americans, 111
visceral fat loss, 4
vision, 215, 282
visual cueing, 217
visual impairment, 125
vitamin A, 4, 5, 54, 190, 231
  drug interactions, 156
vitamin B, 190
vitamin B-6, 5, 6, 36, 159, 231
vitamin B-12, 4, 5, 6, 36, 76, 77, 159, 231
  drug interactions, 156
  lab test, 74, 148
vitamin C, 3, 4, 5, 6, 159, 190
  Alzheimer disease and, 8
  side effects, 6
vitamin D, 4, 5, 6, 54, 82, 231
  drug interactions, 156
vitamin-deficiency disease, 85
vitamin E, 3, 4, 5, 6, 36, 54, 231
  Alzheimer's disease and, 8
  drug interactions, 156

vitamin K, 5, 158, 231
    drug interactions, 156
vitamins, 5, 59, 221
    absorption, 54, 75, 159
    drug interactions, 156
    liver disease, 54
    megavitamins, 162
    multivitamin supplements, 205
vomiting, 252

warfarin, 3, 158
weighted utensils, 215
weight loss, 9, 100, 101, 106, 116, 267–268
    anabolic agents, 208
    conditions associated with, 202
    downward weight trend, 203
    ethical considerations, 208

food-drug interactions, 205, 206
    involuntary, 202–209
    run chart, 275
    stress response, 203
weight maintenance, 4
weight wellness, 271, 273
Wernicke-Korsakoff syndrome, 85, 159
wheelchair-bound clients, 215
wrist weights, 215

xerostomia, 94, 98

Zantac, 3
zinc, 3, 4, 5, 54, 159, 190, 231
    drug interactions, 157
Zoloft, 3